Brain and Early Behaviour

development in the fetus and infant

CENTRE FOR ADVANCED STUDY IN THE DEVELOPMENTAL SCIENCES

Brain and Early Behaviour

development in the fetus and infant

Edited by

R. J. ROBINSON

Institute of Child Health,
London University, England

Proceedings of a C.A.S.D.S. Study Group on "Brain Mechanisms of Early Behavioural Development" held jointly with the Ciba Foundation, London, February 1968, being the second study group in a C.A.S.D.S. programme on "The Origins of Human Behaviour"

ACADEMIC PRESS

1969

LONDON
NEW YORK

ACADEMIC PRESS INC. (LONDON) LTD.
Berkeley Square House,
Berkeley Square,
London, W1X 6BA

U.S. Edition published by
ACADEMIC PRESS INC.
111 Fifth Avenue,
New York, New York 10003

Library of Congress Catalog Card Number: 71–109027
Standard Book Number: 12–590050–3

PRINTED IN GREAT BRITAIN BY
The Whitefriars Press Ltd., London and Tonbridge

Contents

The Infant: development of sleep

The Infant: development of vision

The Infant: learning and conditioning

Primate Studies

Attempts at Synthesis: organization in the development of behaviour

Attempts at Synthesis: structure-function relationships

Attempts at Synthesis: summing up

Membership

Study Group on Brain Mechanisms of Early Behavioural Development held at the Ciba Foundation, London, February 12th–16th, 1968.

R. M. BERGSTRÖM
Department of Physiology, University of Helsinki, Helsinki, Finland

T. G. R. BOWER
Department of Psychology, Harvard University, Cambridge, Mass., U.S.A.

G. BRONSON
Department of Psychology, Mills College, Oakland, California, U.S.A.

J. DITTRICHOVÁ
Institute for the Care of Mother and Child, Prague, 4 Podoli Nabr. K Marxe 157

T. HUMPHREY
Department of Anatomy, Medical Center, University of Alabama in Birmingham, Alabama, U.S.A.

I. C. KAUFMAN
Department of Psychiatry, University of Colorado Medical Center, Denver, Colorado, U.S.A.

L. P. LIPSITT
(Chairman II)
Department of Psychology, Brown University, Providence, Rhode Island, U.S.A.

H. PAPOUŠEK
Institute for the Care of Mother and Child, Prague, 4 Podoli Nabr. K Marxe 157

O. PETRE-QUADENS
Department of Developmental Neurology, Born-Bunge Research Foundation, 59 Filip Williot str., Antwerp, Belgium

D. PLOOG
Manx-Planck-Institute for Psychiatry, 10 Kraepelin St., Munich, West Germany

H. F. R. PRECHTL
Department of Developmental Neurology, University of Groningen, Oostersingel 59, Groningen, The Netherlands

R. J. Robinson
(Chairman I)
Institute of Child Health,
Hammersmith Hospital, Du
Cane Road, London, W.12

L. W. Sander
Division of Psychiatry, Boston
University School of Medicine,
80, East Concord St., Boston,
Mass., U.S.A.

F. J. Schulte
Department of Paediatrics,
University of Göttingen,
34 Göttingen, Humboldtallee 38,
West Germany

P. H. Wolff
Judge Baker Guidance Center,
295, Longwood Avenue, Boston,
Mass., U.S.A.

Centre for Advanced Study in the Developmental Sciences

The Centre for Advanced Study in the Developmental Sciences is being established, near Oxford in England. It is an international Centre for promoting the growth of knowledge about the development of human behaviour and the factors that influence it. It is controlled by the Developmental Sciences Trust, which is a charitable educational trust founded in 1967 under the chairmanship of Lord Adrian.

The Centre's activities relate to all those sciences and disciplines that can contribute to greater knowledge of the biological, social and psychological principles that govern the development and functioning of human behaviour over the life-cycle. The aims of the Centre are, first, to stimulate and coordinate research in directions where it is most needed and to foster among scientists and teachers in these fields a developmental and multi-disciplinary perspective on human nature; second, to encourage the application of knowledge from the developmental sciences by those, in all sectors of society, engaged in coping with or preventing human problems.

The Centre will implement its aims by means of a number of problem-oriented programmes. For each of these it will organize international study groups and training courses, provide facilities for sabbatical or study leave, and publish books and reports on research findings. The Centre will also provide a specialist library in the developmental sciences, run an information service, and provide facilities for other organizations concerned with human development to hold study groups.

The Centre is due to open at Minster Lovell Mill in September 1970. The 3-year preparatory period has been occupied with the building of suitable premises, setting up the administrative and financial organization, and planning the scientific programme. At the same time a preliminary programme of five international study groups was undertaken, with the generous collaboration of the Ciba Foundation, London, on the general theme of the origins of human behaviour. Groups of leading scientists came together, each for five days, to examine in depth the effects of biological and environmental factors on the origins and early development of a number of aspects of behaviour that are basic to the effective functioning of human beings. The present volume represents the proceedings of the second of these study groups.

Developmental Sciences Trust

310 Edgware Road, London, W2

Tel: 01-723 6623

Preface

The fifteen contributors to this volume met for a week to discuss "Brain mechanisms of early behavioural development". The programme for the study group included only eight invited papers, and the major part of the time was free for discussion. The group was left to plot its own course and to pursue whatever topics seemed most relevant to the main task, sometimes inviting particular members to make longer contributions. The book therefore contains three main kinds of material. First there are papers prepared before the meeting—those of Prechtl (both papers), Bergström, Humphrey, Schulte, Wolff, Lipsitt, and Ploog. Secondly there are papers given *ad hoc* at the request of the group during the discussion periods. In two cases the authors have recast these more formally (Petre-Quadens and Sander); the others are changed very little from what the author actually said (Dittrichová, Bronson, Bower, Papoušek, Robinson, and the second papers by Schulte and Bergström). Finally there are the discussions: the majority relate to particular papers and explore the issues they raised, but two of them—"Social Smiling" and "Organization in the Development of Behaviour"—deal with topics or concepts which were not covered by any of the papers but which the group felt a need to examine. The discussions were recorded and occupied over half the total time. They were so stimulating and enjoyable that it was tempting to think the printed version should try to convey their atmosphere as well as their content. However, in the interests of space and readers' time, I abandoned this attempt, and the discussions have been edited into as concise a form as was consistent with keeping the relevant and important matter.

I do not propose to make my own synthesis of or comments on the material. The Introduction, prepared by Heinz Prechtl beforehand, set out the main questions the study group was to tackle, and suggested some methods for answering them. The Summing-Up by Peter Wolff—an extempore *tour de force* which has hardly been altered—brilliantly summarized our successes and our failures. I have only two general comments. First, when picking up books like this which are based on the proceedings of a meeting, one is often misled by a general-sounding title into expecting a broad review of the whole field, and disappointed to find that the papers inside cover very limited ground. In this book, too, some of the papers have rather esoteric titles. However, each author has covered material outside the limits of his title, and related it to the main subject of the study group. As a result, I believe the book gives a reasonable picture of current knowledge and research on early behaviour—especially human—and its brain mechanisms.

My second comment is that this is a multidisciplinary book, based on a multidisciplinary study group. Books based on meetings are often criticized as being simply a medium for publishing more slowly and in a less accessible form papers which would normally appear in scientific journals. That criticism would be justified if each specialist used the book only to refer to the papers in his own particular field. I hope it will be used in just the opposite way. As a paediatrician with a special interest in neonatal neurology, I have learned something from every paper, but most from those of Lipsitt, Bower, and Papoušek, whose approach was totally new to me. I have been interested in the abilities and the perceptual world of newborn babies; these authors have demonstrated a much greater sophistication and complexity of brain function in early human infancy than could ever be shown by the traditional methods of neonatal neurology. I hope, therefore, that other readers will look at papers outside their immediate field of interest, and that some will even find time to read the book as a whole.

I warmly acknowledge the invaluable editorial help of Miss Rena Fenteman, without whose patient and careful work the material would have been far less presentable and readable. However, any errors are my responsibility. I am also grateful to the staff of the Centre for Advanced Study in the Developmental Sciences for their help, and to Mr. W. Hill for preparing the index.

Hammersmith Hospital, London R. J. Robinson
October 1969

Introduction

The Problems for Study

H. F. R. PRECHTL

University Hospital, Groningen

THERE ARE SEVERAL reasons why interest in the ontogeny of the brain and behaviour has greatly increased in the last few years. The most important reason is that we have studied early developmental stages in their own right, and the consequent enrichment of our technical arsenal in brain research and in the recording and analysis of behaviour has done much to facilitate progress. Many data have been accumulated on the structural and functional maturation of the brain, on the ontogeny of its biochemical composition, on the behavioural repertoire of the young organism, and on the capacities of the organism to respond and learn both in natural and in experimental situations.

A second reason, not fully independent from the first, lies in the relatively low degree of complexity of brain mechanisms and behaviour in the early developmental stages—which makes them very attractive for analysis. Moreover, the sequence of changes in the brain can be used as an experimental variable which opens up unique possibilities of exploring the relationship between certain brain structures, neural processes, and overt behaviour, throughout their genesis. One has to keep in mind, however, that this "simple apparatus" and its output is the product of a long evolutionary process of selection and mutual adaptation to the specific ecological conditions of rearing and nursing. It has to be looked upon in its biological context. The infant's brain is by no means a miniature model of the adult brain, but a relatively simple nervous system which has very particular properties at each phase in its development. These properties are determined both by genetically fixed programmes of growth and by environmental factors which influence the function and sometimes even the structure.

A third impetus for developmental studies has come from clinical work. The highest mortality rate of all age groups still occurs in the perinatal period. The clinical problems of prematurity, dysmaturity, and postnatal adaptation have led to a new field, now called neonatology, which includes the study of both normal and abnormal babies. The development of new techniques for early detection of neurological dysfunctions and sensory defects has renewed interest in infantile reflexes and response patterns as well as in the developmental course of sleep-and-awake-cycles and their pathology.

A fourth reason for the increasing interest in developmental studies is the knowledge that early experience may have long-lasting effects and decisive consequences for the life history of man and animals.

Before outlining the particular areas of research which will be discussed at this meeting, I would like to raise some general questions:

1. What is development?
2. What is the nature of the problems we encounter when we study early behaviour?
3. What do we know about the relationship between brain mechanisms and behaviour?

It is difficult to find a definition of the term "development" that would be common to all the fields in which the term is used. However, we are dealing with particular biological processes, and in this much narrower context the term can reasonably be defined as meaning the *sequential changes which continuously transform any biological system of relatively simple organization into one of increasing complexity and differentiation until a final stable stage is reached*. This definition would also fit the term ontogeny.

We also need to define the area covered by the term "early behaviour." There is ample evidence that the onset of activity in the nervous system during embryonic and fetal life is associated with coordinated motor activity which often resembles postnatal behaviour. Whether these motor patterns have a function during prenatal life or whether they are simply the consequences of the structural and functional maturation of the nervous system (with the purpose of being ready to take over at birth) is a matter of dispute, and, more profitably, one for future research.

When an infant is born it has to endure more dramatic changes in the environment than at any time in later life. It is true, of course, that infants are equipped physiologically to meet these problems. Besides physiological regulations which adapt the organism to the new environment, behaviour now plays a crucial role in obtaining regular food, care and protection, and in making social communication. Behaviour thus helps the infant to find and maintain the optimal living conditions and to build up social relations with its caretaker and siblings. It is this kind of phenomenon with which we are concerned when we speak of early behaviour.

The assessment and analysis of behaviour in infancy and childhood creates specific methodological problems. The investigator of the behavioural repertoire of the human infant faces problems similar to those of the ethologist in animal studies. He is dealing with a creature that is initially non-cooperative and non-verbal. Qualitative and quantitative observations of infants' overt behaviour have been carried out but much more work is necessary to complement our knowledge. The application of ethological techniques does not necessarily imply, of course, that ethological theories and hypotheses are immediately applicable as well.

Comparative studies of behaviour during infancy in many species have helped us to understand the correlation of behavioural repertoire with the stage of maturation at birth and with specific environmental conditions. Since animals are born at very different stages of maturation such studies can supply significant information on the genesis of early behaviour.

The third question we asked, and this will be the main topic of the meeting, concerns the relationship between brain mechanisms and early behaviour. Although a mass of descriptive data on early behaviour and its development already exists, comparatively few attempts have been made to analyse behaviour from the point of view of the underlying brain mechanisms. This is surprising, because correlative studies of brain mechanisms and behaviour in adult organisms can claim a long tradition and are connected with the illustrious names of Pavlov, Kleist, Lashley, Luria, W. R. Hess and many others.

Research concerned with the structure-function relation of the brain in birds and mammals has made great progress during the last few years through ontogenetic studies, applying modern electrophysiological and morphological (including electron-microscopical) techniques. The pre-, peri-, and postnatal development of excitatory and inhibitory synaptic mechanisms in the spinal cord and the cortex have been studied in relation to the differentiation of the neuronal substrate in sheep, cats, rabbits, and guinea pigs (Bergström, 1962; Marty and Scherrer, 1964; Purpura *et al.*, 1964, 1965; Scheibel and Scheibel, 1964; Scherrer and Fourment, 1964; Bernhard *et al.*, 1967).

Another blossoming branch of ontogenetic brain research is electroencephalography and evoked potential studies. Since the nature and genesis of these phenomena are still largely obscure their developmental changes are often not more than an interesting concomitant of remote functions of the maturing nervous system.

A new and very exciting approach in ontogenetic brain research is unit recording from immature brain cells in which an analysis is attempted of the spontaneous spike activity of neurones, and their interval distributions and inter-dependency, which may give some insight into the development of the code which the growing brain uses for communication between its various parts. Dr. Bergström will present the data from his own department. Single cell recordings have also been carried out in the cortex of rats and kittens at birth and during the first weeks of postnatal life in order to analyse the correlation of synaptic processes and discharge patterns with the morphological maturation of neurones and glia. Very definite relationships were found, especially with the membrane mechanisms of the dendrites (Purpura *et al.*, 1965). Moreover, Bernhard and his group (Bernhard *et al.*, 1967) have reported on the prenatal development of various gross electrical parameters of the fetal sheep cortex such as steady potentials, evoked somesthetic response, metrazol activation, spontaneous burst activity in the EEG, direct cortical response, and post-stimulation response. They were able to correlate the occurrence of these phenomena with the differentiation of particular components of the morphological substrate.

Another set of neuro-ontogenetic data is concerned with the structural and functional genesis of sensory systems. Well-documented studies are available on the visual system of kittens (Wiesel and Hubel, 1965a, 1965b), on cochlear function in the rabbit (Änggård, 1965), and on proprioceptors (muscle spindles and joint receptors) in kittens (Skoglund, 1960a-e; Skoglund and Romero, 1965; Ekholm, 1967).

In the field of the structural basis of early behaviour the most important contributions have been made by embryologists. Coghill (1940, 1943) spent a lifetime studying this problem in the American salamander, *Amblystoma maculatum*. His work has stimulated many studies in higher species. Experiments and observations in the chick embryo (Hamburger and Oppenheim, 1967; Hamburger, 1968) have contributed a great deal to our knowledge of how prenatal behaviour is produced by the nervous system. There is also a mass of results on mammals, especially rodents and sheep, mostly studies carried out in the 1930s and 1940s by Windle (1940), Barron (1941), and others. Work on the human fetus is inseparably connected with the names of M. Minkowski in Zurich and Hooker and Humphrey in the U.S. They were able to relate the appearance of fetal and postnatal reflexes to the genesis of certain brain structures and their connections. We shall have the pleasure of hearing Dr. Humphrey's exciting results.

Complementary to the studies on human fetuses are recent investigations carried out by means of neurophysiological techniques and behavioural observations, on babies born before term. The prenatal genesis of brain mechanisms in the human infant can thus be studied extrauterinely. Although the relation to the structure is much more difficult to explore because the brain cannot usually be examined morphologically in the same infant, studies of abnormalities of the nervous system are an additional source of such information on structure and behaviour. Dr. Schulte is an expert in this field and he will deal with these aspects.

When we come to discuss brain mechanisms and behaviour in the fullterm newborn infant it is evident that we are dealing with on-going processes which have prenatal antecedents and which continue after birth. For a long time many people looked upon infants' behaviour (mostly examining isolated reflexes and responses to experimental stimuli) as a set of neurological or neurophysiological curiosities. It is only recently that behavioural signs have been used as an analytic tool to study the organization of brain mechanisms. Correlative studies on postnatal brain structure and behaviour are almost completely lacking. With the relation between nervous functions and behaviour we are in a somewhat better position. During the last few years a new method has been introduced which was originally derived from electroencephalography and which is known as the polygraphic technique. The combination of behavioural observation with simultaneous recording of many physiological parameters has made it possible to collect detailed baseline data on spontaneous cycles of physiological and behavioural states under constant environmental conditions. These data form a sound basis, and are even a prerequisite, for investigations of response patterns to experimentally introduced stimuli.

It is evident that such a comprehensive method blurs the traditional distinction between physiology and behaviour. It becomes indefensible to classify the rapid eye movements in a sleeping infant as behaviour when they are observed by the naked eye, yet to consider those very same movements as a physiological phenomenon when they are recorded as an electro-oculogram. Such examples are legion.

New polygraphic techniques are a great advance in the study of very complex phenomena. For their analysis modern automatic data processing techniques are necessary. The stochastic analysis of the statistical properties of observed and recorded phenomena which are, in themselves, probability processes may provide clues about the organization of the underlying brain mechanisms. I shall try to illustrate this point in my subsequent paper.

Studies of brain mechanisms and behaviour in cases in which the nervous system shows distinct pathological conditions such as congenital malformations are of great interest. There are classic descriptions such as that given by Gamper (1925) concerning an anencephalic baby. Dr. Wolff's contribution reports on an arrhinencephalic infant he has studied and his data are an important contribution to our understanding of developing brain mechanisms.

By combining observation of early social communication with studies of neural morphogenesis and the effects of electrical brain stimulation in squirrel monkeys, Dr. Ploog has arrived at fascinating results. Since the monkey infant has a phylogenetic behavioural adaptation to his postnatal ecology which is similar to that of the human infant, comparative studies on primates are especially important and illustrative.

The approach to our problem would be very incomplete if we did not include the process of learning. Recent studies have shown that the brain of the infant is able to store information in memory and alter its responses as a result of previous experience. Dr. Lipsitt, who has made many original contributions to this field, will discuss this topic.

I have tried to outline the problems which will concern us in this meeting, and in doing so have listed the main aspects within a framework which stresses the biological aspects. This framework may need revision, and the data on which it is based might already have been overtaken by the results of more recent work. The importance and significance of developmental studies, however, has been amply demonstrated by the increase in our understanding and by the way in which results have been used.

Modern science is changing its face. The traditional disciplines have generally been oriented to particular techniques and methods. These can no longer deal adequately with a new and complex problem. The study of the development of brain mechanisms and of early behaviour demands a comprehensive approach. We can no longer simply delegate important aspects to colleagues from the other disciplines; we must work in very close contact with them and learn as much as possible of their techniques and their language if we are to make real progress in our research.

REFERENCES

ÄNGGÅRD, L. 1965. An electrophysiological study of the development of cochlear functions in the rabbit. *Acta Oto-laryngol. Suppl.* **203,** 5–64.

BARRON, D. H. 1941. The functional development of some mammalian neuromuscular mechanisms. *Biol. Rev.* **16,** 1–33.

BERGSTRÖM, R. M. 1962. Prenatal development of motor functions. *Annls Chir. Gynaec. Fenn.* **51,** *Suppl.* 112, 48 pp.

BERNHARD, C. G., KOLMODIN, G. M., and MEYERSON, B. A. 1967. On the prenatal development of function and structure in the somesthetic cortex of the sheep. In *Progress in brain research.* Vol. 26. C. G. Bernhard and J. P. Schadé (Eds.), *Developmental neurology.* Elsevier: Amsterdam, London, New York. Pp. 60–77.

COGHILL, G. E. 1940. Early embryonic somatic movements in birds and in mammals other than man. *Child Developm. Monogr.* **5,** 1–48.

COGHILL, G. E. 1943. Flexion spasms and mass reflexes in relation to the ontogenetic development of behaviour. *J. comp. Neurol.* **76,** 463–486.

EKHOLM, J. 1967. Postnatal changes in cutaneous reflexes and in the discharge pattern of cutaneous and articular sense organs. *Acta. physiol. scand.* Suppl. **297,** 29 pp.

GAMPER, E. 1925. Bau und Leistungen eines menschlichen Mittelhirnwesens (Arhinencephalie mit Encephalocele) zugleich ein Beitrag zur Teratologie und Fasersystematik. *Z. ges. Neurol. Psychiat.* **102,** 154–235.

HAMBURGER, V. 1968. The beginnings of co-ordinated movements in the chick embryo. In G. E. W. Wolstenholme and M. O'Connor (Eds.) *Growth of the nervous system.* A Ciba Foundation symposium. Churchill, London. Pp. 99–109.

HAMBURGER, V. and OPPENHEIM, R. 1967. Prehatching motility and hatching behavior in the chick. *J. exp. Zool.* **166,** 171–204.

MARTY, R. and SCHERRER, J. 1964. Critères de maturation des systèmes afférentes corti corticaux. In *Progress in brain research.* Vol. 4. D. P. Purpura and J. P. Schadé (Eds.), *Growth and maturation of the brain.* Elsevier: Amsterdam, London, New York. Pp. 222–236.

PURPURA, D. P., SHOFER, R. J., and SCARFF, T. 1965. Properties of synaptic activities and spike potentials of neurones in immature neocortex. *J. Neurophysiol.* **28,** 925–942.

PURPURA, D. P., SHOFER, R. J., HOUSEPIAN, E. M., and NOBACK, C. R. 1964. Comparative ontogenesis of structure-function relations in cerebral and cerebellar cortex. In *Progress in brain research.* Vol. 4. D. P. Purpura and J. P. Schadé (Eds.), *Growth and maturation of the brain.* Elsevier: Amsterdam, London, New York. Pp. 187–221.

SCHEIBEL, M. and SCHEIBEL, A. 1964. Some structural and functional substrates of development in young cats. In *Progress in brain research.* Vol. 9. W. A. Himwich and H. E. Himwich (Eds.), *The developing brain.* Elsevier: Amsterdam, London, New York. Pp. 6–25.

SCHERRER, J. and FOURMENT, A. 1964. Electrocortical effects of sensory deprivation during development. In *Progress in brain research.* Vol. 9. W. A. Himwich and H. E. Himwich (Eds.), *The developing brain.* Elsevier: Amsterdam, London, New York. Pp. 103–112.

SKOGLUND, S. 1960a. On the postnatal development of postural mechanisms as revealed by electromyography and myography in decerebrate kittens. *Acta physiol. scand.* **49,** 299–317.

Skoglund, S. 1960b. The spinal transmission of proprioceptive reflexes and the postnatal development of conduction velocity in different hindlimb nerves in the kitten. *Acta. physiol. scand.* **49,** 318–329.

Skoglund, S. 1960c. The activity of muscle receptors in the kitten. *Acta physiol. scand.* **50,** 203–221.

Skoglund, S. 1960d. Central connections and functions of muscle nerves in the kitten. *Acta physiol. scand.* **50,** 222–237.

Skoglund, S. 1960e. The reactions to tetanic stimulation of the two-neuron arc in the kitten. *Acta. physiol. scand.* **50,** 238–253.

Skoglund, S. and Romero, C. 1965. Postnatal growth and spinal nerves and roots. A morphological study in the cat with physiological correlations. *Acta. physiol. scand.* **66,** Suppl. 260, 50 pp.

Wiesel, T. N. and Hubel, D. H. 1965a. Comparison of the effects of unilateral and bilateral eye closure on cortical unit responses in kittens. *J. Neurophysiol.* **28,** 1029–1040.

Wiesel, T. N. and Hubel, D. H. 1965b. Extent of recovery from the effects of visual deprivation in kittens. *J. Neurophysiol.* **28,** 1060–1072.

Windle, W. F. 1940. *Physiology of the fetus: origin and extent of function in prenatal life.* Saunders, Philadelphia, Penn.,

Discussion

Bergström: What did you mean by saying the brain processes are quite simple in the beginning?

Prechtl: That brain processes in the early ontogenetic stages are relatively less complex, therefore "simpler", than in the adult organism. I think of the nervous system in terms of a network consisting of units with interconnections and with a certain differentiation. Throughout development the increase in the number of units and in their interconnections, and even the changes in their quality as a result of changes in the membrane properties, are the structural basis of what I described as the increase in complexity of the developing brain.

Ploog: I think this is a very good point at which to start talking about the grade of complexity in the nervous system. Every research worker whether he uses monkeys or *aplysia* says the system he works with is too complicated. Prechtl meant a relatively simple system compared with brain mechanisms in the adult.

Prechtl: In the same species.

Robinson: Prechtl implied that development was necessarily going from increasingly simple things to increasingly complex things. Is this necessarily so?

Prechtl: Yes, based both on embryology and on the repertoire of behaviour. The newborn is not a helpless creature unable to do anything except cry and suck. But compared with a preschool child his repertoire is not only quite different but it is also smaller. Studying the changes throughout development has advantages for attacking certain problems where studies in which you chop pieces off adult brains would not give the answer. At least these two kinds of studies can be complimentary to each other.

WOLFF: This is to define development as a move from a lower to a higher level of differentiation. Might one talk about organization rather than complexity because there are occasions when developmental change leads to simplification. However development is assessed, it is a process which results in something more organized than it was before. So complexity is not simply a greater number of parts. The integration or organization of these parts is what should concern us.

ROBINSON: Do we really define development thus or on a time scale?

WOLFF: Time is irrelevant to development as a concept. The traditional way of thinking about development—in terms of one thing coming after something else—leads to all sorts of contradictions. Many changes with time have nothing to do with development. A disease process is not a developmental process.

LIPSITT: On the other hand, if we consider what we can do with or make out of any given 5-year-old, it may be considerably less than what we can do with or make out of any given newborn. The potential of the newborn child may be more complex, more varied, than the potential of the older child. Perhaps development may be conceived under this view as a gradual suppression of various kinds of responses.

PRECHTL: Did you mean potentialities in the sense that a newborn or an infant can go this way or that way, according to the environment?

LIPSITT: Yes.

PRECHTL: You mean "the programming of the life history"?

LIPSITT: I am thinking in terms of variability of outcome. The variability of outcome is greater for the newborn than for a 5-year-old, who already has a developmental history which imposes certain limitations.

PRECHTL: Have we enough data to make this comparison?

LIPSITT: A great deal is known about the intelligence of the 5-year-old as a basis for the prediction of adult intelligence, but very little is known about the newborn with respect to factors that permit us to predict his adult intelligence. Given any 5-year-old I know better what his intelligence level will be in adulthood than given any newborn child.

PRECHTL: Yes, if the newborn is studied in the first 2 days when he is still in the process of postnatal adaptation. You then get very inconsistent findings. Findings are usually more reliable from the fourth or fifth day on.

MACKEITH: When we discuss the potentialities of the newborn and the potentialities of the 5-year-old, this is mixed up with what we *know* about these potentialities, which is a very different thing.

LIPSITT: Because we know quite a bit about the predictability of intelligence from various previous age levels, I think that it serves as a fair example for the notion that I was presenting about the possible diminution of complexity with increasing age.

WOLFF: It is the fantasy of every patient in psychotherapy who hasn't committed himself to a way of life that he could be anything. It is a kind of verbalism to say that he could become anything until he becomes something, so what we consider as variability is not a statement about the baby, but our idea about what we could do with the baby.

PLOOG: Lipsitt's point of view is much more biological than psychological. In the first periods of gestation the fetus has more potentiality than it has in the fortieth week. Lipsitt took intelligence just as one example because we are able to measure it more accurately than, let's say, personality variables.

PRECHTL: If you think in terms of units with interconnections—a computer network—and you add units and interconnections then you get this thing which you call more complex. But keeping it completely descriptive this means just increase in units and interconnections. Observing the output of such a thing—not what you can do with it—the less complex system will be much more labile and random than the more complex one. An increase in complexity nearly always results in an increase in stability. Perhaps that is what Dr. Lipsitt has in mind: that the potentiality, or in my terms the lability and unpredictability, is greater at the younger stage than at the older one.

The Fetus

Electrical Parameters of the Brain During Ontogeny[1]

R. M. BERGSTRÖM

University of Helsinki

INFORMATION AND ELECTRICAL PARAMETERS

Information

ANY STUDY OF the maturation of the neural structures demands that attention be paid to the capacity of neural tissue to mediate information. This capacity is the most important factor in determining the sensory and motor activity—the animal behaviour—of the developing individual. A study of the early behavioural development of the individual is, therefore, a study of the ontogenetic development of the neural, information-carrying system.

In such a study one may proceed in a classical way with investigation of the three systems: the sensory, the motor, and the integrative functions of the brain. However, this approach does not shed any further light on the most typical processes of the brain, the stochastic phenomena of the neuronal assemblies. From the aspect of information-carrying capacity these processes are of fundamental importance, since they form the basis for definition of the statistical information. A study of the statistical minute processes of the developing neurons themselves is therefore of fundamental importance.

According to the statistical theory of information (Shannon and Weaver, 1949), the information content (I) of a system can be defined as the negative logarithm of probability (p) of the information-carrying process:

(Equation 1) $$I = -\log p$$

In a neural system the processes which mediate information within the

[1] This work was supported by a grant from the National Research Council for Medical Sciences, Finland.

system itself can best be characterized by the electrical parameters which describe the propagating action potentials. Notwithstanding the possibility that other electrical parameters of the brain (steady potentials, EEG, etc.) may be essential for the information flow in brain structures, the binary all-or-none signals seem to form the most useful level of the information-carrying functions at which the process can be handled with exactness.

A distinction must be drawn between three different main categories or groups of parameters which define the binary electrical signalling processes in the brain: (1) the quantity of the binary signals (2) the time pattern and (3) the space pattern of these signals. The first category relates to the number (n) of the propagating action potentials of a given system. The second category indicates the successive pattern of these impulses and the third the spatial pattern of the impulses. As will be seen later, changes occur in all these categories of events in the brain during the ontogenetic development of the individual. Along with these changes there is a change in the information-carrying capacity of the brain during ontogeny.

Probability and Brain Functions

To determine the information content of the developing neural system it is necessary, according to equation 1, to consider the probability of the appearance of the events described by the three groups of parameters. It may thus be concluded that a change (ΔI) in the information content of the brain during ontogenetic development is described by a function (f) of the probabilities of the three types of parameters

(Equation 2) $$I = f(P_n, P_t, P_l)$$

in which (P_n) gives the probability of the appearance of a given number (n) of the binary signals, (P_t) the probability distribution of these signals in time, and (P_l) the probability distribution of these signals in space. I will not attempt an exact formal treatment of the problems of the developing brain but I shall examine in more detail the characteristics of the different types of probabilities, since the purpose of this paper is that of describing the changes in electrical parameters of the developing brain from the aspect of development of the informative processes in the brain structures. Furthermore, the informative processes form the basis of the output and input functions of the neural system, that is, the basis for the behaviour of the developing individual.

Before discussing the different categories of the probability parameters in equation 2 we ought to consider the relationship between the concepts of information, order, and entropy in a system consisting of mutually connected neurons which exhibit binary signals (Bergström, 1967). According to the information theory, information can be understood as negative entropy of the system concerned. As is the case with the physical systems, a neural system may contain an event or a structure which displays a degree of entropy or—as the entropy can be interpreted—a given degree of disorder. If this is put the other way around, a neural system may display events with a given amount of orderliness, or, as it can be termed, negative entropy. This negative entropy of the neural event is a measure of the information content of the behaviour of the system.

However, according to the statistical theory of information (equation 1), the probability of an event determines the information content of that event, whereas by the Boltzmann law of entropy the probability of the event determines the degree of entropy or disorder in the system of which the event is a part. It is thus possible to connect the concepts of information, entropy, and order.

In a developing brain, therefore, the degree of order both in the structural elements and in the function of those elements can be studied; by this means knowledge is gained of the entropy-probability relations and information content of the neural system.

Of the three categories of probability parameters in equation 2, the space factor (P_l) is determined by the geometry of the neural elements and their connections. As will be shown, a change of the neural geometry is discernible during the ontogenetic development of the individual. This change influences the information-carrying abilities of the system. The time factor (P_t) manifests itself as the successive pattern of the binary signals. This pattern, as is demonstrable by study of the unit electrical activity of the developing brain, also changes during development of the individual, along with the development in behaviour. Finally the third factor, the quantity parameter (P_n), which describes the number of signals, is determined by the quantity of excitation contained in the developing system. Evidence also exists that this parameter changes during ontogenetic development.

DEVELOPMENT OF NEURAL GEOMETRIES

Order of Maturation in the Brain

To discover the successive order in which different neural structures become active during the different stages of ontogenetic development, registration of the gross electrical activity provides a suitable measure of the functional ability of the different parts of the brain. Another indicator for this purpose is the ability of the different parts of the brain to respond to electrical stimulation. After experiments of this type have been made it is possible to determine which kinds of neural structure mature first, and which mature subsequently, and in this way to determine the factor P_l in equation 2. In a series of experiments the old concept (*cf.* Windle, 1940), according to which the maturation of the central nervous system begins at the medullary level, and proceeds in the caudal and oral direction, was tested. Registrations of the gross electrical activity and the results of stimulation experiments both reveal that the first signs of functional maturity are observable along the whole brain stem at a relatively early stage of development. Thus, EEG potentials are obtainable from the hippocampal region in the guinea-pig (Fig. 3; Stenberg *et al.*, 1968) at the 35th to 37th day, the normal length of gestation being 65 days. Signs of gross activity appear in the lower brain stem at the same stage (Stenberg, 1967). Similarly, positive registrations of gross activity have been obtained in a 4-month-old human fetus from the corresponding oral part of the brain stem (Stenberg and Bergström, unpublished observations). The first electrical activity was of the same type in all cases, and was described as a primitive wave pattern of irregular frequency, or intermittent wave complexes. In the human fetus, electrical maturation of the lower brain stem begins at the 70th day (Table I; Bergström and Bergström, 1963). Moreover, stimulation experiments show that the oral brain stem is capable of responding with regulative functions at a relatively early stage (Bergström *et al.*, 1966a), as does the lower brain stem (L. Bergström, 1966).

All these results indicate that the first part of the fetal brain which matures functionally is the whole reticular core, extending from the oral to the caudal parts of the brain. Further experiments relating to the beginning of the fetal cortical EEG (for references *see* Bergström, 1962) in the guinea-pig have shown that the peripheral parts of the brain do not mature until later. The direction of functional maturation is accordingly from the reticular core to the periphery.

That the reticular core matures first is interesting because its function exhibits certain characteristics which should be reflected in the over-all performance of the brain, and in the behaviour of the individual. This behaviour should also be typical of the fetus at an early developmental stage. To learn about this early type of behaviour it is necessary to analyse the information flow in reticular neural structures, as compared with that in more geometrically ordered structures. Such neural structures of more ordered type, which are mainly situated in the periphery of the brain, do not become functionally active until later in the course of development.

Structural Relations of Neural Elements

For the purpose of structural analysis it is appropriate to distinguish between two extreme types of neuronal geometries: those organized reticularly and those organized in parallel structures (Fig. 1). With

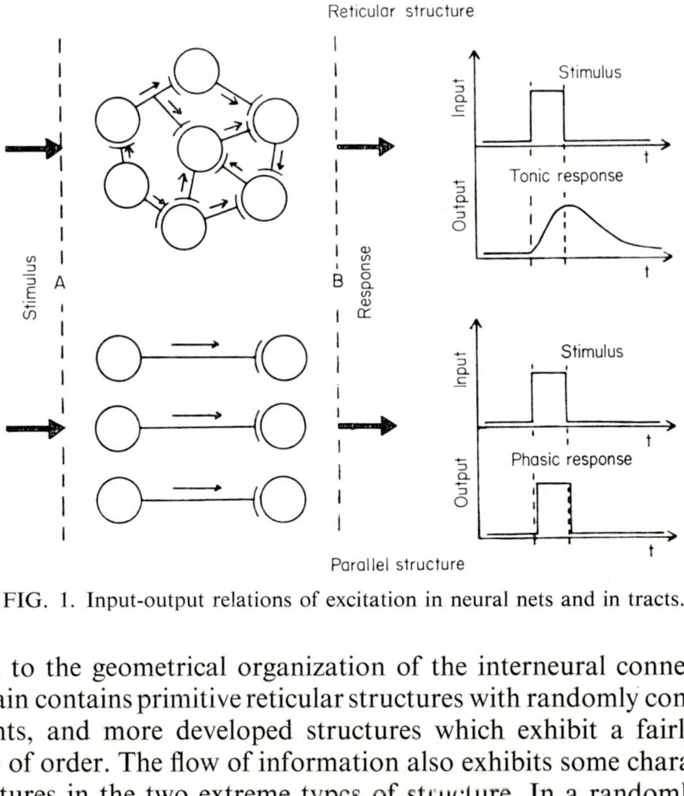

FIG. 1. Input-output relations of excitation in neural nets and in tracts.

regard to the geometrical organization of the interneural connections, the brain contains primitive reticular structures with randomly connected elements, and more developed structures which exhibit a fairly high degree of order. The flow of information also exhibits some characteristic features in the two extreme types of structure. In a randomly connected reticular net, the input-output relation of the information flow displays what can be called "tonic" characteristics, whereas the relation is "phasic" in the structure connected in parallel. In other words, a randomly connected reticular net shows diffuse time relations between the stimulus and response, but in the parallel structure the relation is more exact. The space relations also differ in both structures: in the reticular net the spread of signals does not follow a specified direction as it does in the parallel structure.

In reality, of course, the brain contains neural geometries which are intermediate between these extremes, although both types do exist in the extreme form—the randomly connected structures in the core substance of the brain, and the parallel structures in the brain tracts. The main point is that the most primitive structures exhibit more randomness in their geometry than do more developed structures. In respect of information flow, the most primitive structures show diffuse time and space relations in the transmission of signals; in the more developed structures, transmission is more exactly defined in relation to time and space.

Experiments concerned with both the unit electrical activity of the developing brain and the spontaneous and stimulated motor activity of the developing organism indicate a change during ontogeny from the kind of information flow typical of randomly connected neural geometries to that typical of more ordered neural geometries.

DEVELOPMENT OF TIME STRUCTURES OF ELECTRICAL ACTIVITY

Gross Electrical Activity

There is extensive literature concerning ontogenetic development of the EEG, particularly in regard to the beginning of cortical activity in various animal species and in man. However, relatively little is known about the development of the gross electrical activity of subcortical structures (Schwartze, 1966), and almost nothing about the statistical parameters which describe the wave pattern in the developing brain (Stenberg, 1967).

It is known that cortical EEG potentials appear in the human premature infant at about 5–6 months as a discontinuous wave pattern which becomes continuous at 8 months (Dreyfus-Brisac, 1962). In the pontine brain stem, electrical waves are discernible from the 70th day, and they grow to a fixed amplitude between the 70th and the 112th day (studied in a series obtained from Caesarean sections, Bergström and Bergström, 1963; Fig. 2 and Table I). In the hippocampus of the human fetus, electrical waves appear about the 4th month (Stenberg and Bergström, unpublished observations). Initially the potentials appear to be of irregular type in the cortex (Dreyfus-Brisac, 1962), and in the oral brain stem the activity is intermittent. Intermittent activity was not observed in the lower brain stem.

TABLE I. BRAIN AND MUSCLE ACTIVITY IN THE HUMAN FETUS (Bergström and Bergström, 1963)

Case No.	*Age (days)*	*Spontaneous movements*	*Leg flexor reflex*	*Gastrocnemius stretch reflex*		*Reflex irradiation*	*Electrical activity in brain stem*		*Respiratory movements*
				Appearance	*Inhibition*		*Spontan.*	*Response*	
17	59	−	−	−			−	−	−
4	61	−	−	−			−	−	−
2	70	+	+	−			+	−	+
19	71	+	+	−			+	−	−
10	80	−	+	+?			+	−	−
6	84	+	+	−			+	+	−
21	88	+	+	−			+	+	−
8	93	+	+	−					+
20	94	+	+	−			+	−	−
14	98	+	+	+	−	+	+	−	−
12	98	+	+	+	−	+	+	+	+?
18	101	+	+	+	−	+	+	−	−
11A	105	+	+	+	−	+	+	+	−
11B	104	+	+	(+)					
5	108	+	+	+	−	+	+	+?	−
16	112	+	+	+	−	−	+	+	+
1	112	+	+	+	+	−			−
9	121	+	+	+	+	−	+	+	+
15	122	+	+	+		−	+	+	+
3	133	+	+	+	+?	−			+
13	140	+	+	+	+	−	+	+	+
7	158	+	+	+	+	−	+	+	+

Corresponding observations on the development of gross activity in the brain during ontogenic development have been made in animals (Fig. 3). In the guinea-pig, studies have also been made of the changes in the frequency spectrum of the gross activity during the fetal period (Stenberg, 1967). A clear fixation of the main frequency of the waves in the lower brain stem from an original dysrhythmic pattern is observable. Similar findings have been made in respect of the cortical potentials.

Although we know nothing about the connection between the gross electrical wave pattern of the brain and the unit electrical activity—so observations on the EEG cannot be related directly to the information processing of the units—there are certain aspects of the immature EEG

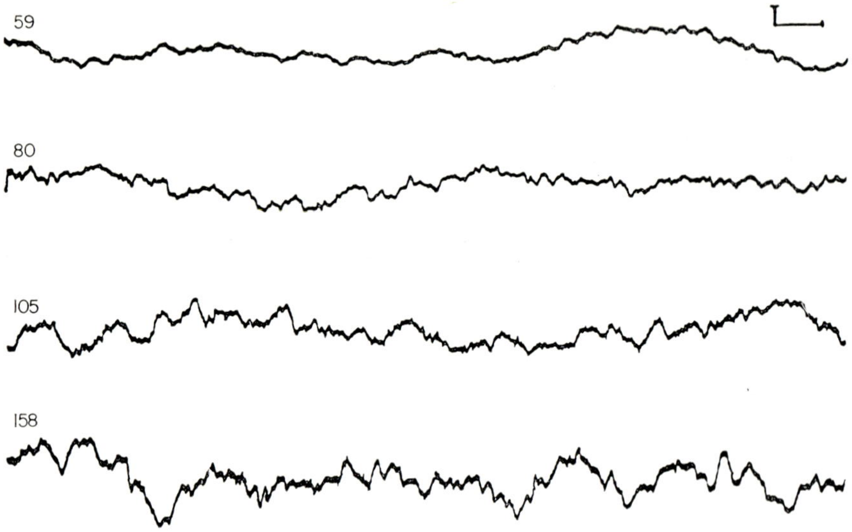

FIG. 2. Gross electrical activity in the pontine brain stem of the human fetus. Figures are age in days. Calibration: 50 uV, 1 sec (Bergström and Bergström, 1963).

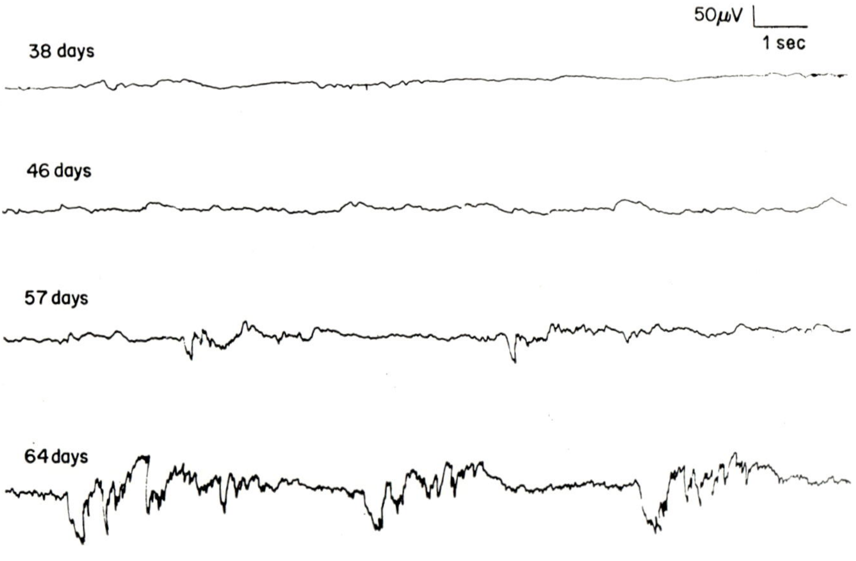

FIG. 3. Gross activity from hippocampus in the guinea-pig fetus.

which are of interest from the standpoint of the entropic relations of the developing brain. Consequently the appearance of certain fixed frequencies from an original, primitive dysrhythmic wave pattern in the EEG can be interpreted as an increase in the orderliness of the waves or of the corresponding neuronal functions. This implies that the entropy of this particular function—which is of course unknown—diminishes during maturation of the brain.

Study of the gross electrical activity of the brain is valuable not only because it gives us the opportunity to learn about the maturation of the different sites (*see* Fig. 7), but also because it is an indicator of the over-all state, the "macrostate" (Bergström, 1967), of the central nervous system. This over-all state, again, influences the information flow in central structures, for example, as it operates in the different degrees of arousal. The significance of this influence is discussed later in this paper.

Unit Electrical Activity

It can be assumed that the electrical activity of the single units of the brain is more closely related to the intracerebral information flow. However, studies of the statistical properties of the spike potentials in the developing brain are almost lacking. Only such statistical relations of the unit potentials, including time series analysis, could provide knowledge of the data processing of these units and assist in comprehension of the ontogenetic development of the information-carrying system. The time series analysis would contribute to the determination of the factor P_t in equation 2.

It is known that unit activity in the rabbit cerebral cortex appears between the 5th and 10th days of postnatal age (Schadé, 1960). Action potentials of long duration, together with synaptic potentials, have been observed in newborn kitten cortex (Purpura *et al.*, 1965). Spontaneous unit impulse activity from subcortical structures in the newborn rabbit has been demonstrated by Bergström *et al.*, (1966a). Cells from the striatum, the hippocampus and the hypothalamus exhibited a resting membrane potential of the order of 5—20 mV, and the extracellular action potentials had a duration of up to 10 msec. The observed impulse interval histograms resembled the gamma distribution (Fig. 4), but differed from the theoretical gamma-distribution. In a more advanced study of the spontaneous unit activity of the sub-cortical structures in the postnatal rabbit Hyvärinen (1966) demonstrated a negative correlation between the duration of the action potential and the age of the animal. The impulse frequency increased with age (thus contri-

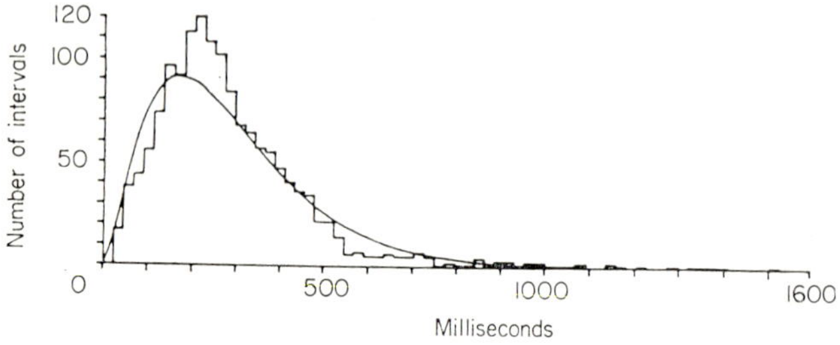

FIG. 4. An impulse interval histogram of a cell in the globus pallidum of an 8-day-old rabbit. Stationary sample of 1,448 impulse intervals lasting 4 min 45 sec; mean impulse frequency 5·2 imp/sec. The curve shows the best fitting theoretical gamma distribution for the same material (Bergström *et al.*, 1966).

buting to the amount of binary signals in the brain and influencing the factor P_n in equation 2), and exhibited a decrease in dispersion with age. Statistical analysis of the impulse interval trains showed histograms of mono-, bi- and multimodal distributions (up to six peaks). The monomodal distributions were of normal, and also of gamma, and exponential types. The normal distributions of Gaussian type were most frequently observed in the globus pallidus, capsula interna, and zona inserta. No systematic association of the gamma or of the exponential distributions with age or brain region was apparent in this study. The multimodal distributions were most frequent in the non-specific nuclei of the thalamus, and their number increased with age.

The time series analysis indicated that the intensity functions and the renewal densities increased with age. During puberty a transient diminution occurred in these parameters.

It was possible to show some of the same features in the cortex of kittens, from the age of 1 week (Jokinen *et al.*, unpublished studies). Initially the action potentials occurred at a slow rate, and were of long duration. The histograms also exhibited a relatively large spread initially.

The time relations in single unit activity thus show a distinct correlation with age. As Hyvärinen (1966) concluded, certain relations indicate that the long duration of the action potentials is correlated with a Poissonian tendency. Nevertheless, the long duration exhibited a reduction to approximately adult values at the age of 2 weeks in the rabbit. These characteristics indicate a diminution in the random features of the spontaneously active brain cells during ontogenetic development; a connection is discernible between this finding and the capacity of the brain structures to mediate information. The results of the study indicate that the informative state of the brain becomes more effective with increasing age.

MOTOR OUTPUT

Stimulated Output

The motor output of the individual, that is, the motor behaviour, reflects the events in the central nervous system. Examination of the processes connected with the motor phenomena can therefore be used for studies on the intrinsic functions of information processing in the central nervous system, and thus for research into the changes that take place in this processing during ontogenetic development.

A systematic study of the motor responses which follow electrical stimulation of the mesencephalic brain stem structures in the guinea-pig fetus has been made by Lea Bergström (1966). The first types of movement (Fig. 5) obtained in this manner were in the fore limb, shoulder

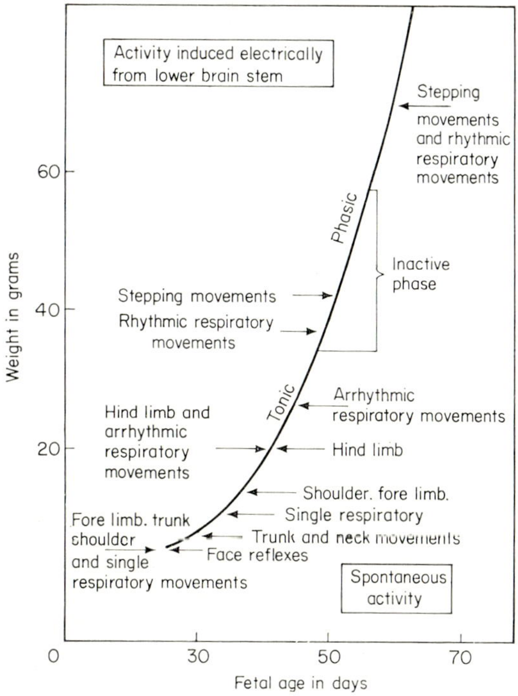

FIG. 5. Spontaneous and electrically induced motor activity in the guinea-pig fetus (L. Bergström, 1966).

and upper trunk at a gestational age of 28 days. These motor responses were highly tonic in nature. Moreover, single respiratory movements appeared at this age after the stimulation. Tonic movements of the limbs, including the hind limbs, and of the whole trunk, were discerned at 40 days. At this stage the stimulation could also produce short series of arrhythmic respiratory movements. Not until about 50 days were clearly phasic muscle responses obtained. These appeared mainly in the limbs, and included series of stepping movements. A common observation at this stage was that the limb movements were connected with corresponding trunk contractions. The phasic nature of the responses became more apparent after this developmental period; in parallel, the limb movements were obtained without corresponding contractions of the trunk muscles. After the 50th day clearly rhythmic respiratory movements were observable after stimulation.

In the experiments with electrical stimulation there was a clear change in the muscular responses from tonic to phasic type at an age of approximately 50 days. Simultaneously with this change the regulatory connection between trunk and limb movements was broken.

Studies of muscle reflexes during the fetal period in sheep (Änggård *et al.*, 1961), in the guinea-pig (Bergström *et al.*, 1961), and in the human being (Bergström and Bergström, 1963), show that when reflex behaviour begins there is pronounced irradiation of the reflexes elicited from the skin in different regions; the first reflexes were obtained from the face and the neck. In the studies of the sheep fetus (gestation period 150 days), it was found that from the 60th day a "fetal myotatic reflex" induced by stretch of the gastrocnemius muscle was obtained. This reflex was characterized by a spread of the excitation to antagonistic muscle (the anterior tibial muscle) and a lack of antagonistic inhibition; the latter occurred later, at the 72nd day. This type of fetal reflex, which shows a lack of balance between the excitatory and inhibitory mechanisms, was also demonstrable in the guinea-pig fetus (between the 45th and 56th day), and in the human fetus (between the 98th and 112th day, Fig. 6).

Furthermore, in the reflex studies a more or less gradual change was observed in the reflex responses, from a tonic to a phasic type. This change is apparent roughly during the same period as that in which the fetal stretch reflex dominates, and irradiation of the excitation ends. It has been pointed out (Änggård *et al.*, 1961) that the absence of the inhibition, which results in the tonic and widespread character of the reflex activity, is of central origin.

Experiments on the stimulated motor output functions, carried out both electrically and by means of reflexes, indicate that at an early fetal

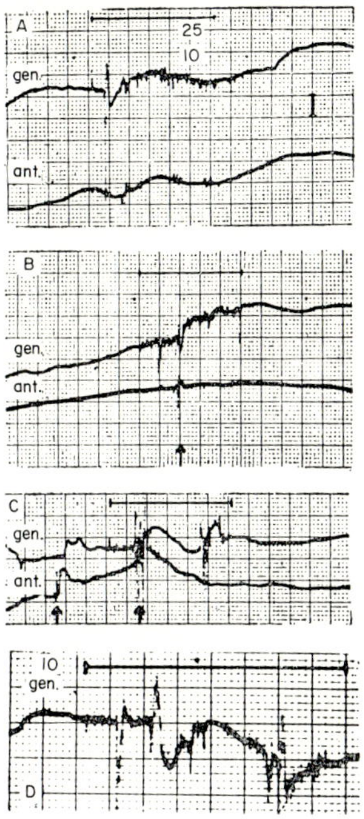

FIG. 6. Electromyogram recordings from the gastrocnemius muscle (gen) and tibialis anterior muscle (ant) in human fetuses during stretch of the gastrocnemius (shown by horizontal bars) and ipsilateral plantar skin stimulation (shown by arrows). A: age 105 days, B: 108 days, C: 158 days, D: 158 days. Vertical bar in A, 200 uV. Horizontal intervals in squares: 0·5 sec (Bergström and Bergström, 1963).

stage the motor output is random to the extent that the different muscular elements are functioning without observable order. It seems possible that the appearance of ordered time and space sequences of performance during later development is connected with the appearance of inhibitory mechanisms, probably of central origin.

Spontaneous Output

Along with these studies of the stimulated and reflex behaviour of the immature central nervous system the spontaneous behaviour of the fetuses was also observed. An additional study was made of the spontaneous motor behaviour of the intra-uterine guinea-pig fetus with intra-uterine placement of EMG and EEG leads (Bergström, 1962). These studies partly supported the concept of the early tonic mode of activity of the muscular apparatus, and the irradiation of this activity in the initial motor development of the fetuses.

TABLE II. FETAL DEVELOPMENT OF THE CNS AND THE EPS FUNCTIONS IN THE HUMAN

Developmental stage	*Age in months*	*Type of motor activity*	*Highest matured EPS-centre*	*Electrical maturation of CNS*	*Typical motor behaviour*	*Primitive reflexes*
I	1·5	INACTIVE	—	—	—	—
II	2	TONIC ACTIVE	Bulbopontine	Appearance in pons	Tonic, lateral movements of upper trunk	Tonic, irradiating reflexes to neck and mouth, "Hautschutz-, Saug-, Handgreif-, Rückgrat-Reflexe".
III	4		Tegmental	Maturation in pons	Tonic, proximal limb muscles with trunk	Tegmental reactions, head and body righting, compensatory eye movements, "Schnappatmung"
IV	4·5	PHASIC ACTIVE	Diencephal	Matured in pons	Proximal limb muscles independent of trunk, beginning of phasic activity	"Bauchdeckenreflexe", extension of the limbs, Moro(?), "Schreckreflex", rigidity
V	5–8		Pallidal	Thalamus (?), appearance in cortex	Phasic activity of distal limb muscles	"Pallidumwesen"
VI	8–postnatal 3	LETHARGIC ACTIVE	Striatal	Maturation in cortex	Relatively inactive	Arousal reaction
VII	postnatal 3 onwards	VOLUNTARY ACTIVE	Cortical	Matured in cortex	Voluntarily active	Disappearance of primitive reflexes, appearance of conditioned reflexes

In Lea Bergström's study (1966) the different types of fetal motor performance were obtained by means of electrical stimulation of the brain slightly earlier during the course of development than the point at which they appeared spontaneously. This indicates that the application of electrical current, that is, neural excitation, moves the state of the motor system of the brain to a later development stage. In view of the above, this implies that the application of stimuli to the brain diminishes the randomness of the function of the neuronal elements of the central nervous system. A diminution in the randomness of the neural elements would, by virtue of the theoretical considerations already presented, also increase the order or the informational content of the system.

By way of conclusion to this part of my paper I suggest that the motor behaviour of the immature individual can be separated into stages that are directly linked to its motor output functions (Table II and Bergström, 1963b). In the first stage no motor activity is discernible. The second and

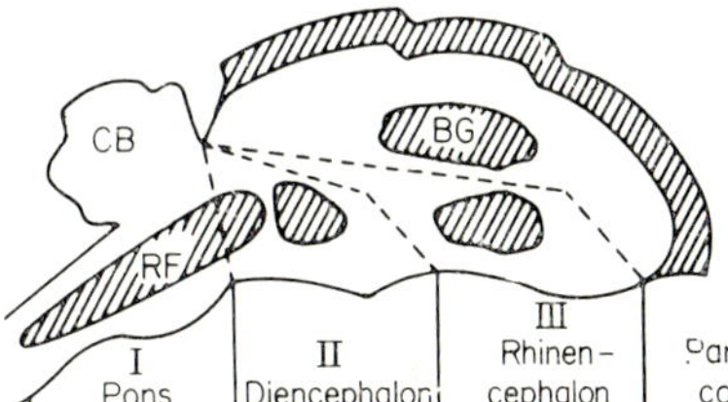

Maturation of EEG and motor activity	I Pons	II Diencephalon	III Rhinen-cephalon	IV Parietal cortex
Human	70–120	140	129	170 →
Guinea-pig	35–52	45	35	47–65
EEG maturation	Growth of amplitude	Appearance		Growth of amplitude
Motor behaviour	General, tonic	Local, phasic		Inhibited

FIG. 7. Motor activity and gross electrical activity of different parts of the brain in human and guinea-pig fetuses. The numbers are the gestational age in days at which electrical activity appears in different parts of the brain. BG: basal ganglia. RF: reticular formations. CB: cerebellum. (Data on human EEG maturation from Dreyfus-Brisac, 1962.)

third stages are a tonic active period characterized by tonic spontaneous and reflex motor behaviour, at first of bulbo-pontine, and later of tegmental, nature. The fourth and fifth stages are the phasic active period, also characterized by distinct activity in the limbs—first in the proximal parts and then in the distal—and a lack of primitive irradiation of the motor performance. These stages are followed by a relatively inactive period, ranging in the human fetus from the 8th prenatal month to the 3rd postnatal month. This stage is also clearly discernible in the guinea-pig fetus between the 50th and 60th day. At this stage spontaneous movements are few, although it is possible to obtain responses to electrical stimulation of the lower brain stem (Lea Bergström). The next stage could be termed a voluntarily active period, characterized by willed motor activity. A connection is discernible between these developmental periods and the maturation of the EEG, as is illustrated in Table II and in Fig. 7.

ENTROPY AND ELECTRICAL DEVELOPMENT

Structural Entropy

Experimental findings enable us to make a geometrical model of the brain for study of its behaviour during ontogeny. This model can be based upon studies of the motor output of the brain by Monnier and Lévy (1961), and upon the description of the organization of the extra-pyramidal system in a mature central nervous system by Jung and Hassler (1960), works which have been considered with respect to the ontogenetic aspects (Bergström, 1963a). This brain model (Fig. 8) comprises a reticular core substance (RF), along with shells of neural structures organized in reflex circuits through the cerebral nuclei. The first circuit is situated nearest the core, and consists of a subthalamo-pallido-rubral pathway; the next is the centromedian-striatal-nigral pathway, and the third, lying nearest the periphery, is the thalamo-cortico-spinal pathway. Each of these shell circuits possesses an input and an output to and from the reticular core, which acts in part as a common input and output channel. There may also be an additional circuit nearest to the reticular core through the tonic mesencephalic nuclei, commisura posterior, nucleus interstitialis and nucleus prestitialis. These nuclei are known to regulate the tonic movements of the head and upper trunk (Jung and Hassler, 1960, on the basis of findings made by Hess). This mesencephalic circuit is not indicated in Fig. 8. The importance of the pallidal and striatal reflex arcs in the pathogenesis

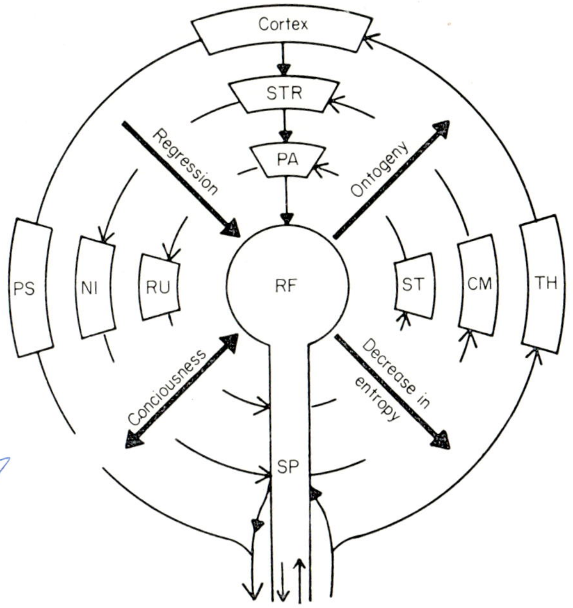

FIG. 8. A structural and functional model of the brain consisting of a reticular core surrounded by shell reflex circuits.
RF: reticular substance. ST: subthalamus. Pa: pallidum. RU: nucleus ruber. CM: centrum medianum. STR: striatum. NI: substantia nigra. TH: thalamus. SP: spinal cord. PS: pyramidal system.

of extrapyramidial disorders has been pointed out by Monnier and Lévy. The significance of the other circuits from the aspect of the pathogenesis of involuntary movements has been described by Bergström (1963a), who considered these symptoms to be signs of a regression of the brain function to a level which is genetically more primitive.

The geometrical organization of the neural elements in the different parts of the model exhibits features of considerable interest. As was mentioned earlier, the reticular formation, which forms the core substance, presents a random geometrical order of the connections between the elements. The nearer a circuit is to the periphery, the more order it has. The outermost shell circuit, that is, the pathway going through the cortex, possesses the maximum degree of geometrical order and the minimum degree of randomness. The cortical mass itself contains distinct geometrical relations with respect to the intracortical fibres. Possibly the dendritic masses of the cerebral cortex and the other nuclei of the shell circuits, which also seem to possess random connections between the elements, act as a "storehouse" for excitation in the form of reverberating circuits. Nevertheless, the ordered elements prevail in the over-all function of the circuit concerned.

Functional Entropy

The geometrical organization of the brain—in a reticular core substance, and peripheral, more ordered shell circuits—permits the use of a model from which we can draw conclusions about the way in which the different parts of the brain function. Such conclusions may be important to our understanding of the ontogenetic development of the central nervous system.

In view of my earlier statements about the tonic nature of the input-output relations of randomly connected networks, and the phasic nature of more ordered geometrics, it is obvious that the different parts of the model will function differently. The inner reticular core acts in a tonic way, whereas, the nearer the outer shell, the more phasic is the action. The highest degree of phasicity should be displayed by the cerebral cortical pathway with the pyramidal output system and the specific sensory input system. These considerations seem to be in close accord with reality, since the output of the cortico-pyramidal system is a phasic system, as opposed to the typically tonic system of the mesencephalic reticular systems (the reticular core and the circuits through the tonic mesencephalic nuclei). The circuit through the subthalamus and pallidum and ruber is known to regulate motor functions of a medium degree of tonicity (Monnier and Lévy, 1961; Bergström, 1963a).

Adequate evidence of this main distribution of tonic and phasic functions in the brain mechanisms has been gained by experience in the study of extrapyramidal disorders, and in their surgical treatment. It is known that dystonic syndromes, including pathological tonic alteration of the motor functions, result from impairment of the innermost shell circuits (Monnier and Lévy, 1961). Syndromes consisting of medium degree tonic behaviour (ballismus) result from impairment of the subthalamic pathway, and syndromes of a phasic nature (choreoathetotic movements) result from interruption of the striatal circuit. It seems that the impairment of the outermost cortical circuit results in apraxia—a different kind of motor syndrome—which can be regarded as a disease of the voluntary function itself.

Experience obtained both in physiological experiments on normal brain mechanisms and in the study of pathological functioning, supports the concepts used in constructing the model. If the function of the circuits and of the core of the model is now considered from the point of view of the distribution of entropy in those parts, more evidence is derived for employment of the model as a tool for study of the dynamics of ontogenetic development.

Schlesinger (1962) has pointed out that the primitive brain stem centres exhibit a higher degree of probability in their functions than do the more developed brain centres. This finding is supported by the fact that the autonomic and highly stable regulatory centres of circulation and respiration are situated in the lower reticular brain stem. Nevertheless, the higher and psychological functions of the brain, related to the centres of the cerebral cortex, are unstable, and therefore exhibit less probability in their functions. Identical properties of these structures can also be deduced from the geometrical organization of the elements in the corresponding structures; this follows from the high degree of entropy displayed by the geometrical organization of the reticular core, as was seen above. By the Boltzmann law of entropy this high degree of entropy corresponds to a high probability.

It is clear that the organization of the brain in different shells surrounding a reticular core explains some of the functional properties of its parts. Knowledge of these properties can now be used in a study of the ontogenetic development.

Dynamics of the Brain in Ontogeny

We know that the reticular core of the brain is the first part of the central nervous system to be developed during ontogeny, and that the more peripheral parts develop later. Study of the information flow in neural geometries of the random type which are typical of the reticular substance, and of the ordered type typical of the peripheral circuits, reveals that the first mode of information transmission to be developed at an early fetal stage is that characterized by diffuse time and space relations. This stage is followed by modes of information flow which are characterized by increasingly exact time and space relations. Such a pattern of information flow development is in fact reflected in the behaviour of the developing individual, as well as in the results of experiments concerned with the unit electrical activity of the brain. The change in motor behaviour of the developing individual from a tonic to a phasic type, together with the appearance of inhibition in the reflex pattern and the disappearance of the reflex irradiation, can be interpreted as the result of such a change in the intracerebral information flow. This is demonstrated more directly by the decreasing Poissonian character of the binary signal trains of the brain units.

The change in the type of information flow is also connected with some aspects of the information content itself. Together with the development of the peripheral brain circuits with highly unstable, that is, improbable functions (low entropy), the over-all state of the brain is turned towards higher informative content; this is reflected in the appearance of the voluntary type of motor behaviour, closely connected with conscious behaviour. Against this, the earliest and most primitive modes of information flow are connected with over-all states of the brain, characterized by highly stable and highly probable subconscious non-voluntary behaviour (with low information).

It is well known that the individual who is in a mature state can exhibit regressive behaviour either during normal life (this is especially true of children) or in neurological diseases. During such a regression there is a repetition of the ontogenetical stages. In some extrapyramidal disorders this is certainly the case (Bergström, 1963a) and it is said that all extrapyramidal syndromes, if they are chronic, lead to a severe tonic state of the whole muscular system. It seems that the regression constitutes a major response of the central nervous system to disturbances of many kinds. If that is so we can formulate a common entropic law, verifiable also from physical systems, that a neural system tends to move towards the most probable state if disturbed. The brain functions of the highest probability are those carried by the reticular core, which possesses the highest degree of entropy even in the geometrical organization of its elements.

In normal life, also, the central nervous system tends to move towards the most probable states, in which the reticular core—which is the most primitive structure ontogenetically—dominates the behavioural patterns. This is the case in oscillation of the consciousness between a waking state and sleep. In children, where the most peripheral, highly improbable functioning brain circuits are poorly developed, the oscillation is balanced towards the most probable side, that is, to the lower degrees of consciousness and to sleep.

SUMMARY

Studies concerned with the gross electrical activity of different parts of the brain during ontogenetic development lead to the conclusion that the functional development of the brain proceeds outwards from the whole reticular core (both parts of which, the oral and caudal, mature at the same developmental stage) to the periphery. Structurally, the core consists of elements which are mutually connected in a random way and thus display a high degree of geometrical entropy. The geometrical organization of the units shows an increase in order towards the periphery. The structural organization corresponds to an information flow which exhibits poor time and space relations (tonic) in the random structures, and far more exact time and space relations (phasic) in the ordered structures. This corresponds to low information-carrying capacity in the former, and high capacity in the latter. Studies of the unit electrical activity of brain neurons, and of the motor behaviour, both reflex and spontaneous as well as electrically stimulated, indicate that during ontogeny the randomness of these functions diminishes with age (an increase in order). This leads to the deduction that the brain exhibits a diminution in the Poissonian tendency (Table III) of the

TABLE III. CHANGES IN BRAIN STRUCTURE AND FUNCTION DURING ONTOGENY

Structural relations	Networks with RANDOM GEOMETRY (reticular substance)	→	STRUCTURES WITH NON-RANDOM GEOMETRY (higher brain centres)
Gross electrical relations	RANDOM EEG ACTIVITY	→	FIXED EEG PERIODICITY
Motor output relations	TONIC, NON-COORDI-NATED ACTIVITY (spontaneous, reflexive)	→	PHASIC, COORDI-NATED BEHAVIOUR
Unit discharge relations	SERIAL INDEPENDENCE OF IMPULSE INTERVALS	→	SERIAL DEPEND-ENCE OF IMPULSE INTERVALS
Entropy relations	POISSONIAN CHARACTER OF EVENTS (high entropy, low information)	→	NON-POISSONIAN CHARACTER OF EVENTS (low entropy, high information)

function of its elements, corresponding to an increase in information content. A structural and functional model of the brain is developed, consisting of a reticular core with random structure (high entropy and low informational content) and of surrounding shell circuits with structures which are more ordered (lower entropy and higher informational content) the nearer a circuit is to the periphery. In sequence ontogenetic development exhibits the different functional properties of the core and the shell circuits, the most primitive state reflecting a tonic, highly stable and unconscious behaviour, and the most developed state reflecting phasic, highly unstable, and willed (conscious) behaviour. Normal and pathological regression to and oscillation between different ontogenic states can be observed, particularly in children.

REFERENCES

ÄNGGÅRD, L., BERGSTRÖM, R. M., and BERNHARD, C. G. 1961. Analysis of prenatal spinal reflex activity in sheep. *Acta physiol. scand.* **53,** 128–136.

BERGSTRÖM, L. 1966. Foetal development of mesencephalic motor functions in the guinea-pig. *Acta physiol. scand.* **68,** Suppl. 277, 22.

BERGSTRÖM, R. M. 1962. Prenatal development of motor functions. A study on the intra-uterine guinea pig foetus in the conscious pregnant animal. *Annls Chir. Gynaec. Fenn.* **51,** Suppl. 112, 1–48.

BERGSTRÖM, R. M. 1963a. On the physiology of the meso-diencephalic extra-pyramidal system, with special reference to the pathogenesis of involuntary movements. *Acta neurol. scand.* **39,** Suppl. 4, 52–60.

BERGSTRÖM, R. M. 1963b. On the pathophysiology of the extrapyramidal syndromes. *Duodecim* **79,** 200–213.

BERGSTRÖM, R. M. 1967. Neural macrostates. *Synthese.* **17,** 425–443.

BERGSTRÖM, R. M. and BERGSTRÖM, L. 1963. Prenatal development of stretch reflex functions and brain stem activity in the human. *Annls Chir. Gynaec. Fenn.* **52,** Suppl. 117, 1–21.

BERGSTRÖM, R. M., HÄLLSTRÖM, P. E., and STENBERG, D. 1961. Prenatal stretch reflex activity in the guinea-pig. *Annls Chir. Gynaec. Fenn.* **50,** 458–466.

BERGSTRÖM, R. M., HIRVONEN, J. I., and KARLSSON, L. K. J. 1966a. Respiratory changes during electrical stimulation of rhinencephalic structures in the foetal guinea pig. *Nature, Lond.* **210,** 1176–78.

BERGSTRÖM, R. M., HYVÄRINEN, J., and KURENIEMI, E. 1966b. Spontaneous impulse activity in immature rabbit brain. *Acta physiol. scand.* **66,** 383–384.

DREYFUS-BRISAC, C. 1962. The electroencephalogram of the premature infant. *Wld. Neurol.* **3,** 5–15.

HYVÄRINEN, J. 1966. Analysis of spontaneous spike potential activity in developing rabbit diencephalon. *Acta physiol. scand.* **68,** Suppl. 278, 1–67.

JUNG, R. and HASSLER, R. 1960. The extrapyramidal motor system. In F. Field (Ed.), *Handbook of physiology.* Vol. 2. Sect. 1. Neurophysiology. American Physiological Society, Washington, D.C. Pp. 863–927.

MONNIER, M. and LÉVY, A. 1961. Die physio-pathologischen Mechanismen der Dystonien und Dyskinesien. *Schweizer Arch. Neurol. Neurochir. Psychiat.* **85,** 100–139.

PURPURA, D. P., SHOFER, R. J., and SCARFF, T. 1965. Properties of synaptic activities and spike potential of neurons in immature neocortex. *J. Neurophysiol.* **28,** 925–942.

SCHADÉ, J. P. 1960. Origin of the spontaneous electrical activity of the cerebral cortex. In *Recent advances in biological psychiatry.* Grune & Stratton, New York. Pp. 23–42.

SCHLESINGER, B. 1962. *Higher cerebral functions and their clinical disorders.* Grune & Stratton, New York.

SCHWARTZE, P. 1966. Ontogenetische Entwicklung der bioelektrishen Aktivität des Gehirns mit besonderer Berücksichtigung der durch weckende Reize und Pharmaka hervorgerufenen Veränderungen. *Sb. Prací přir Fak. palack. Univ. Olomouci.* **41,** 161–172.

SHANNON, C. and WEAVER, W. 1949. *The mathematical theory of communication.* Univ. of Illinois Press, Urbana.

STENBERG, D. 1967. The ontogenesis of the spontaneous electrical activity of the lower brain stem. *Acta neurol. scand.* **43,** Suppl. 31, 162.

STENBERG, D., BERGSTRÖM, R. M., and VEHASKARI, M. 1968. Gross electrical activity in hippo-campal regions in the guinea-pig fetus. *Scand. J. clin. Lab. Invest.* **21,** Suppl. 101, 62.

WINDLE, W. F. 1940. *Physiology of the fetus.* Saunders, Philadelphia and London.

Discussion

SCHULTE: Estimating gestational age from intra-uterine growth is inaccurate. Is it really true that the human fetal brain does not produce detectable bio-electric brain activity before age 170 days—24 weeks' conceptual or 26 weeks' postmenstrual age? Preterm infants of this age live for a while, and certainly have EEG activity.

BERGSTRÖM: The date I quoted for cortical activity in the human fetal brain is taken from Dreyfus-Brisac (1962. *Wld. Neurol.* **3,** 5).

SCHULTE: If you put a needle into the brain of a human fetus, you would surely detect activity in the parietal region earlier than 170 days' conceptual age. In fact, at that age EEG activity can be detected from the scalp.

PLOOG: What does Dr. Bergström mean by "tonic"?

BERGSTRÖM: We define it as an input/output relationship: thus, in a tonic model of response an input lasting a precise time interval gives a response which grows slowly and lasts for a long time after the end of the stimulation.

PLOOG: This is not true for all networks. For instance you have a very tonic response from a receptor . . .

BERGSTRÖM: Receptors differ in their input/output relationship. There are tonic receptors and also phasic receptors. It is possible that the micro-organization of a receptor differs in both types. Engineers know quite well that there are such different systems in the technical sense; it appears that there are these different types of transfer functions in biological systems too. I like this definition because it's the same as the one the engineers use.

PLOOG: The engineering type of thinking is sometimes far removed from the biological facts.

BERGSTRÖM: It's dangerous to go too far in this mode of thinking, but it will enable us to use formal and quantitative descriptions. For instance, it is difficult to define formally and quantitatively the concept "integrated activity", often used by physiologists in connection with brain development. What is meant when we say there are "integrative functions" in the brain?

PLOOG: Does Shannon's definition of information apply to the biological systems? Your signal is a purely technically defined one, not a signal such as the nervous system receives. Therefore, the Shannon type of information is not the type we ought to consider in biology. The same is true with the Boltzmann equation—in this case it would mean that the increase in entropy ought finally to lead to the highest disorder, if you take the whole life span. But what really occurs is that there is an increase and then there is a decrease of order and so we finally have the highest degree of disorder: death.

BERGSTRÖM: According to physical laws all systems tend to go to the maximum entropy, to a minimum of order. So the whole life, in spite of its showing high degrees of order, will always have a tendency to go to disorder or maximum entropy. In that sense, biological systems are similar to physical systems. Only there is some transient force in the developing individual which drives the whole thing to a greater order.

ROBINSON: The biological system is not a closed system. The organism is altering the entropy of the universe.

BERGSTRÖM: Yes.

PRECHTL: Brain engineering helps tremendously to describe nervous processes in more concrete terms. You then have measurable entities which you can formalize in a mathematical sense. What is the evidence that we cannot apply information theory to living systems?

PLOOG: We can take engineering models as brain models. My reservation concerns only the inadequacy of the Shannon definition of information. If we use these words like "coding" and "decoding", ignorant of the underlying processes, we may gloss over our ignorance. We should be careful in using these terms and make it clear that we have to find out what really happens in the biological system.

WOLFF: You may not like "integration", but you use the words "order" or "organization". Did you mean simply to define order in terms of your pictorial model, or have you some other less mathematical conception of what that order would be?

BERGSTRÖM: Neurophysiology shows that the reticular formation is truly a randomly organized net. The tracts going through the reticular formation do not belong to it. By the physiological concept "reticular formation", physiologists mean only the neural net. Nearer the periphery you have more ordered tracts and structures, and also in the more developed nuclei you have more ordered mutual connections between the elements. In the cortex, finally, you may have some randomly connected elements, but they are not so typical in the cortex, with its high degree of structural order.

WOLFF: How do you describe whether something is ordered or not ordered?

BERGSTRÖM: We are looking at all kinds of order, not only geometrical order. In connection with the unit impulses, for instance, we may talk about dependency and independency. Independency does not show any order, it's a random process; dependency means a certain amount of order, so that order and disorder are only alternative words for negative entropy and entropy. But we also use the term "geometrical order". It's an important concept, because we believe that if the channel consists of elements which are randomly organized, or disordered, then the physiological point of view is that such structures with no order function tonically. The more there is order, the more there will be phasicity of the output, according to the definition of the concept.

KAUFMAN: Your concept of the tonic or sustained response, which outlasts the stimulus, is based on a functional net in which the messages continue to go in a variety of side-chains as well as forward-chains. At what point may structure be replaced by patterned or functional organization in the development of the nervous system, and to what extent are characteristics of response determined purely by structural considerations? Even a reticular structure could be so organized that messages travelled in parallel fashion and not sideways.

BERGSTRÖM: That is possible. If you have another organized structure more complex than the parallel structure, let's say organized nets, perhaps you can get quite other types of response. Those responses from complicated organized systems are not fully tonic, they are nearer the phasic system, because there is a clearly organized pattern of the response. It differs from long-lasting sustained and non-organized activity

SCHULTE: Was it in the guinea-pig that you had tonic activity up to 50 days and from then on more phasic activity?

BERGSTRÖM: Yes.

SCHULTE: Skoglund in his work with kittens found almost the reverse kind of development. He had phasic activities first and it was very hard to get any tonic activity in the very young kittens. Only after some days or even weeks could he get mild tonic activity in the kitten by stretching the muscle. Are you describing another type of tonic muscle?

BERGSTRÖM: Those results concern the peripheral motor system. Our studies were at a much earlier—prenatal—stage of development than Skoglund's in the kitten. Perhaps the newborn animal shows some reverse function when it is adapting to a new environment. Birth may have a strong influence on neural processes. We have studied development in uniform, intra-uterine conditions.

PRECHTL: One function certainly connected with the reticular formation is body posture. This can't work phasically; if it did, an organism would just jerk continuously. Therefore this system really is organized to give a tonic output and sustain it.

PLOOG: Yes, because of all cranial nerve nuclei the vestibular nucleus is closest to the reticular formation. Phylogenetically it is derived from the large reticular elements which progressively become differentiated into a large mass. Here occurs the tonic production of impulses and a very distinct phasic type of interaction. How does this occur in development? There is not just a core with net functions; there is already a type of nervous system which should give phasic responses. The idea of interaction right from the beginning might be more appropriate.

BERGSTRÖM: Yes, perhaps we could make this difference softer, but I must add just one qualification: those responses of the vestibular nuclei which are phasic are mostly responses to stimuli from the outside world. The amniotic fluid provides a fetal environment where there is relatively speaking no gravity. So I suspect those experiments where the fetus is first removed from the amniotic fluid where it doesn't need any posture. For instance, Lea Bergström (1966. *Acta physiol. scand.* **68,** Suppl. 277, 22) has observed that, if electrical stimuli are applied to the brain of the fetus, one can get the electrical responses and the behaviour earlier, which later on appear spontaneously. So can you say that the vestibular nuclei are functionally developed early. The nucleus is there but it doesn't function.

PLOOG: All non-human primates would die if they didn't have a very well developed postural system at birth.

BERGSTRÖM: At birth, yes. But before? They don't need any postural mechanism because they are like men in space.

HUMPHREY: In human embryonic material I found that the lateral vestibular nucleus had neurones developed to a functional level—if one can judge by the staining of the Nissl material—as early as 35 to 37 millimetres crown-rump length, or 9½ to 10 weeks of menstrual age. Although these neurones have reached a functional level, I do not know whether the remainder of the vestibular system is capable of functioning also.

BERGSTRÖM: We don't know if it functions in reality.

HUMPHREY: I suspect that it does, or at least that it is sufficiently developed to function. Minkowski thought the vestibular system functioned at this time. We have seen activity that is suggestive of a response to a change in position. We have also observed movements of small hamster fetuses that were interpreted at the time as of vestibular origin.

Postnatal Repetition of Human Prenatal Activity Sequences with some Suggestions of their Neuroanatomical Basis[1,2]

TRYPHENA HUMPHREY[3]

University of Alabama in Birmingham

INTRODUCTION

On various occasions brief reference has been made to the observation that the sequence in which an activity develops during fetal life is repeated during early postnatal development (Gesell and Amatruda, 1945; Hooker, 1952, 1954, 1958; Hooker and Humphrey, 1954; Humphrey, 1964a; Humphrey and Hooker, 1959). Some of this sequential repetition occurs perinatally as well as postnatally, especially for actions that have their origin extremely early in the course of embryonic development.

Three outstanding examples of this repetition of fetal activity sequences have been selected for consideration. Various others might

[1] This investigation was supported by Public Health Service Research Career Program Award NB–K6–16716 from the National Institute of Neurological Diseases and Blindness.

[2] It was aided by Research Grant HD–00230 from the National Institute of Child Health and Human Development, National Institutes of Health. The present paper is Publication No. 53 in a series of physiological and morphological studies on human prenatal development, begun in 1932 under the direction of Dr. Davenport Hooker. The collection of cinematographic records of human fetal activity on which this paper is based has been supported in the past by grants to Dr. Hooker from the Penrose Fund of the American Philosophical Society, the Carnegie Corporation of New York, the University of Pittsburgh, and the Sarah Mellon Scaife Foundation of Pittsburgh, as well as by Grant B–394 to Dr. Hooker and the author from the National Institute of Neurological Diseases and Blindness, National Institutes of Health.

[3] The author is deeply appreciative of the excellent assistance of Mrs. Catherine P. Glazner and Mrs. Edith N. Vaughn in the preparation of the manuscript and the illustrations. She is also most grateful for the criticisms and helpful suggestions of Professor Elizabeth C. Crosby, and for the aid rendered in various ways by other members of the Department of Anatomy of the University of Alabama in Birmingham.

have been chosen, but these three include the earliest reflex sequence executed by the human fetus, as well as reflex sequences appearing later in development. They have the further advantage of being both well known and involving movements of widely different parts of the body—the head, the hand and the foot.

COMPARISON OF OBSERVATIONS ON THE FETUS AND THE INFANT

Head Movements Elicited by Perioral Stimulation

Fetal head movements. Bending the head to one side in response to stroking the perioral area with a hair esthesiometer is the earliest reflex thus far observed in human fetuses. When it begins at 7·5 weeks of menstrual age[4] the reflex consists only of bending the head and upper trunk away from the site of the stimulus (Hooker, 1952, 20·7 mm; Fitzgerald and Windle, 1942, 20·0 mm). The action soon becomes much more extensive, however, and at 26·0 mm (8·5 weeks) this contralateral flexion reflex (Fig. 1)[5] consists of neck, trunk and pelvic flexion with extension of the arms and sometimes pelvic (or rump) rotation (Hooker, 1952, 1958; Humphrey, 1964a, 1968b, 1969b). The movement of the lower extremities separates the soles of the feet (8, Fig. 1).

These contralateral flexion reflexes (Figs. 1 and 2) have been referred to as avoiding reactions, because the region stimulated is moved away from the stimulating agent (Hooker, 1952, 1958, 1960; Hooker and Humphrey, 1954; Humphrey, 1952, 1964a, b). The term was employed by Coghill (1916, 1929) in amphibian behavioural studies and by Angulo (1932) in his observations on reflexes in the fetal rat. In slightly more mature fetuses, the reflex includes a greater degree of extension at the shoulders, slight extension at the elbows, flexion of the hands, and spreading apart of all digits (7, 8, Fig. 2.). The rump rotation becomes more marked, the soles of the feet separate more, and the toes spread apart also.

The reflexes just described (and similar ipsilateral ones) have been known as total pattern reflexes because they involve all the neuromuscu-

[4] All ages given in this paper are menstrual ages, based on the tables of Streeter (1920) and taken from the records of Dr. Davenport Hooker. The crown-rump length (CR) is given in millimetres (mm) for each fetus.

[5] In each figure containing photographs from the motion picture records, frame numbers are used as follows. Number 1 designates the frame immediately preceding the beginning of the action; higher numbers indicate the succeeding frames in their correct order. Thus 8 on Fig. 1 illustrates the 7th frame of the action and 11 the 10th. The motion pictures in Figs. 1 and 10 were taken at 24 frames per second; those in all other figures were photographed at 16 frames per second.

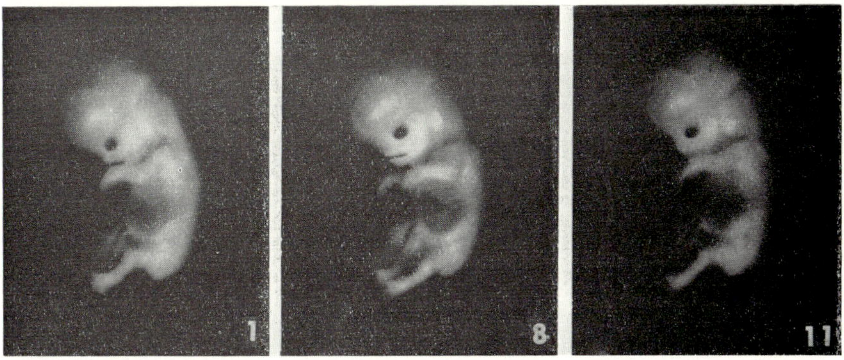

FIG. 1. Contralateral flexion reflex of the total pattern type in response to stroking the skin of the left side of the face lateral to the nose and mouth area with a 100 mgm hair esthesiometer. In frame 1, immediately preceding the beginning of movement, the stimulator overlies the nose and adjacent area of the cheek. Frame 8 illustrates the height of the reflex with the head, trunk, and rump flexed contralaterally, the arms extended at the shoulders, the soles of the feet pulled apart, and the mandible lowered to open the mouth. In frame 11 the fetus has returned almost to the original position. 26·0 mm fetus, CR length; 8·5 weeks' menstrual age. Photographs at about 1·2 times natural size.

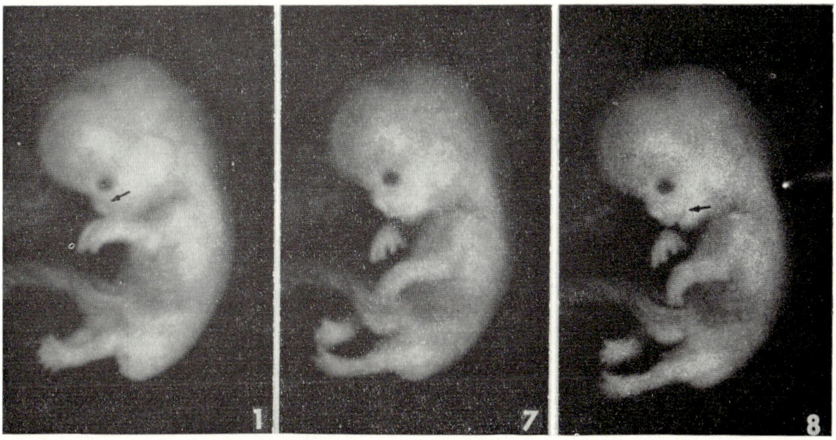

FIG. 2. A contralateral flexion reflex of the total pattern types elicited by stroking the left side of the face from the mouth area to the bridge of the nose. In frame 1, preceding the beginning of the action, the stimulator is overlying (but not touching) the area from the ala nasae to the bridge of the nose (at arrow). In frames 7 and 8 there is marked head and trunk flexion and rump rotation. In this vigorous reflex, neither the two arms nor the two lower extremities move symmetrically and all digits are spread apart. At the peak of the reflex (frame 8) the ipsilateral hand is markedly flexed. The mouth, already open when uncovered by the hands, (as in frame 7), is open wider (arrow on frame 8) at the height of the reflex. 27·1 mm fetus, CR length, 8·5 weeks' menstrual age. Photographs at approximately 1·6 times normal size.

lar mechanisms capable of responding to stimulation at the time when they are elicited (Coghill, 1916, 1929; Hooker, 1944, 1952, 1958, 1960; Humphrey, 1964a, 1968b,). In the recent frame-by-frame examination of all motion picture films recording these reflexes, the more forceful reactions were found to include incomplete, but active, mouth opening at 26·0 mm (Humphrey, 1968b). When the reflex is vigorous enough to produce spreading of the digits, separation of the soles of the feet (8, Fig. 1), and asymmetrical upper extremity movements (7, 8, Fig. 2) the mouth almost always opens. Thus mouth opening develops as an integral part of the total pattern reflexes.

In a few reflexes the mouth has already begun to open completely by 27·1 mm (as indicated by the arrow on 8, Fig. 2). By 9·5 weeks complete mouth opening is fairly constant (Humphrey, 1968b). During the 8·5- to 9·5-week age period, when mouth opening is part of the vigorous contralateral flexion reflexes, the tongue moves to the floor of the mouth and the palatal shelves change from the vertical position lateral to the tongue to the horizontal one superior to it and begin to fuse. Recently I have suggested (Humphrey, 1968a,b, 1969a,b) that fetal mouth opening at this age provides a dynamic force which is significant in bringing about these changes in the position of the tongue and the palatal processes.

Ipsilateral flexion reflexes have not been observed so early in development as contralateral ones, and they occur much less frequently. A recent tabulation based only on the motion picture records of the 8–10 week period showed 95·1 per cent of the 198 lateral flexion reflexes to be contralateral and only 4·9 per cent ipsilateral (Humphrey, 1968b,c). The earliest ipsilateral reflex photographically recorded was noted at 8·5 weeks, a week after the first contralateral response was seen. At this age a forceful ipsilateral reflex (Fig. 3) includes extensive lateral head and trunk flexion, rump rotation and separation of the soles of the feet equal to that found in the contralateral reflexes of the same fetus. However, it is not possible to determine whether the mouth opens, for the ipsilateral hand covers the mouth even more completely during the peak of the response (11, Fig. 3) than when the fetus is at rest (1, 40, Fig. 3).

By 10·5 weeks the contralateral flexion reflexes are being replaced by head and trunk extension (Hooker, 1958; Humphrey, 1968). This reflex is the predominant reaction to perioral stimulation by 11 weeks (Fig. 4), especially when the stimulus is near the midline (Hooker, 1952, 1958). Like the contralateral flexion reflex, head and trunk extension are avoiding in type, for, as shown in the photographs,

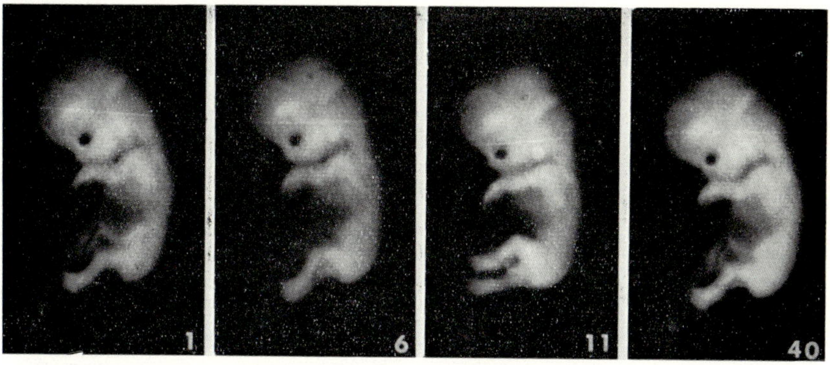

FIG. 3. A vigorous ipsilateral flexion reflex elicited from the fetus illustrated in Fig. 1. The stimulator touches the area lateral to the mouth (frame 1), but is hidden by the left hand. The ipsilateral bending of the head, trunk and rump, already evident in frame 6, is more marked in frame 11 when rump rotation has been added. In frame 40, the return to a resting position is complete. With such ipsilateral flexion reflexes the hands cover the mouth, so opening, if present, cannot be seen. 26·0 mm fetus CR length; 8·5 weeks' menstrual age. Photographs at about 1·2 times normal size.

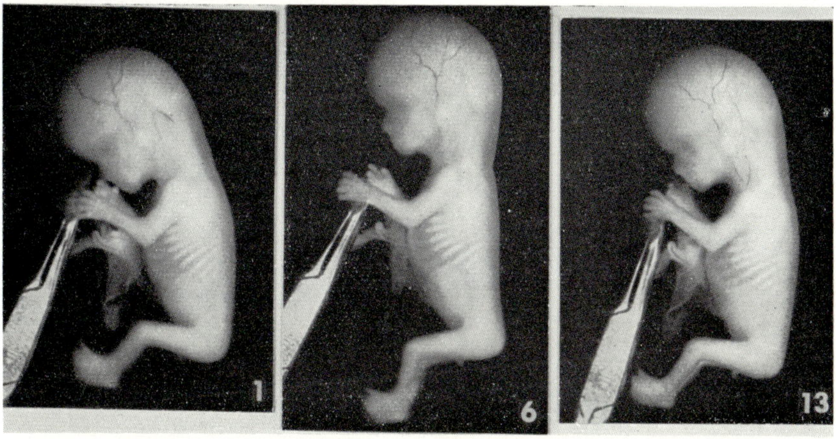

FIG. 4. An extension reflex elicited by touching the face near the midline (just lateral to the nose) with the clamp on the umbilical cord. The position of flexion immediately before the beginning of movement (frame 1) changed to marked extension of the head, trunk and pelvis in frame 6. The fetus has returned to the resting position in frame 13. Extension reflexes are numerous at this age. At the peak of the movement the lips often appear compressed, but usually otherwise there is no additional movement. 48·7 mm fetus, CR length; 11 weeks' menstrual age. Photographs at about 0·9 of normal size.

the area stimulated is rapidly moved away from the source of stimulation (6, Fig. 4).

Ventral head flexion, a reflex that brings the area touched towards the stimulus, has not been seen so early in development as head extension and is rare until after 11 weeks. It has been observed in combination with swallowing at 12·5 weeks and later (Hooker, 1952, 1958; Humphrey, 1964a, 1968b). Ventral head flexion is illustrated here (Fig. 5) as part

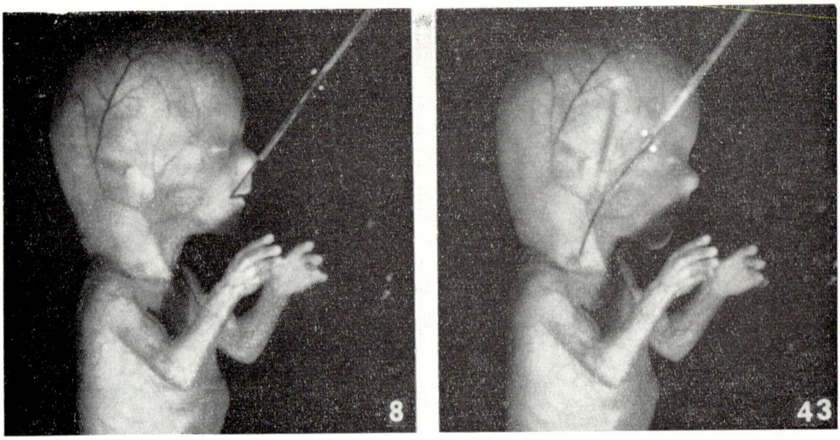

FIG. 5. Two frames, 8 and 43, showing ventral head flexion as part of a swallowing reflex of a 14-week fetus. The 2 gram stimulator used to elicit this reflex was drawn along the upper lip from the midline to the right corner where it is seen in frame 8, the 7th frame of the action. The mouth was open when the stimulation began, then closed as the head extended slightly. The head flexed ventralwards as the fetus swallowed, and remained flexed (frame 43) when the mouth reopened at the end of the reflex. There were no movements of the trunk or extremities with this reflex. Head flexion involved about two-thirds of the total time (more than 2 seconds) for this reflex. 88·5 mm fetus, CR length, illustrated at approximately 0·8 normal size. The remainder of this reflex is shown in the 1939 *Atlas* of Hooker and in Humphrey (1968b, 1969b).

of a swallowing reflex at 14 weeks (illustrated elsewhere at 13 weeks also; Humphrey, 1968b, 1969b). When ventral head flexion is combined with swallowing, it is preceded by a limited but rapid head extension, as the larynx is elevated (8, Fig. 5). The ventral flexion accompanies the completion of the swallowing act when the larynx is lowered (43, Fig. 5).

With additional differentiation of the neuromuscular system, rotation of the head becomes possible. At first the rotation is accompanied by lateral head and trunk flexion or by head and trunk extension. Later there is rotation of the head alone. In these movements the face is rotated away from the stimulus at an earlier stage in development than that at which it turns towards the stimulus (Hooker 1958, Humphrey, 1964a). Indeed, rotation of the face towards a stimulus about the lips cannot always be elicited from the newborn infant (*see* below).

Perinatal and postnatal head movements. The reactions of the normal newborn infant to stimulation about the mouth have received much attention (André-Thomas and Saint-Anne Dargassies, 1952; Prechtl, 1958; Peiper, 1963; Prechtl and Beintema, 1964; Illingworth, 1966). Customarily four points are touched along the border of the lips—the upper and lower lips at the midline region and the corners of the mouth. The response is usually reported only as present or absent; other reactions are rarely mentioned. The normal fullterm infant turns towards the stimulus and opens the mouth, then closes it on the stimulating finger if the finger enters the mouth (Fig. 6C and D). The reflex is most easily elicited when the infant is hungry, and difficult to obtain when it is asleep (Stirnimann, 1937; Prechtl, 1958; Peiper, 1963).

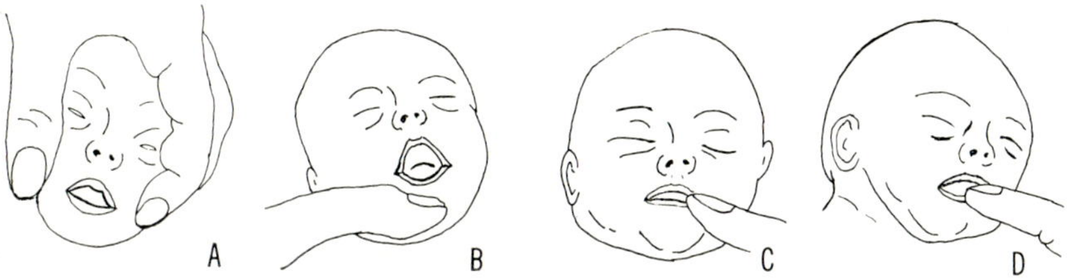

FIG. 6. A and B show the methods used to open the mouth in feeding premature infants that do not turn towards a stimulus and open the mouth. A: pressing on the cheeks; B: pulling down the mandible. [Based on Figs. 39 and 41 in Lundeen and Kunstadter (1958) by courtesy of Lippincott.] C and D show the head-turning and mouth-opening customarily seen in the fullterm newborn infant. [Based on Fig. 40 in Prechtl and Beintema (1964) published by the Spastics Society's Medical Education and Information Unit. William Heinemann Medical Books Ltd.]

Premature infants usually react by turning the face away. Because the mouth often remains closed, techniques such as pressing on the cheeks (Fig. 6A) or pulling down the mandible (Fig. 6B) are sometimes used in feeding (Hess and Lundeen, 1949; Lundeen and Kunstadter, 1958). Some fullterm infants also fail to respond in the normal manner shortly after birth. Thus Stirnimann (1937) found that on the first postnatal day 56 of 73 infants lacked this response from one or more of the four points customarily tested, and 8 infants lacked the reflex from all four points.

Correlations between fetal and postnatal head movement sequences. When the developmental sequences for fetal head movements are considered in relation to the perinatal and postnatal order of development, certain similarities are immediately evident. First, movement away from an agent touching the perioral area precedes movement towards it, both in fetal life and perinatally. In fetal life this is true whether the motions are contra- and ipsilateral head flexion, head extension and ventral flexion, or rotation of the oral region towards or away from the stimulus. In postnatal life lateral flexion of the head does not ordinarily occur and rotation is the common action for side-to-side motion. Rotation towards a stimulus (the directed head-turning response of Prechtl, 1958) develops later than rotation away from the stimulus. After turning towards the stimulus has become a well established reaction, the earlier developing avoiding movements often recur if the infant is not hungry or is under stress (crying, for example).

In fetal life head extension appears before ventral head flexion. Extension of the head during the early fetal period (Fig. 4), like bending the head away from a stimulus, is an avoiding movement, whereas forward flexion brings the area touched towards the stimulating agent. Avoidance of the stimulus on extension is present at this age regardless of which lip is touched. When the extension reflex is forceful the lips are compressed, probably passively (Humphrey, 1968b). Opening the mouth on stimulation of the lips and closure on the stimulator begins later, but it has been observed by 15·5 weeks (Humphrey, 1968b). Postnatally mouth opening is accompanied by very little head extension and when the upper lip is touched by the examiner's finger the finger enters the open mouth (Prechtl, 1958).

Hand Movements Elicited by Palmar Stimulation

Fetal hand movements. The earliest response to stimulation of the palm of the hand was noted by Hooker (1952, 1958; Humphrey, 1964a) at 10·5 weeks. Both at 10·5 and 11 weeks this reflex consists of incomplete finger closure without movement of the thumb (Fig. 7). All four fingers move in the same manner and there is usually flexion of the hand and sometimes flexion and pronation of the forearm as well. At this age the palms of the hands face medially when at rest, but the hands are not symmetrically positioned as they are earlier (Figs. 1–3) or later (Fig. 9). The action is extremely rapid (Hooker, 1938) and cinematographic recording is necessary to show that a fist is not formed (5, Fig. 7).

By 13 weeks finger closure is variable and often there is greater flexion of digits 3 to 5 than of the index finger (4, Fig. 8). The thumb begins to participate in the flexion by 12 to 12·5 weeks (Hooker, 1938) by moving across the palm, as it does later (Fig. 16). Hooker (1958)

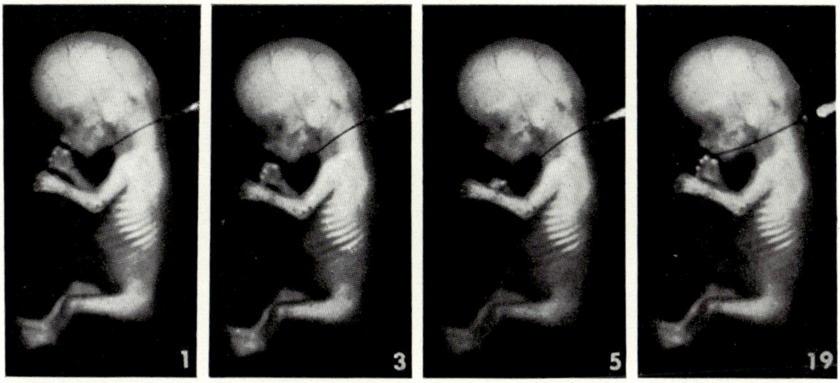

FIG. 7. A finger closure reflex following stimulation of the palm of the right hand with a 25 mgm hair esthesiometer at 11 weeks, menstrual age. This reflex was illustrated by Hooker in his 1939 *Atlas* where additional frames show the slow return of the fingers to the original position. Note that all the fingers flex to the same degree, that the thumb does not participate in the reflex and that both the hand and forearm flex. 48·5 mm fetus, CR length; 11 weeks, menstrual age. Photographs at approximately 0·8 natural size.

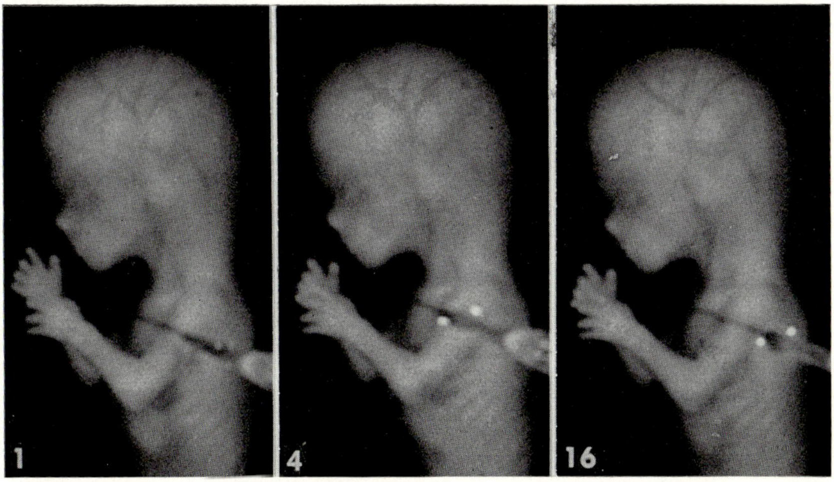

FIG. 8. Flexion of the digits elicited by stroking the palm of the right hand of a 13-week fetus. The 3rd to 5th fingers flex more than the index finger (compare frames 1 and 4) and the thumb does not move. The flexed position was maintained for close to a second. 75·0 mm fetus, CR length; 13 weeks, menstrual age. Photographs at about the size of this fetus.

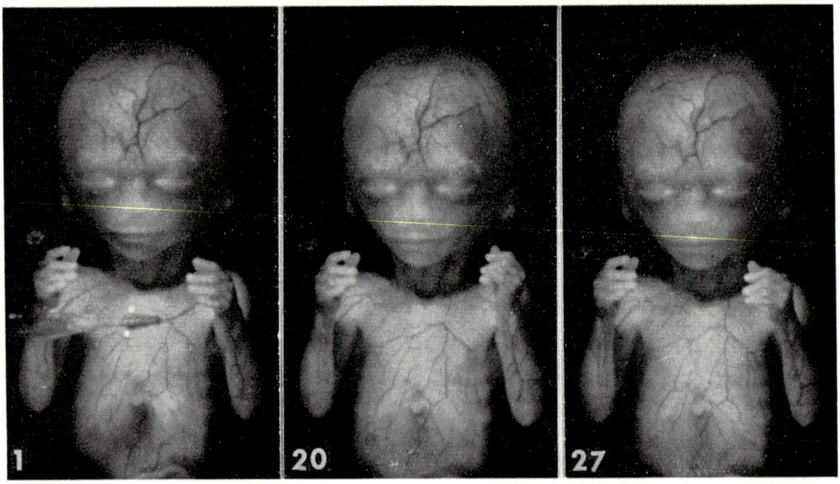

FIG. 9. Finger flexion following stimulation of the palm of the left hand of a 15·5-week fetus. At this age only the middle and ring fingers move exactly alike as a rule. At rest also, these digits are in the same position (right hand in all three frames and left in frame 1). On finger closure at this age the movements are variable, as seen in frames 20 and 27 where the little finger overlaps the ring finger and the index finger has moved less than the others. Two similar finger flexions followed each other rapidly on a single stimulation in this case; the first one is shown in frame 20 and the second in frame 27. 112·0 mm fetus, CR length; 15·5 weeks, menstrual age. Photographs at approximately 0·6 natural size.

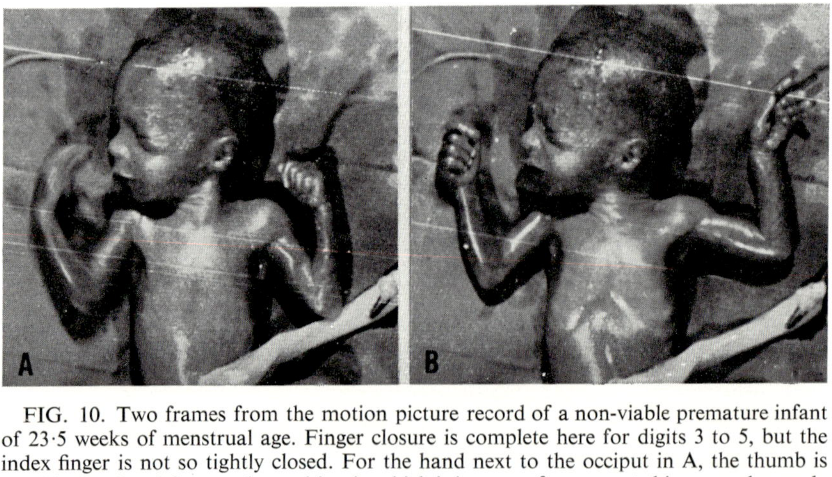

FIG. 10. Two frames from the motion picture record of a non-viable premature infant of 23·5 weeks of menstrual age. Finger closure is complete here for digits 3 to 5, but the index finger is not so tightly closed. For the hand next to the occiput in A, the thumb is outside the closed fingers, the position in which it is most often seen at this age and as early as 20 weeks (Humphrey, 1968b, 1969b). For the hand near the face in B, the thumb is caught under the index finger with the tip of the thumb between the index and middle fingers. In B, also, the fetus has just taken a deep inspiration and the mouth is open ready to cry. 205 mm fetus, CR length. Photographs at about 0·3 of the size of the fetus.

found that finger closure on the stimulator might be maintained at 15·5 weeks. Finger movements vary during this period and the actions of the individual fingers may differ greatly (Figs. 9 and 16). The reflex illustrated at 15·5 weeks (Fig. 9) has little, if any, thumb movement, but that at 14 weeks includes distinct thumb action (Fig. 16). By 18·5 weeks, Hooker (1958) found grasp present, although still weak. The position of the thumb with the hand closed as in grasping is shown at 23·5 weeks (Fig. 10). Although neither hand is holding an object, the photographs show the variable position of the thumb in grasping at this age—either at the side of the fist (Fig. 10A), or caught under the fingers (Fig. 10B). Grasp is stronger than at 18·5 weeks, and at 27 weeks Hooker (1958) found it nearly sufficient to support the weight of the fetus for a brief interval.

Postnatal hand movements. To illustrate the development of voluntary hand movements four of Halverson's (1943) drawings showing the infant's hand holding a rod are reproduced (Fig. 11). There is uniform

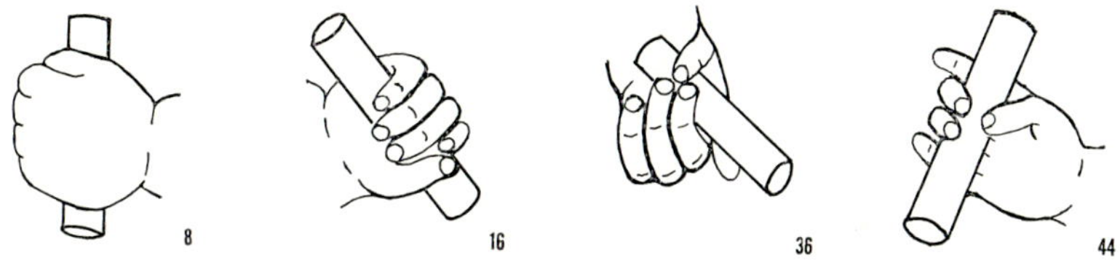

FIG. 11. Illustrations from Fig. 2 of Halverson (1943) to show the development of voluntary movements of the hand. The numbers on the drawings give the age of the infant in weeks. [From R. G. Barker, J. S. Kounin, and H. F. Wright (Eds.), *Child behaviour and development.* Copyright 1943 by McGraw-Hill Book Co., Inc. Used by permission of McGraw-Hill Book Co.]

finger closure on the rod without thumb participation at 8 postnatal weeks, finger closure with thumb action at 16 weeks, independent action of the index finger and primitive opposition of the thumb at 36 weeks, and variable finger flexion with thumb opposition at 44 weeks. The fine thumb and forefinger movement that enables the infant to pick up a small pellet is not present until 60 weeks (Halverson, 1943).

Correlations between fetal and postnatal hand movement sequences. Hooker (1958) pointed out that the two elements which Halverson (1937, 1943) found in the development of prehension—finger closure and grasp—appear during fetal life in the same sequence. Finger closure and grasp, in that order, occur on an automatic basis perinatally and postnatally (Gesell and Amatruda, 1945, 1947; Gentry and Aldrich, 1948). In the voluntary movements of prehension that enable the child to reach out at will and take the rod when he sees it (Fig. 11), there is still another sequential repetition: first of uniform finger closure shown at 11 weeks of menstrual age (Fig. 7), then of beginning thumb opposition and independent finger action illustrated at 13 to 15·5 weeks (Figs. 8 and 9) and finally of the characteristic movements of grasping (Fig. 10).

The automatic grasp that is normally elicited from newborn infants (Prechtl and Beintema, 1964) by pressure at the base of the fingers cannot be elicited by light touch. Pressure is usually classified as a proprioceptive stimulus, not as an exteroceptive one. Because the fetal reflexes are all exteroceptive, the reflex elicited by pressure is not considered in the present paper.

Reflexes Elicited by Plantar Stimulation

Plantar stimulation of fetuses. The earliest reflex elicited by stroking the sole of the foot with a hair esthesiometer was noted by Hooker (1958) at 10·5 weeks, but plantar reflexes are not readily elicited before 11 weeks. Thus in age of appearance the plantar and palmar reflexes overlap slightly. The initial reaction to this stimulus is plantar flexion of all the toes, according to Hooker (1958). This observation is in agreement with the report in Minkowski's paper of 1923, but later Minkowski (1928) decided that dorsiflexion of the great toe with toe fanning appears at the same age as plantar flexion. Plantar flexion of all the toes was illustrated by Hooker (1939) at 11·5 and 12 weeks, and this reflex is shown here at 13 weeks (Fig. 12). Although easily seen in the motion pictures, plantar flexion is difficult to demonstrate satisfactorily with photographs because the movement is so limited.

Hooker (1958) found dorsiflexion of the great toe and toe fanning at 11·5 to 12 weeks and reported that, by 12·5 weeks, the same fetus might respond to one stimulus with dorsiflexion of the hallux and toe fanning and to another stimulus with plantar flexion of all toes. Either reflex may be accompanied by flexion at the knee and hip (also sometimes rotation and abduction of the thigh). The characteristic movements accompanying dorsiflexion of the great toe and toe fanning, that is, flexion at the ankle, the knee and the hip, are shown at 14 weeks (Fig. 13).

Hooker (1952, 1958) found that, beginning at about 12·5 weeks, stroking the sole of the foot frequently elicited dorsiflexion of all the toes, also with toe fanning and flexion at the ankle, knee and hip joints (Fig. 14). This reaction continued up to about the same period as dorsiflexion of the great toe and toe fanning, that is, 18·5 to 20 weeks.

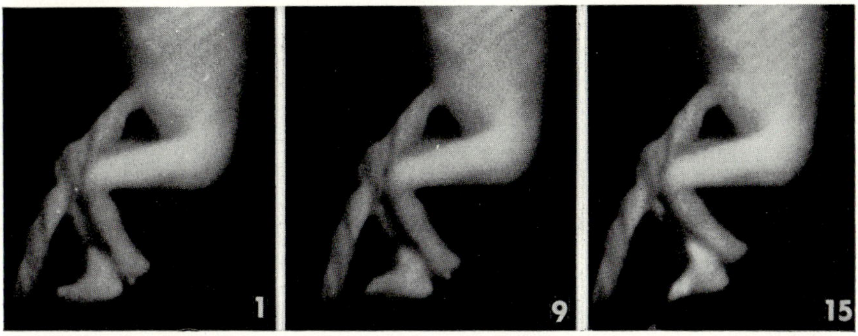

FIG. 12. Plantar flexion of all the toes of the right foot of a fetus of 13 weeks' menstrual age, following stroking the lateral aspect of the sole with a 25-mgm stimulator (frame 1, stimulator not visible). In frame 9 the toes are flexed distally. At the height of the reflex (frame 15) the flexion included the proximal joints as well. The return to position was not yet complete on frame 20. 75·0 mm fetus, CR length; 13 weeks, menstrual age. Photographs at slightly less than actual size.

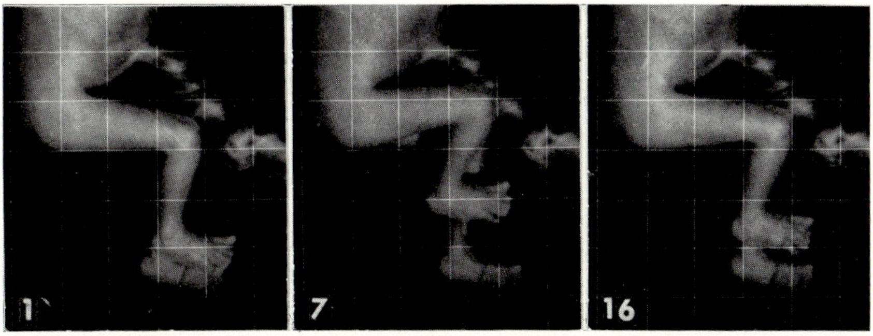

FIG. 13. Dorsiflexion of the great toe and fanning of the other toes of the right foot of a 14-week fetus following stimulation of the lateral side of the sole by a 2 gram hair esthesiometer (dark line, frame 1). At the height of the reflex, six frames after it began (frame 7), the great toe was dorsiflexed and the other toes slightly dorsiflexed and spread apart (especially the 5th toe) in a Babinski reflex like that of the adult. In this fetal reflex, the foot and thigh are somewhat flexed also and there is marked flexion at the knee joint. In frame 16, the great toe is no longer dorsiflexed, but the little toe is still widely separated, and digits 2–5 are plantar flexed. Other frames from this reflex were included by Hooker in his 1939 *Atlas*. To complete the return to position, 3 seconds were required. 88·5 mm fetus, CR length, 14 weeks, menstrual age. Photographs at approximately 0·8 the size of the fetus. The grid in these photographs made for Dr. Hooker was used in an attempt to show small changes in position.

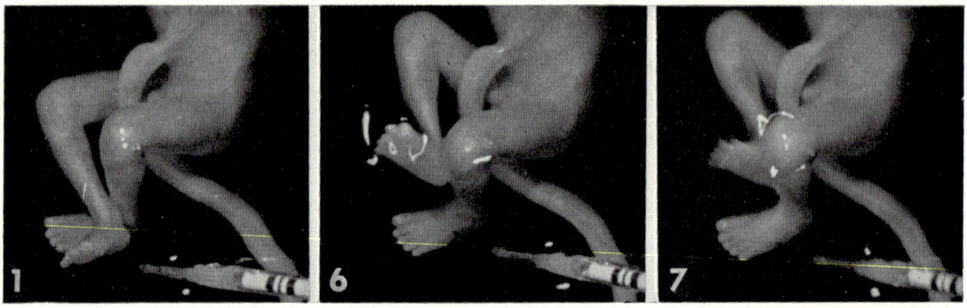

FIG. 14. Reflex following stimulation of the sole of the right foot (frame 1) of a 16·5-week fetus with a 2 gram esthesiometer, the strength of which is indicated by the pattern of wide and narrow bands at the lower right. In this reflex there was marked dorsiflexion of the foot, with sharp flexion also at the knee and the hip (frame 6). All the digits dorsiflexed. The action is rapid toe in frame 7. 121·0 mm fetus, CR length; 16·5 weeks, menstrual age. Photographs at about half the size of the fetus.

The tabulations of Hooker from the motion picture records demonstrate the plantar flexion reflex even at 18·5 to 20 weeks, although it decreases in frequency, whereas dorsiflexion of the great toe with fanning of the other digits becomes more common. According to Minkowski (1928) dorsiflexion is present most often when conditions are good, but it may revert to plantar flexion when they become poor. The reappearance of plantar toe flexion under adverse conditions is evidence of its earlier development. Indeed, contralateral head and trunk flexion, the earliest reflex that develops, is usually the last that can be elicited before all reflexes cease (Hooker, 1952, 1954, 1958; Humphrey, 1953, 1964a).

Perinatal and postnatal plantar stimulation. The two essential parts of the Babinski reflex (or sign), according to DeJong (1967), are the dorsiflexion of the toes, especially the great toe, and the separation, or fanning, of the toes. To elicit the reflex in an adult, DeJong recommends stimulation with "a blunt point, preferably a match stick, a tooth pick, wooden applicator, or a broken tongue blade" and states that some examiners use a finger tip, the thumb nail or even a pin. This neurologist considers that the stimulus should be made from the heel forward only as far as the metatarsophalangeal joints and that it should be light. Although the reflex is more readily elicited from the lateral aspect of the sole, DeJong suggests that both the inner and outer aspects should be tested.

In the examination of infants, Prechtl and Beintema (1964) elicit the Babinski reflex by scratching the lateral aspect of the sole of the foot "from the toes to the heel". Illingworth (1966) illustrates the "correct method of eliciting it" as scratching the distal half of the lateral aspect of the sole with a safety pin. André-Thomas and Saint-Anne Dargassies (1952) point out that the character of the reflex elicited depends upon the area and the type of stimulation.

Peiper (1963) emphasizes the variability of the plantar responses of infants as compared with those of adults. He also comments on the differences between the reactions to successive stimuli, as had Bryan (1930). The variability is also emphasized by André-Thomas *et al.* (1960, Fig. 48d) who report that with simultaneous stimuli one foot may react with a dorsiflexion reflex and the other with plantar flexion.

In reviewing the plantar responses of infants, Richards and Irwin (1935) mentioned the variability in the site and direction of the stimulus and in the pressure used. Probably many of the contradictions in the literature concerning plantar flexion of the toes are due largely to the variations in the site stimulated and to the use of pressure that may elicit the proprioceptive tonic foot grasp reflex instead of the plantar toe flexion response to exteroceptive stimulation.

Although some investigators report that plantar flexion of the toes is the more common response at birth (Bersot, 1920; Lantuejoul and Hartmann, 1923; Langworthy, 1933; Gentry and Aldrich, 1948) and for the first few days postnatally (Waggoner and Ferguson, 1930), many others mention dorsiflexion of the great toe and fanning of the other digits as the typical reaction of the newborn infant to plantar stimulation (Engstler, 1905; Wolff, 1930; Brain and Wilkinson, 1959; Prechtl and Beintema, 1964). However, André-Thomas *et al.* (1960) mention that stimulating the lateral border of the sole of a newborn infant's foot may produce flexion of the toes. Likewise Bryan (1930) never found a Babinski sign on the first postnatal day, but did on the second day and thereafter for white infants, but not until the 8th day, or even later, for negro infants. This investigator used a blunt pencil for the stimulus and a stroke from near the great toe almost to the heel. In premature infants, Feldman (1922) and Pratt (1960) stated that plantar flexion is the prevailing response. Both Feldman (1921) and Minkowski (1922) mentioned plantar flexion as the more common response during the later part of fetal life although both found the Babinski reflex present before birth.

A plantar grasp reflex, elicited by pressure on the ball of the foot (André-Thomas *et al.*, 1960; Paine, 1960; Prechtl and Beintema, 1964; Illingworth, 1966) has been described by Galant (1931), the Stirnimanns (1940) and others (for further references *see* Peiper, 1963). This tonic foot grasp reflex (Fig. 15D), described and discussed for infants by Brain and Curran (1932), Gentry and Aldrich (1948), Brain and Wilkinson (1959), Paine (1960) and others, is not the same reaction as that elicited by stroking the sole of the foot. In the correlations between fetal and postnatal responses to stimulation of the plantar surface, therefore, this tonic foot grasp is not considered.

Correlations between fetal and postnatal plantar reflexes. Plantar flexion of the toes has been demonstrated earlier in fetal life than has dorsiflexion of the great toe with toe fanning (the Babinski sign), but the latter reflex appears very shortly. After it develops the Babinski reflex may be elicited in response to one stimulus, and plantar toe flexion in response to others. Both reflexes have been recorded throughout the same period, but plantar flexion of the toes occurs less often than the Babinski types of reflex in the later part of the period.

From comparison with the reports in the literature it is clear that reflexes in response to superficial plantar stimulation, like those elicited by palmar stimulation, develop during fetal life in a sequence that is repeated during later development. Plantar flexion of the toes (Fig. 15A),

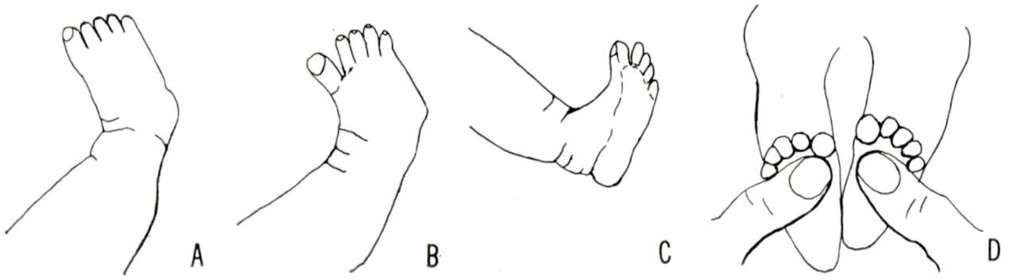

FIG. 15. Three types of reflex elicited by stimulation of the sole of the foot of newborn infants. A: plantar flexion of the toes; B: dorsiflexion of the great toe and fanning of the other toes; C: dorsiflexion of all the digits of the foot. [Sketched from the positions at rest shown in Fig. 1 in Wolff (1930) *Am. J. Dis. Child.* **39,** 1176–1185]. D: the plantar grasp reflex that is elicited by pressure at the base of the toes rather than the cutaneous stimulation used for the reflexes of the Babinski type. [From Fig. 35 in Prechtl and Beintema (1964) published by the Spastics Society's Medical Education and Information Unit/William Heinemann Medical Books Ltd.]

the reflex which develops earlier in fetal life, is the more frequent reflex in premature infants and sometimes immediately after birth, whereas the Babinski types of reflex (Fig. 15C and D), which appear slightly later in fetuses, are not often seen in premature infants and cannot always be elicited in normal newborn infants. The overlap in time of development of the plantar flexion and of the dorsiflexion reflexes in fetal life, like the order of their later appearance, is also recapitulated.

It is often mentioned in the literature on human fetal behaviour that the Babinski reflex does not make its appearance until after birth. In consequence this reflex has been referred to in the literature on fetal behaviour as "Babinski-like" or as a "fetal Babinski reflex" (Hooker, 1958; Humphrey, 1964a). Therefore, it should be emphasized that the reflex illustrated in this paper at 14 weeks (Fig. 13) meets all the usual requirements for the sign of Babinski. Moreover, variations of the Babinski reaction, like that illustrated at 16·5 weeks (Fig. 14), are also present during fetal life. Beginning at about 19 to 20 weeks of menstrual age, the fetuses become sluggish and react to stimulation less often (Hooker, 1944, 1952). Consequently these reflexes are rarely seen later in fetal life. In the postnatal period, and sometimes earlier, the Babinski reflex reappears.

In the perinatal period, as in fetal life, there is an overlap in the ages at which the Babinski reactions and the plantar toe flexion reflexes can be elicited, but at earlier ages the toe flexion reflexes tend to be present more often than do the Babinski reflexes. Failure to recognize or to consider this overlap undoubtedly adds to the confusion in the literature covering this period of infant life.

Hand-mouth Reflex Relationships

Fetal hand-mouth reflexes. At 14 weeks eyelid stimulation may elicit a sneer-like reflex in which the corner of the mouth is pulled back, the upper lip is elevated near the corner, and the ala of the nose is raised on the ipsilateral side. As a part of such a reflex, the orbicularis oculi may contract ipsilaterally and produce a squint-like appearance, the head may flex to the contralateral side, then extend, and finally the face may rotate to the opposite side (*see* the illustrations of Hooker, 1939; and Humphrey, 1968b, 1969b).

Stimulation of the hand elicited similar movements from the 88·5 mm fetus from which these reflexes were secured (Fig. 16). The stimulator was drawn across the left palm from the base of the fingers over the thenar eminence. The mouth, already open (1, Fig. 16), opened wider (11, Fig. 16). Next the upper lip was lifted a trifle ipsilaterally, medial to the corner (11 and 21, Fig. 16), and the angle of the mouth was retracted. The lower lip was raised a little at this time, thus narrowing the mouth medial to the corner (21 and 31, Fig. 16). Before the stimulus was applied the head was flexed towards the hand about to be touched. During the lip movements, the head tilted towards the midline and appeared to extend slightly. The force produced by the movement rolled the fetus from a full face to a profile view, so interpretation of the head

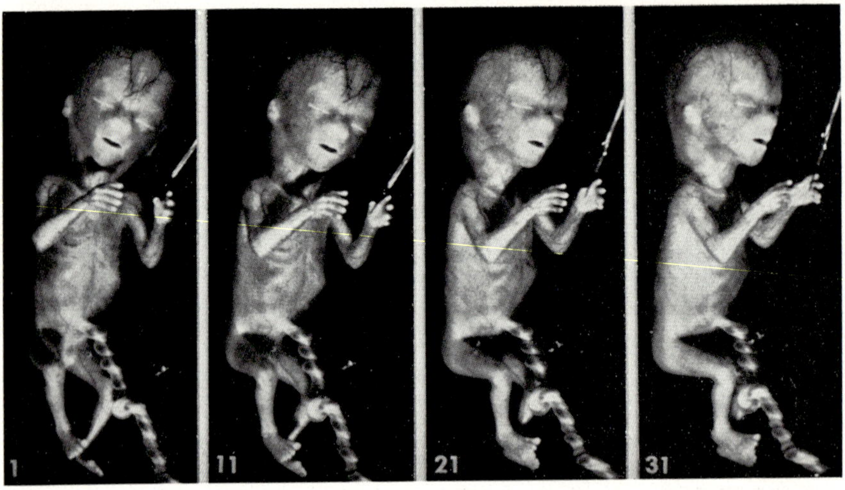

FIG. 16. A reflex elicited from stimulating the palm of the left hand of a fetus of 14 weeks. The stimulator was drawn across the palm of the hand from the base of the fingers (frame 1) to the thenar eminence (frames 11 and 21) then back to the base of the ring finger near the end of the reflex (frame 31). The mouth was open before the stimulation began, and the head was flexed towards the stimulated hand (frame 1), with the chin rotated slightly to the opposite side. The action shown in the photographs consisted of a slight elevation of the ipsilateral upper and lower lips near the corner (frames 11 and 21), movement of the head towards the midline and slight extension (frames 21 and 31), opening the fingers of the stimulated hand with flexion of the thumb, and flexion of digits 3–5 of the contralateral hand. In addition, the tongue appeared to be elevated in frame 11, but a greater magnification is needed to show this satisfactorily. 88·5 mm fetus, CR length; 14 weeks, menstrual age. Photographs at about half the true size.

movement is hazardous. The profile view also shows the sneer-like lip movements less satisfactorily than for the comparable oral reflexes which followed stimulation of the eyelids. As part of the reflex elicited by palmar stimulation, the fingers of the ipsilateral hand extended partially, but the thumb flexed at the distal joint and moved a little towards the palm (21 and 31, Fig. 16). Digits 3 to 5 of the contralateral hand also flexed. Similar oral area reflexes have been photographed three times following palmar stimulation at 18 weeks (140 mm, CR length). The muscles involved in the lip movements have been reported by both Futamura (1906) and by Gasser (1967) to be well delineated at 14 weeks and, according to Gasser, capable of contraction. In many respects this reflex resembles the palmomental reflex discussed on p. 62.

As early as 12·5 weeks stimulation of the volar surface of the forearm elicited mouth opening combined with tongue elevation, ipsilateral head and forearm flexion, and extension and abduction of the arm, followed by mouth closure and a return to the original position (Humphrey, 1968b). The mouth was opened by lowering the mandible, not by lip movement. When the cinematographic records for this age period have been completely studied a similar action may be found to result from palmar stimulation.

In one fetus of 14 weeks (85·5 mm crown-rump length) stimulation of the palm of the hand evoked a different oral reflex that included more extensive tongue movements (Fig. 17). Prior to stimulation the head

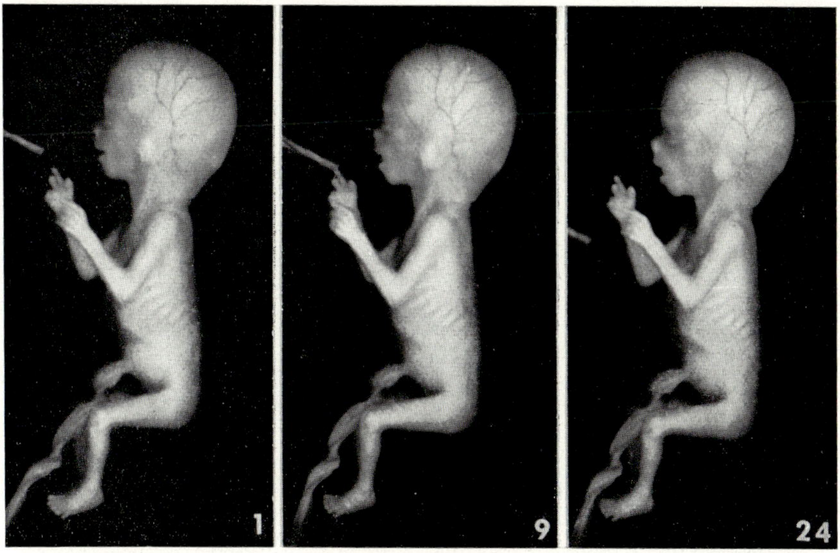

FIG. 17. A reflex elicited by stimulation of the left palm of a fetus of 14 weeks. In frame 1, where the mouth was open and the head turned away from the stimulated hand, the stimulator began pulling a bit of tissue out of the left hand. Following this palmar stimulation, the mouth opened wider, the tongue was elevated and protruded, and the head turned towards the midline and flexed slightly ventralwards (compare frames 1 and 24). Later the stimulated hand closed and flexed and the tongue was retracted (Humphrey, 1968b, 1969b). 85·5 mm fetus, CR length; 14 weeks, menstrual age. Photographs at approximately 0·6 the natural size.

was extended and bent a little to the right side, with the face also turned to the right (1, Fig. 17). When the left hand was stimulated (by pulling a bit of the amnion from between its fingers) the mandible lowered and the mouth opened much wider (9 and 24, Fig. 17). The tongue was lifted and was thrust forward somewhat, then was retracted while the mouth was still open (Humphrey, 1968b). The face rotated towards the hand stimulated, which in this case was also towards the midline of the fetus, and the head flexed forward slightly. After the tissue was pulled away from the left hand there was flexion at the elbow and extension at the wrist. The third to fifth fingers closed tightly, but the index finger remained extended longer. These two reflexes include the essential features of the Babkin reflex described on p. 64.

Postnatal hand-mouth reflexes. It is well known that reflexes of two types can be elicited postnatally by stimulating the palm of the hand. One of these, the palmomental reflex, was described by Marinesco and Radovici (1920) and the other by Babkin (1960; *see* also Peiper, 1963).

Various methods have been recommended for testing the palmomental reflex. Reis (1961) states that, in the adult, the palmomental reflex is elicited by "a stimulus to the thenar eminence of the hand, usually the dragging of a sharp object". In the adult, also, DeJong (1967) mentions that tapping the thenar eminence, as well as scratching it in either direction with a blunt point, will elicit the reflex. August and Miller (1952) recommend a "brisk scratch". Reis (1961) used an electrical stimulus for his investigation.

In the examination of infants, Peiper (1963) states that the palmomental reflex may be elicited by scratching the hypothenar eminence as well as the thenar eminence. Parmelee (1963a) used "gentle scratching" of the thenar eminence or, if the reflex was not elicited, "the blunt end of a straight pin" and tested the two hands in succession in his study

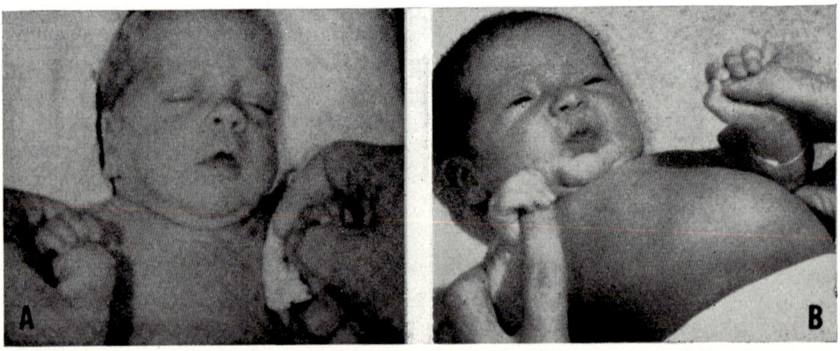

FIG. 18. Two illustrations of the palmomental reflex, elicited in normal infants by stimulating the thenar eminence. A: the reflex is present only on the left side of the face. [Fig. 2 in Parmelee, Jr. (1963a) by courtesy of the author, the publishers of *Developmental Medicine and Child Neurology*, Spastics Society's Medical Education and Information Unit/William Heinemann Medical Books Ltd.] B: the palmomental reflex was elicited bilaterally. In addition to contraction of the mentalis muscles, the action of the upper lip is well shown bilaterally. The palmomental and grasp reflexes were both elicited in this case. [From Fig. 34 of Prechtl and Beintema (1964) published by the Spastics Society's Medical Education and Information Unit/William Heinemann Medical Books Ltd.]

on premature infants (Fig. 18A). An illustration of this reflex from the paper of Prechtl and Beintema (1964) is reproduced in Fig. 18B. Bilateral palmar stimuli (apparently applied simultaneously) elicited a bilateral reflex.

The actions included in descriptions of the palmomental reflex also differ. All observers mention contraction of the ipsilateral mentalis muscle. August and Miller (1952) and DeJong (1967) include contraction of the orbicularis oris with retraction and elevation of the angle of the mouth in the adult. August and Miller (1952) and Reis (1961) state that the reflex may be bilateral.

In his study of 50 infants, 43 of which were premature, Parmelee (1963a) mentioned only the ipsilateral response (*see* Fig. 19A). He found the reflex absent more frequently in the younger premature infants. The smallest from which it was elicited weighed 1,175 grams. The palmomental reflex was found in all newborn infants by Lippmann (1958), and in 73 per cent of infants in the early postnatal weeks by Magnusson and Wernstedt (1935).

Schachter-Nancy (1937) found the palmomental reflex present in only 28 per cent of the 1,207 children that he examined between 6 and 12 years of age. However, the palmomental reflex was reported in normal adults by Marinesco and Radovici (1920), Blake and Kunkle (1951), and August and Miller (1952). By using electrical stimulation Reis (1961) elicited this reflex in normal adults from many widely

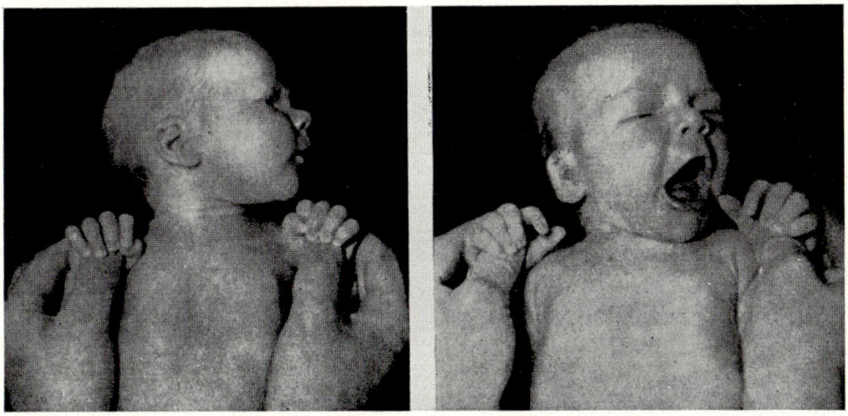

FIG. 19. The reflex of Babkin in the newborn infant, produced by pressure bilaterally on the palms of the hands. The mouth is opened, the tongue elevated and the head turned towards the midline. [From Fig. 14 in Peiper (1963) by courtesy of the author and Consultants Bureau, New York].

spread areas of the body surface, including the sole of the foot. Its presence in the adult in response to the customary methods of testing for it, however, has often been considered to be a sign of pathologic change in the central nervous system (Blake and Kunkle, 1951; August and Miller, 1952; Reis, 1961; DeJong, 1967).

The Babkin reflex (Fig. 19) is elicited by pressure applied bilaterally on the palms of the infant's hands (Peiper, 1963; Prechtl and Beintema, 1964) and is difficult to secure by unilateral palmar pressure (Lippmann, 1958; DeJong, 1967). The reflex is described by Peiper (1963) as consisting of mouth opening, forward bending of the head and closing of the eyes. Lippmann (1958) found rotation of the head to the midline, head flexion forward, and mouth opening; eye closure was not always present. Babkin himself (1960) reported flexion of the forearm with the reflex. In the response of premature infants Parmelee (1963b) included tongue elevation immediately after the stimulus, but did not mention closure of the eyes.

The Babkin reflex is suppressed after birth. Thus both Babkin (1960) and Lippmann (1958) found that it disappeared by the third or fourth postnatal month. Babkin, Lippmann, and Parmelee (1963b) all reported the Babkin reflex to be readily elicitable in premature infants. Parmelee even obtained this reflex in one weighing only 580 grams. All these investigators consider the reflex to be a very primitive one.

Relation of fetal and postnatal hand-mouth reflexes. In the mouth opening reflex elicited by stimulating the palm of one 14-week fetus (Fig. 17) the lowering of the mandible, the elevation of the tongue, the turning of the head towards the midline (also towards the hand stimulated), and the slight ventral head flexion are all parts of the Babkin reflex (Fig. 19) as reported in the literature. For the oral area reflex illustrated for another 14-week fetus (Fig. 16), the thenar site of stimulation, the type of head movements, and the action of the facial muscles in moving the lips all resemble the main actions reported for the palmomental reflex (Fig. 18).

Both hand-mouth reflexes, then, may occur during fetal life and both are repeated perinatally and postnatally. One of them, the Babkin reflex, has been demonstrated very early in premature infants and disappears early in childhood. Although, as yet, its fetal precursor has not been demonstrated satisfactorily before 14 weeks, mouth opening by lowering the mandible—a characteristic part of the reflex (Figs. 17 and 19)—is the earliest of all oral reflexes to appear in fetal life.

The other reflex from palmar stimulation, the palmomental reflex, evidently develops a little later in premature infants (Fig. 18), is commonly present later in childhood, and is often seen in normal adults. Because of the later morphological and functional development of the muscles which produce the characteristic movements of this reflex (mentalis, orbicularis oris and others that aid in moving the lips), it is unlikely that this reflex will be found much earlier in fetal life than is reported here (Fig. 16). Thus the evidence to show that the sequence of prenatal development of these two hand-mouth reflexes is comparable to that found postnatally is incomplete, but the trend in that direction is clear.

SUGGESTIONS ON THE NEUROANATOMICAL BASIS FOR THE POSTNATAL REPETITION OF FETAL ACTIVITY SEQUENCES

All skeletal muscle activity is initiated by nervous impulses transmitted over the motoneurones of cranial and spinal nerves. Consequently the arrangement of these neurones in the longitudinal plane of the brain stem and spinal cord is in itself a major factor in determining the manner in which motor activity develops. Closure of the human neural tube begins at about midcervical levels and proceeds both cervicocaudally and cervicorostrally (Kingsbury, 1924). Consequently cervical motoneurones mature and function earlier than either those caudally located in the spinal cord or those more rostrally situated in the brain stem. Because the spinal cord motoneurones differentiate in the general cervicocaudal order just mentioned, the reflexes mediated by them likewise appear in a comparable order, that is, they begin in the cervical region with head movements and spread caudalwards to upper-extremity, trunk and then lower-extremity activity. The development of the total pattern lateral flexion reflexes as outlined in the present account and in greater detail by Hooker (1952, 1958) demonstrates this fact.

In the cervicorostral maturation of reflex connections the upper cervical location of those spinal cord motor nerve cells that function in depressing the mandible (at C1 and C2; Humphrey, 1954, p. 148) is undoubtedly the most significant factor in the early addition of partial mouth opening to the total pattern contralateral flexion reflexes. As differentiation of the motor nerve cells spreads farther rostralwards into the brain stem, no doubt the limited mandibular action itself contributes in some fashion to the selective differentiation of the trigeminal and facial motoneurones that then function in depressing the lower jaw and so change partial to complete lowering of the mandible.

The order followed in the distribution of the fibre tracts that inhibit, regulate, and activate the motoneurones is also dependent upon the longitudinal arrangement of the motoneurones in the brain stem and spinal cord. These fibre systems are descending pathways almost exclusively. As they grow caudalwards, therefore, the fibres destined for cervical levels establish functional connections earlier than those that pass to lumbosacral spinal cord levels. Therefore, unless other factors intervene, the secondarily developing activities that are initiated by the descending fibres from higher levels will appear in the same general order, as development proceeds, as that already established in the development of the reflex arcs. As a result, the motor activity initiated by them will repeat this order.

Finally, when the motor cortex differentiates, the corticospinal fibres that arise from it reach the motoneurones of the spinal cord in a comparable order (Humphrey, 1960). Therefore, synaptic connections will be established with them in a similar order and voluntary activity will again be manifested in essentially the same sequence. The course of differentiation of the neurones of the motor cortex at birth and one month postnatally (Conel, 1939, 1941) is also essentially the same inasmuch as the neurones in the neck and shoulder areas are better developed than those of either the upper or lower extremity areas. With a few exceptions the neurones of the face area are the least well differentiated. Likewise, the aberrent corticobulbar tracts, at least, develop relatively late (Humphrey, 1960). Moreover, in their outgrowth all corticobulbar fibres reach the midpons location of the motor trigeminal neurones that act in mouth opening and closing before they arrive at the caudal pontine levels of the motor facial neurones that govern facial expression. The order of differentiation of the muscles supplied by these two nerves peripherally is also essentially the same, for most of the muscles related to mandibular activity develop earlier than those concerned with facial expression (Futamura, 1906; Gasser, 1967). Thus from the development of the muscles peripherally to the differentiation of the related neurones of the motor cortex, the functional order established by the reflex arcs is repeated.

As each region of the central nervous system in turn becomes dominant over motor activity the movements may change somewhat, but the general sequence in which they appear will be maintained. As each succeeding brain level (for example, midbrain, striatal region, cortex) becomes dominant over activity, the one previously regulating movements will be brought under control by inhibition, then activated. So long as function of the efferent limb of the reflex arc is retained it will be inhibited for the most part, but sometimes facilitated, and will always remain under the influence of descending fibre systems.

It is probable that, in addition to anatomical factors, several functional factors contribute to the repetition of fetal activity sequences. The most likely agent is the oxygen requirement of fetal reflex arcs. Those that have functioned longest require the least oxygen and the reflexes mediated over them can be elicited with less stimulation than can those more recently matured (Angulo, 1932; Windle, 1944; Hooker, 1944, 1952, 1958; Humphrey, 1953, 1964a). Thus when the oxygen supply is decreased or conditions are unfavourable for other reasons, the reflexes that develop earliest are the most readily elicited. Since recently developed centres require a higher oxygen level, motoneurones that have been active for a longer time are more easily fired than newly functioning motor nerve cells, and so become regulated earlier by descending fibre systems than do those that mature later.

SUMMARY

Three specific examples of the postnatal repetition of fetal activity sequences are described, illustrated and discussed. These are: (1) the avoiding or negative types of head movement in response to perioral stimuli, and the positive reactions that move the area touched towards the stimulus; (2) the maturation of finger movements into grasping; (3) the development of plantar reflexes. In addition two complex reactions that appear during fetal life, the palmomental and the Babkin reflexes, are described and compared with these actions in premature and newborn infants.

Like the fetal reflex sequences, the perinatal and early postnatal reactions are automatic in nature, but the specific movements in a postnatal developmental sequence differ somewhat from those of the comparable fetal reflexes. When voluntary actions appear during postnatal life the order in which the activity develops recurs again as the infant learns to execute movements in response to visual and other types of stimuli.

Finally, suggestions are made concerning the neuroanatomical basis for the postnatal repetition of fetal activity sequences. Some of the factors involved are: (1) the longitudinal arrangement of the motoneurones in the spinal cord and brain stem; (2) the onset of neural tube closure at upper cervical levels; (3) the cervicocaudal and cervicorostral directions in which the motor nerve cells mature and begin functioning; (4) the almost exclusive regulation of motor activity by descending fibre tracts; (5) the differentiation of the neurones in the motor cortex in the same general order as that in which the cranial and spinal motoneurones become functional; (6) the development of the muscles innervated in a manner consistent with the order in which reflex function develops.

REFERENCES

André-Thomas and Saint-Anne Dargassies, S. 1952. *Études neurologiques sur le nouveau-né et le jeune nourrisson.* Masson, Paris.

André-Thomas, Chesni, Y. and Saint-Anne Dargassies, S. 1960. *The neurological examination of the infant.* Heinemann, London.

Angulo y Gonzáles, A. W. 1932. The prenatal development of behavior in the albino rat. *J. comp. Neurol.* **55,** 395–442.

August, B. and Miller, R. B. 1952. Clinical value of the palmomental reflex. *J. Am. med. Ass.* **148,** 120–121.

Babkin, P. S. 1960. The establishment of reflex activity in early postnatal life. In *The central nervous system and behavior.* pp. 24–31. [A translation from Fiziologii Zhurnal USSR 44 (10), 922–927.] Russian Scientific Translation Program, National Institutes of Health, Bethesda, Md.

Bersot, H. 1920. Développement réactionnel et réflexe plantaire du bébé né avant terme à celui de deux ans. *Schweiz. Arch. Neurol. Psychiat.* **7,** 212–239.

Blake, J. R. and Kunkle, E. C. 1951. The palmomental reflex: a physiological and clinical analysis. *A.M.A. Archs Neurol. Psychiat.* **65,** 337–345.

Brain, W. and Curran, R. D. 1932. The grasp-reflex of the foot. *Brain* **55,** 347–356.

Brain, R. and Wilkinson, M. 1959. Observations on the extensor plantar reflex and its relationship to the functions of the pyramidal tract. *Brain* **82,** 297–320.

Bryan, E. S. 1930. Variations in the responses of infants during the first ten days of post-natal life. *Child Develop.* **1,** 56–77.

Coghill, G. E. 1916. Correlated anatomical and physiological studies of the growth of the nervous system of Amphibia. II. The afferent system of the head of Amblystoma. *J. comp. Neurol.* **26,** 247–340.

Coghill, G. E. 1929. *Anatomy and the problem of behaviour.* Cambridge Univ. Press, London. Reprinted 1964: Hafner, New York.

Conel, J. L. 1939. *The postnatal development of the human cerebral cortex.* Vol. I. *The cortex of the newborn.* Harvard Univ. Press, Cambridge, Mass.

Conel, J. L. 1941. *The postnatal development of the human cerebral cortex.* Vol. II. *The cortex of the one-month infant.* Harvard Univ. Press, Cambridge, Mass.

DeJong, R. N. 1967. *The neurologic examination.* 3rd ed. Harper & Row, New York and London.

Engstler, G. 1905. Ueber den Fussohlenreflex und das Babinski-Phänomen bei tausend Kindern der ersten Lebensjahre. *Wien. Klin. Wschr.* **18,** 567–569.

Feldman, W. M. 1921. The nature of the plantar reflex in early life and the causes of its variations. *Br. J. Child. Dis.* **18,** 24–27.

Feldman, W. M. 1922. The nature of the plantar reflex in early life and the causes of its variations. *Am. J. Dis. Child.* **23,** 1–40.

Fitzgerald, G. E. and Windle, W. 1942. Some observations on early human fetal movements. *J. comp. Neurol.* **76,** 159–167.

FUTAMURA, R. 1906. Über die Entwicklung der Facialismuskulatur des Menschen. *Anat. Hefte* **30,** 433–516.

GALANT, J. S. 1931. Über die rudimentären neuropsychischen Functionen der Säuglinge. *Jb. Kinderheilk.* **133,** 104–108.

GASSER, R. F. 1967. The development of the facial muscles in man. *Am. J. Anat.* **120,** 357–376.

GENTRY, E. F. and ALDRICH, C. A. 1948. Toe reflexes in infancy and the development of voluntary control. *Am. J. Dis. Child.* **76,** 389–400.

GESELL, A. and AMATRUDA, C. S. 1945. *The embryology of behavior.* Harper, New York.

GESELL, A. and AMATRUDA, C. S. 1947. *Developmental diagnosis: normal and abnormal child development.* 2nd ed. Harper, New York.

HALVERSON, H. M. 1937. Studies on the grasping responses of early infancy. *J. genet. Psychol.* **51,** 371–449.

HALVERSON, H. M. 1943. The development of prehension in infants. In R. G. Barker, J. S. Kounin, and H. F. Wright (Eds.), *Child behavior and development.* McGraw-Hill, New York. Pp. 49–65.

HESS, J. H. and LUNDEEN, E. C. 1949. *The premature infant, medical and nursing care.* 2nd ed. Lippincott, Philadelphia, Pa.

HOOKER, D. 1938. The origin of the grasping movement in man. *Proc. Am. phil. Soc.* **79,** 597–606.

HOOKER, D. 1939. *A preliminary atlas of early human fetal activity.* Published privately by the author.

HOOKER, D. 1944. *The origin of overt behavior.* Univ. of Michigan Press, Ann Arbor.

HOOKER, D. 1952. *The prenatal origin of behavior.* Univ. of Kansas Press, Lawrence.

HOOKER, D. 1954. Early human fetal behavior, with a preliminary note on double simultaneous fetal stimulation. *Res. Publs Ass. Res. nerv. ment. Dis.* **33,** 98–113.

HOOKER, D. 1958. Evidence of prenatal function of the central nervous system in man. James Arthur Lecture for 1957 on The Evolution of the Human Brain. American Museum of Natural History, New York.

HOOKER, D. 1960. Developmental reaction to environment. *Yale J. Biol. Med.* **32,** 431–440.

HOOKER, D. and HUMPHREY, T. 1954. Some results and deductions from a study of the development of human fetal behavior. *Gaz. méd. Port.* **7,** 189–197.

HUMPHREY, T. 1952. The spinal tract of the trigeminal nerve in human embryos between 7·5 and 8·5 weeks of menstrual age and its relation to early fetal behavior. *J. comp. Neurol.* **97,** 143–210.

HUMPHREY, T. 1953. The relation of oxygen deprivation to fetal reflex arcs and the development of fetal behavior. *J. Psychol.* **35,** 3–43.

HUMPHREY, T. 1954. The trigeminal nerve in relation to early human fetal activity. *Res. Publs Ass. Res. nerv. ment. Dis.* **33,** 127–154.

HUMPHREY, T. 1960. The development of the pyramidal tracts in human fetuses, correlated with cortical differentiation. In D. B. Tower and J. P. Schadé (Eds.), *Structure and function of the cerebral cortex.* Elsevier, Amsterdam. Pp. 94–103.

HUMPHREY, T. 1964a. Some correlations between the appearance of human fetal reflexes and the development of the nervous system. *Prog. Brain Res.* **4,** 93–135.

HUMPHREY, T. 1964b. Embryology of the central nervous system, with some correlations with functional development. *Ala. J. med. Sci.* **1,** 60–64.

HUMPHREY, T. 1968a. The dynamic mechanism of palatal shelf elevation in human fetuses. *Anat. Rec.* **160,** 369.

HUMPHREY, T. 1968b. The development of mouth opening and related reflexes involving the oral area of human fetuses. *Ala. J. med. Sci.* **5,** 126–157.

HUMPHREY, T. 1969a. The relation between human fetal mouth opening reflexes and closure of the palate. *Am. J. Anat.*, **125,** 317–344.

HUMPHREY, T. 1969b. Reflex activity in the oral and facial area of human fetuses. In J. F. Bosma (Ed.), *Oral sensation and perception* (Second Symposium). Thomas, Springfield, Ill., in press.

HUMPHREY, T. and HOOKER, D. 1959. Double simultaneous stimulation of human fetuses and the anatomical patterns underlying the reflexes elicited. *J. comp. Neurol.* **112,** 75–102.

ILLINGWORTH, R. S. 1966. *The development of the infant and young child, normal and abnormal.* 3rd ed. Williams & Wilkins, Baltimore, Md.

KINGSBURY, B. F. 1924. The significance of the so-called law of cephalocaudal differential growth. *Anat. Rec.* **27,** 305–321.

LANGWORTHY, O. R. 1933. Development of behavior patterns and myelinization of the nervous system in the human fetus and infant. *Contr. Embryol.* **24,** 1–57.

LANTUEJOUL, P. and HARTMANN, E. 1923. Note sur le réflexe cutané-plantaire, chez le jeune enfant, notamment au moment de la naissance. *Revue Neurol.* **1,** 387–398.

LIPPMANN, K. 1958. Über den Babkinschen Reflex. *Arch. Kinderheilk.* **157,** 234–238.

LUNDEEN, E. C. and KUNSTADTER, R. H. 1958. *Care of the premature infant.* Lippincott, Philadelphia and Montreal.

MAGNUSSON, J. H. and WERNSTEDT, W. 1935. The infantile palmo-mentalis reflex. *Acta paediat., Stockh.* **17,** Suppl. 1, 241–245.

MARINESCO, G. and RADOVICI, A. 1920. Sur un réflexe cutané nouveau à réflexe palmomentonnier. *Revue Neurol.* **27,** 237–240.

MINKOWSKI, M. 1922. Über frühzeitige Bewegungen Reflexe und muskuläre Reaktionen beim menschlichen Fötus, und ihre Beziehungen zum fötalen Nerven- und Muskelsystem. *Schweiz. med. Wschr.* **52,** 721–724, 751–755.

MINKOWSKI, M. 1923. Zur Entwicklungsgeschichte, Lokalisation und Klinik des Fussohlenreflexes. *Schweiz. Arch. Neurol. Psychiat.* **13,** 475–514.

MINKOWSKI, M. 1928. Neurobiologische Studien am menschlichen Foetus. In E. Abderhalden (Ed.), *Handbuch d. biol. Arbeitsmethoden.* Abt. V, Teil 5B, Heft 5, Ser. 253, 511–618.

PAINE, R. S. 1960. Neurologic examination of infants and children. *Pediat. Clin. N. Am.* **7,** 471–510.

PARMELEE, A. H., Jr. 1963a. The palmomental reflex in premature infants. *Devl Med. Child Neurol.* **5,** 381–387.

PARMELEE, A. H., Jr. 1963b. The hand-mouth reflex of Babkin in premature infants. *Pediatrics, Springfield* **31,** 734–740.

PEIPER, A. 1963. *Cerebral function in infancy and childhood.* [A translation J. Wortis (Ed.), of *Die Eigenart der Kindlichen Hirntätigkeit*, 3rd ed., 1961. Thieme, Leipzig.] Consultants Bureau, New York.

PRATT, K. C. 1960. The neonate. In L. Carmichael (Ed.), *Manual of child psychology.* Wiley, New York and London. Pp. 215–291.

PRECHTL, H. F. R. 1958. The directed head turning response and allied movements of the human baby. *Behaviour* **13,** 212–242.

PRECHTL, H. F. R. and BEINTEMA, D. 1964. *The neurological examination of the full-term newborn infant.* Heinemann, London.
REIS, D. J. 1961. The palmomental reflex. *Archs. Neurol., Chicago* **4,** 486–498.
RICHARDS, T. W. and IRWIN, O. C. 1935. Plantar responses of infants and young children: an examination of the literature and reports of new experiments. *Univ. Iowa Stud. Child Welfare* **11,** 1–146.
SCHACHTER-NANCY, M. 1937. Le réflexe palmo-mentonnier (Marinesco-Radovici) chez l'enfant. *Revue fr. Pédiat.* **13,** 180–186.
STIRNIMANN, F. 1937. Die Einstellreaction beim Neugeborenen. *Jb. Kinderheilk.* **149,** 326–339.
STIRNIMANN, F. and STIRNIMANN, W. 1940. Der Fussgreifreflex bei Neugeborenen und Säuglingen. Seine diagnostische Verwendbarkeit. *Annln Paediat.* **154,** 149–265.
STREETER, G. L. 1920. Weight, sitting height, head size, foot length, and menstrual age of the human embryo. *Contr. Embryol.* **111,** 143–170.
WAGGONER, R. W. & FERGUSON, W. G. 1930. The development of the plantar reflex in children. *Archs Neurol. Psychiat., Chicago* **23,** 619–633.
WINDLE, W. F. 1944. Genesis of somatic motor function in mammalian embryos: a synthesizing article. *Physiol. Zoöl.* **17,** 247–260.
WOLFF, L. V. 1930. The response to plantar stimulation in infancy. *Am. J. Dis. Child.* **39,** 1176–1185.

Discussion

Nature of the Reflex Arc

PLOOG: What is the nature of the reflex arc involved in the early reflexes?

HUMPHREY: The earliest reflex arc is polysynaptic, not monosynaptic. The sensory fibres of the trigeminal nerve are stimulated when the stimulator is drawn across the skin of the perioral area. The naked, growing nerve tips have not yet reached the basement membrane underlying the epithelium at that time. These trigeminal fibres enter the brain stem and descend into the second cervical segment of the spinal cord by the time the first reflexes have been seen. We have traced this tract (spinal tract or descending root of trigeminal nerve) this far at 7½ weeks and at 8½ weeks. When mouth-opening is added to the reflex we have followed the fibres into the upper part of the fourth cervical segment. Interneurones that send their axons through the ventral commissure transfer the impulses to the motoneurones on the opposite side of the spinal cord. Both the commissural fibres and the motoneurones develop very early. Development proceeds from these upper cervical spinal-cord levels in both caudal and rostral directions.

At the beginning of reflex action, therefore, I believe that the reflex arc is of a three-neurone type consisting of the trigeminal nerve fibres (sensory limb), commissural neurones (interneurones), and motoneurones (ventral horn cells and neurones of the spinal accessory nucleus). Figure 20 shows such a reflex arc. The heavy lines outline the surfaces of the spinal cord and brain stem.

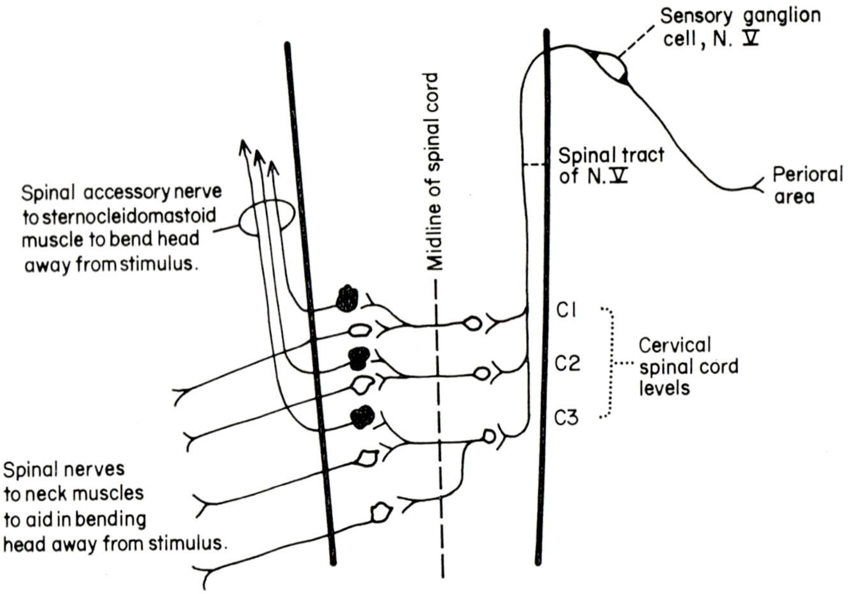

FIG. 20

As soon as the action extends beyond cervical levels, however, additional neurones participate. In the spinal cord the fibres that interconnect different spinal-cord segments and the reticulo-spinal fibre systems will take part. In the brain stem, connecting nerve cells transfer the nervous impulses to reticulo-spinal pathways which descend through the brain stem and into lower levels of the spinal cord. These paths will function in the activity of the lower extremity and lower trunk. By the time the mouth opens (8·5 weeks) the interneurones will also transfer the impulses to the neurones which supply the muscles that open the mouth. I shall not add these fibres to the diagram because to do so would make it too complex.

Effects of Repeated Stimulation

LIPSITT: What about repetitive observations under repeated stimuation?

HUMPHREY: Repetitive stimulation of the same area elicits the reflex two, three, or even more times, but it becomes weaker. Then you can no longer get the reflex. The reflex arc is no longer functioning. On turning the fetus over and trying the same area on the other side of the face, probably the same reflex will be elicited.

LIPSITT: That would rule out the baby's death process as being the determinant of the fatigue or what might be habituation. There must be some sort of practice effect that you are getting. Let's make a case for learning in the fetus!

HUMPHREY: I am sure that there is summation in connection with some of these reflexes before we can get a reaction, because sometimes two or three stroking stimuli of an area are needed, or even more, before there is a response.

LIPSITT: That seems to be the opposite effect. You were first talking about a diminution of response with repetitive stimulation, now you are talking about some sort of a recruitment phenomenon.

HUMPHREY: Both occur, but under different circumstances, of course. You may have a reflex arc which is temporarily no longer functional after you have elicited the same reflex repeatedly. Under other circumstances, when the reflex arc has not been stimulated before, for example, you may not get a response to the first stimulus, or even to the second one, but elicit a reflex on the third stimulus. Then you have had summation or recruitment.

PRECHTL: Is the low excitatory state of the nervous system of the fetus responsible for recruitment at the beginning, followed by a very rapid decline?

LIPSITT: One possible explanation for a recruitment-type phenomenon is that the infant is becoming increasingly aroused with repetitive stimulation and when he is aroused beyond a certain point then the next stimulus is sufficient to elicit a response.

BRONSON: We have talked about these very early fetal reactions to stimulation as simple reflex arcs. Is there a possibility that later on in fetal life, when you get a reticular system of networks at a functional level, some kind of "zero-level" habituation to the chronic prenatal sensory input establishes a neural pattern, and that after this has been established, the responses to stimulation are not from an essentially resting nervous system which is suddenly excited by something, but are responses to sensory input which disrupts this "zero-set" pattern of activity?

It has been suggested that maternal rhythm, maternal heartbeat, is setting the neural system to some kind of expected environment, and that this would account for some of the quieting effects on infants after birth when they are rocked, and perhaps more questionably, to heartbeat sounds. The prenatal environment is providing sensory input to the primitive parts of the nervous system and setting a kind of tonic background so that after birth we can't think of a stimulus-response arc as simply going through a simple input-output channel.

ROBINSON: Is the intra-uterine period a critical period then?

BRONSON: In this sense, yes. The question becomes: What kind of patterns are being codified as a result of tonic prenatal stimulation which then get disrupted by discordant characteristics of the postnatal environment?

LIPSITT: We must not ask, is there learning in the newborn or in the fetus; but rather, what kind of information is codified by the newborn and by the fetus and to what effect.

BRONSON: Might the quieting effect of swaddling, for instance, be due to tactile stimulation which in a sense replicates the chronic situation before birth? If so it is replicating the "zero set" established in certain neural systems before birth.

WOLFF: One kind of stimulation the baby is not getting before birth is light; yet flashing light has an effect quite similar to that of rocking, mother's heartbeats, Securitone, Slumbertone, and the rest. It is the repetitiveness of the input which matters, not its specific nature.

Effect of Hypoxia

ROBINSON: Hypoxia would be one factor producing diminution of response in your observations?

HUMPHREY: Unquestionably hypoxia is the biggest factor in the decrease of the response, although, like other reflex arcs, a reflex can be elicited only so many times before you can no longer secure it.

PLOOG: This is obviously not true for the monosynaptic reflex.

HUMPHREY: But these are multisynaptic or polysynaptic reflexes.

PLOOG: Since adult brains suffer after only one minute of lack of blood supply, how many minutes after an embryo has been taken out is it worked with?

HUMPHREY: As a rule it is between a minute and a minute and a half after the fetus has been removed in the operating room before the photography starts. With the smallest fetuses ($7\frac{1}{2}$ to $8\frac{1}{2}$ weeks), it is 5 or 6 minutes more before the oxygen supply has been used up. With the older ones it may be 10 minutes or more before reflexes cease. The time becomes longer as the fetus approaches a viable age. The heart beats for some time after the reflexes cease.

ROBINSON: There is very good evidence that the neonatal brain is less susceptible to hypoxia than the adult brain; is it possible that the brain of these fetuses is even less susceptible to hypoxia?

HUMPHREY: Probably it is. If the oxygen gradient in the central nervous system of the fetus is like that in the adult, then the lower levels of the nervous system require less oxygen. Certainly the spinal cord and brain stem are the levels functioning during the early fetal period.

ROBINSON: The bath is oxygenated saline?

HUMPHREY: No, it does no good to oxygenate the bath. Hooker tried oxygenating the placenta also and we could see practically no difference. It was a lot of trouble and so was abandoned.

PLOOG: But neuro-pathology shows pretty well whether the cells have suffered hypoxia. When you cut these brains did you get any correlation between the reflex patterns observed and the degree of hypoxia?

HUMPHREY: No; the differences would be too minute to detect with the histological techniques used.

ROBINSON: This is a general problem about acute hypoxic changes. They take some time to produce changes in the neurones so that if the animal dies shortly after the acute hypoxia it is unlikely to show in the neuro-pathology.

SCHULTE: Many newborn infants finally die from hypoxia but the pathologists find little in the brain of these cases.

HUMPHREY: You would have to use histo-chemical methods to demonstrate anything.

WOLFF: It's the capacity for anaerobic metabolism, which makes some of the difference.

ROBINSON: Probably, but it is not fully understood why the neonatal brain is less susceptible to hypoxia. One idea is that there are many fewer dendrites in the neonatal brain and therefore less membrane to be kept functioning than in the adult, and that this is the limiting factor in resistance to ischaemia and hypoxia (K. C. Dixon, 1967. *Lancet* **ii,** 289).

HUMPHREY: That fits in with the fact that the immature cell which is nonfunctional really requires less oxygen to stay alive and undamaged than a mature cell. Immature neurones can survive a hypoxic state that will destroy mature ones.

PRECHTL: Schwartze in Leipzig examined the pO_2 in newborn guinea-pigs. Guinea-pigs raise their heads suddenly some 10 to 20 minutes after delivery either to a stimulus or spontaneously. You can't get the response before that or in the fetus. When the head-raising response occurs the pO_2 jumps up. There is obviously a correlation between a certain critical pO_2 and the motor performance, admittedly a rather complex one. Now when they raised the pO_2 in the fetus they were also able to elicit the response.

ROBINSON: There is certainly evidence from other species that the arterial pO_2 in the fetus is much lower than immediately after birth: of the order of 40 millimetres or less (F. C. Battaglia *et al.* 1968, *J. clin. Invest.* **47,** 548).

PAPOUŠEK: These fetuses are good experimental models for observing hypoxia. For example, you said that around 11 weeks the contralateral contraction is replaced by an ipsilateral one, but with increasing hypoxia the contralateral response reappears. Is it always the less mature response, or the one that appears later in development, which is more sensitive to hypoxia?

HUMPHREY: Yes. This is true all of the way through the first half of fetal life, at least. What it means is that the reversal to early maturing responses on the development of anoxia and asphyxia is because newly functional reflex arcs require more oxygen than those that are longer established. For any particular age level, the fetus must be adequately supplied with oxygen to perform the developmentally latest bit of his reflex repertoire. Unless the oxygen supply is good, the reflexes that have most recently matured cannot be elicited.

Effects of Intra-uterine Posture

BRONSON: In all of your sequences the fetus returned to a previous position. Does this imply some kind of tonic feedback in the neural system which is bringing it back to a defined position or is it entirely due to the effect of the fluid in which it is floating?

HUMPHREY: It is simply relaxation of the muscles that contracted, with a passive return to position in younger fetuses.

BRONSON: I believe the normal position of a newborn infant varies according to the intra-uterine position taken before birth. If this is the case it would imply some kind of learning—in the sense of setting the neural parameters of the feedback for muscle position to the zero position in the uterus, which then after birth will programme what is the zero position for the infant when he is lying in his bassinet.

PRECHTL: For example, babies born in breech presentation tend to continue the intra-uterine position for days and weeks after delivery.

So do babies born in face presentation. The effect of intra-uterine position is not only on postnatal posture, but also on responses. We found that in the extended-leg breeches there may be a reversal of the withdrawal response, so that the baby moves its foot towards the stimulus, sometimes after a very brief jerky flexion of the leg (H. F. R. Prechtl and A. R. Knol. 1958. *Arch. Psychiat. Z. Neurol.* **196,** 542). There have been cases, however, without these changes in posture and reflex pattern. In all these cases a change of the intra-uterine position was found in the weekly obstetric examination shortly before delivery. The abnormal intra-uterine position has to be prolonged, actually throughout the last 4 weeks or so, in order to influence posture and responses postnatally.

PLOOG: In monkeys the position changes even a few days before birth so it is not so easy to establish for how long they really have been in the breech presentation before birth.

Spontaneous Movement: Inhibition

PRECHTL: Your film showed spontaneous movements which occur without stimulation and even perhaps at a time when there is no anatomical connection of the afferent system with the spinal cord.

HUMPHREY: No, there is already an anatomical connection. Both the cervical dorsal roots and the sensory fibres of the trigeminal nerve have entered the central nervous system of embryos only 5 millimetres long. Reflexes following stimulation begin when the fetus is about 20 millimetres long. The spontaneous movements in the motion pictures were made by a 26-millimetre fetus. You have a completely different situation with the chick, where contraction of the amnion gives rise to rocking movements. In cat fetuses, too, spontaneous movements appear before reflex activity. For the human material, the reaction to touch occurs before there are any spontaneous movements that we have ever seen. This sequence illustrates the general line of phylogenetic development. In fishes the skeletal muscle contracts before any motor nerve fibres have grown into it. Then there is activity over the motor nerve fibres to the muscle, and still later you have activity regulated by the reflex arcs.

ROBINSON: Is the period of about 18 to 22 weeks really a period of scarce movement or of scarce fetuses? You had many fewer fetuses at that time than earlier or later.

HUMPHREY: Yes, the relative scarcity of fetuses at that period is true enough. However, when you compare the human studies with other mammalian studies like those of Barcroft and Barron on the sheep, scarcity of material should not have been a problem and they reported the same decrease in activity. Barcroft and Barron felt that this change was due to the difference in oxygen supply—with the greater amount of oxygen required by the larger fetuses. Another relevant point, brought up by Bergström, is the matter of inhibition of reflexes. Inhibition of activity begins long before this period, but becomes a big factor in reducing activity during it. The total-pattern contralateral flexion reflex reaches its peak of performance around 35 millimetres. Then parts of the action disappear—in a specific order, not just haphazardly. Movements of the lower extremities and lower trunk are lost first, then activity of the upper trunk and next the upper extremities, although there is a tendency for the hand to remain responsive. The last part of the total pattern that is retained with a local reflex is movement of the head. The head movements remain and become part of the reflex arcs that are functional postnatally. There is a definite order in which the parts of the total pattern disappear, just as there is a definite order in which they develop.

SCHULTE: Are data available about the development of inhibitory interneurones in the spinal cord or of Golgi tendon organs in the muscles, which have an inhibitory influence on the spinal motoneurones?

HUMPHREY: I do not know about the functional development of the Golgi tendon organs or interneurones. Bodian is doing electron microscopy of fetal monkey spinal cords that shows two types of terminal boutons on the motoneurones early in development. He correlates one type with inhibition of activity and the other with activation.

PLOOG: Fink and Heimer (*Brain Res.* **4,** 369, 1967) have developed a new version of the Nauta method to stain the boutons so that this distinction could be made even more easily than by Bodian's method of recognizing the excitatory and inhibitory types of synapse. These methods may establish how early inhibition really starts.

Contralateral Before Ipsilateral

WOLFF: Whenever something new happens the contralateral seems to come first and then the ipsilateral?

HUMPHREY: This sequence really is significant. Psychiatrists in particular have been much interested in whether we are predominantly negativistic creatures in our reactions or the opposite. The two questions Hooker was asked most often by them were whether the fetus followed the Freudian sequence in the development of skin sensitivity and whether it first acted negatively or positively.

WOLFF: Denny-Brown has proposed this kind of a scheme: first the contralateral and then the ipsilateral reflexes develop as if this sequence were built into the programme.

KAUFMAN: Has this anything to do with the crossed nature of our nervous system?

HUMPHREY: I think that the crossed fibre system is related to survival. In lower forms, like Amblystoma for instance, if the organism uniformly turned towards the stimulus it would not survive long. The human embryo *in utero* is protected, but the phylogenetic neuronal pattern that resulted in survival (the crossed interneuronal connection) is retained and functions embryologically.

PLOOG: The nature of the stimuli which you are applying is important. Movies of a birth show that turning-towards and turning-away movements are present at the same time. As long as you use only tactile stimulation and even a stimulation with a hair you can expect that certain types of responses will be preferred.

HUMPHREY: The literature indicates that the strength of the stimulus may make the difference. Nevertheless, with the same strength of stimulator and applying it as nearly equally as possible, there is a preponderance of the contralateral over the ipsilateral responses during early development.

Postnatal Repetition

ROBINSON: Humphrey's observations were mainly on fetuses and she referred to other people's work on postnatal repetition of these sequences. Will Prechtl comment on the postnatal aspect?

PRECHTL: Humphrey mentioned the sequence of finger closure to tactile stimulation of the palm, in the order 3, 4, 5 and then 2. The thumb does not yet work. I found the same sequence in fullterm infants. In slow motion you see it quite clearly. The same sequence occurs in voluntary grasping in the 4-month-old when he grasps an object in his visual field. So this is something which persists in the first postnatal months. Another example of the repetition may be the flexor posture of the arms. The embryo has a flexed posture, but the preterm born baby tends to extend the arms. This may be simply because he is now in the field of gravity, but then gradually, as Franz has shown electromyographically, there is an increase in the tonic biceps activity and the arms go into flexion. I had thought that this was simply a matter of muscle bulk, since the biceps are much more developed than the triceps, but there is obviously real activity. When does the flexor posture go into an extensor posture in the fetus? Have you ever seen this or did all the fetuses you examined stay in this flexed posture?

HUMPHREY: As far as I know, the preponderance of flexure remains. Unless you elicit activity, the posture at rest is a variable degree of flexure.

BERGSTRÖM: Does this repetition of the pattern of development occur over a very long time?

HUMPHREY: I was referring particularly to the perinatal period when there is a tendency towards repetition of the sequences of movements. Part of the activity is eliminated as development progresses. The repetition that we see perinatally is particularly striatal in origin. Later the activity becomes cortical. The striatal activity is automatic, or reflex, if you wish. (I prefer "automatic" because it avoids the misconceptions that arise from association with less complex neural arcs.) Ultimately the comparable activity sequence is on a voluntary basis. After the child sees an object, for example, and reaches for it, his primitive finger closure and then his grasp repeat the early sequence of reflex and of automatic hand closure and grasp, but they then become more specific and coordinated.

WOLFF: Here is a general problem in development: when a new behaviour pattern appears analogous to a previous one, do we assume that pieces of the previous one are used as building blocks for the subsequent one?

HUMPHREY: If we remember that the motoneurones involved are the same in all cases, then at least the early behaviour pattern must be a precursor. Unless it were possible to develop new motoneurones to add to or replace those functioning from the beginning, I don't see how parts of the previous pattern can fail to be retained.

WOLFF: Is walking built out of the reflex stepping movements?

HUMPHREY: The walking movements are activated from the cortex and the stepping movements from the level of the striatum.

WOLFF: So they use the same instrument, as it were?

HUMPHREY: Yes, but one is stopped for a time, then utilized in another fashion. The striatal activity is suppressed, then regulated and activated from the cortex.

PRECHTL: This is exactly what I meant by different complexity. And in this connection you really have a concrete example where you have more units involved.

HUMPHREY: Yes, more units are involved and more neuronal circuits with them—associations in the cortex, between the parietal cortex and the extrapyramidal areas and the motor cortex. Sensations reach the cortex from the muscles, so that the child knows the position of his hand. Otherwise he cannot move the hand where he wants to, for he lacks the knowledge of its location.

KAUFMAN: Aren't we getting into the problem of organization now? If A controls B and then it comes to pass that C can take over control of B regardlesss of A, then you have a new organization, whereas if C takes over control of B by taking control over A, then you have a kind of development in which organization has proceeded into greater complexity. Obviously the final common pathway is the same in all motions involving the flexion of the foot, but how that pathway gets activated is really the question.

Response to Tickle. Respiratory Movements.

ROBINSON: How early do your fetuses make respiratory movements?

HUMPHREY: As early as 13 weeks. At 14 weeks, when a stimulator was drawn up the back, the fetus appeared ticklish and, as part of the response, there was an inspiratory gasp and a movement of the ribs cage, just as the adult may react when tickled.

ROBINSON: Apart from this do they make apparently spontaneous rhythmical respiratory movements?

HUMPHREY: Not until later. The 23½-week non-viable fetus had to be resuscitated with a respirator. Then there were rhythmical respiratory movements, but respiration couldn't be maintained for more than a few hours even with oxygen.

BERGSTRÖM: There is evidence that the real rhythmical breathing begins when inhibitory functions are appearing in the brain. Rhythmical respiratory movements begin at the same time as one can see the first signs of inhibition in the reflexes. But there are earlier respiratory movements of the mouth region called *Schnappatmung*. Did you observe this type of behaviour?

HUMPHREY: There are some quick mouth reactions as early as 11 weeks of menstrual age. The mouth is very quickly snapped open and shut. The whole reflex phenomenon takes less than one-half of a second. I have never thought of it as part of a respiratory pattern. One ought to have accompanying diaphragmatic or rib cage movements in order to link the mouth action with respiration.

KAUFMAN: Behavioural observation of young infants indicates that the mouth is a primary organ for tactile processing. So it certainly makes sense that any tactile stimulation should activate the mouth for processing behaviour. But that doesn't rule out the relationship to feeding behaviour or possible respiratory behaviour.

AMBROSE: I am interested in the respiratory gasp which occurs in response to tickle. This may be one of the origins of the laughing behaviour pattern which begins to occur in the fourth month of life, and it is interesting to see this component of it *in utero*.

HUMPHREY: As soon as there is reflex action of the muscles of facial expression (innervated by the seventh cranial nerve), you have some of the background movements for smiling and laughing, but the movements are very crude because the muscles themselves are not well differentiated. In some instances the fetus looks pleased with itself; in others it looks distressed. Of course, there is no emotion, for we usually relate emotion to higher nervous system levels that are not yet functioning, but the motor manifestations of emotion appear before there is any possibility of emotion.

PRECHTL: Is the tickle response homologous to what in the fullterm infant we call the Galant response or the incurvation of the trunk?

HUMPHREY: Perhaps. Is there any facial expression on the infant's face at the time that you get the incurvation?

PRECHTL: No, there is little change in facial expression.

MACKEITH: My impression was that the response in the fetus was a symmetrical extension of the back which puts it more as a Carbonell-Perez response rather than a Galant response. You scratch their back and they lift their bottom up.

ROBINSON: I agree that the fetuses may be showing a Galant reflex. This reflex is already present in prematurely born infants of about 26 weeks' gestation which suggests that it probably has continued from the age at which Humphrey observed it. Most of the reflexes observed in the fetuses are also present in prematurely born infants. (R. J. Robinson. 1966. *Archs Dis. Childh.* **41,** 437).

HUMPHREY: Have they been elicitable continuously from the stage at which we have seen them to the premature stage when you see them or has there been a period of quiescence during which they would not have been elicitable? Has the activity been inhibited for a time during maturation? There is some evidence that activities which appear early and function at lower brain stem and spinal cord levels are regulated later from higher levels of the brain stem. The upper levels take over by first inhibiting and then facilitating, but always regulating, the activity at the lower level. But as activity is regulated from still higher nervous system levels and eventually by the cortex, the type of reaction changes—movements become finer, new combinations appear, and there is more coordination.

PLOOG: Since the lungs don't function and no breathing movements are present. I was interested that you already got swallowing at 11 weeks.

HUMPHREY: More clearly a little bit later at about 12½ to 13 weeks.

PLOOG: That means that the highly coordinated interaction between the glottis and the swallowing movement is already in action at this time, otherwise you would find water in the lungs.

HUMPHREY: Some investigators report that the fetus inspires amniotic fluid and that it expands the lungs. That could be an example of activity *in utero* serving a purpose in development.

SCHULTE: Does the fetus really perform respiratory movements *in utero*? This was believed for 100 years, but it is very much questioned now. Contrast material in the amniotic fluid only enters the lungs if the fetus is in bad condition, which was true in all the old experiments. If the fetus suffers from hypoxia or from acidosis then, of course, it makes respiratory movements. Under other circumstances Adams has shown just the reverse: the lung produces amniotic fluid. We have also got some clinical evidence for this new theory in the last few years: in cases of intra-uterine transfusions on fetuses with erythroblastosis, as part of the technique, a catheter is put into the amniotic fluid and contrast material injected in order to determine the position of the fetus. The fetus always swallows this contrast material, but provided the conditions are good and the fetus tolerates the procedure well, the contrast material never enters the lungs.

ROBINSON: I agree. There is also evidence that inhalation of amniotic fluid is probably harmful and predisposes to hyaline membrane disease.

Function of Fetal Reflexes

ROBINSON: I like your idea of these fetal reflexes having a function and in particular the idea of the mouth opening being essential to the formation of the palate. I suppose there is an experiment of nature over this. In the baby with the Pierre-Robin syndrome, the lower jaw is small and the palate is defective. The tongue is pushed up through the cleft in the palate and of course this is liable to cause great difficulty with respiration after the baby is born. Is there anything we ought to look for in these babies in the postnatal sequence of reflexes—would you expect perhaps that their Babkin or palmo-mental reflexes would be defective?

HUMPHREY: I won't guess about that. It might be valuable to look into the history of drugs taken by the mother early in pregnancy, particularly those that influence the fetus and might prevent or reduce its activity at a crucial time. If my concept is correct, the drugs taken early in pregnancy may become an increasingly important factor in prenatal care.

ROBINSON: There are other suggestions of fetal reflexes having a function: that the walking and crawling reflexes help the baby to move around the uterus until it gets into the right position for a vertex presentation and that babies with paralysis of the limbs are more likely to have abnormal presentations at birth (W. Langreder. 1949. *Z. Geburtsh. Gynak.* **131,** 236).

HUMPHREY: I believe that even good prenatal development of the muscles of the infant is dependent upon their movement. If the fetus did not kick around a bit it would not develop strong muscles before birth. Do you people in paediatrics find any correlation between the amount of movement before birth—which the mother can tell you—and the developmental state of the muscles at birth?

ROBINSON: Mothers of babies with the congenital forms of muscular dystrophy very often give a history that the child has moved very little, at least in the latter stages of pregnancy but that is a different situation.

HUMPHREY: Mothers who have fraternal twins sometimes report that one moves much more than the other before birth. The difference is enough to distinguish between them, and postnatally one twin may be hyperactive and the other one lethargic.

The Infant:

physiological and behavioural studies

Excitation, Inhibition, and Impulse Conduction in Spinal Motoneurones of Preterm, Term and Small-for-dates Newborn Infants[1]

F. J. SCHULTE, ILONA LINKE,
R. MICHAELIS, and RENATE NOLTE[2]

University of Göttingen

INTRODUCTION

EMBRYOLOGISTS HAVE ALWAYS assumed that structural development is dependent on conceptional age. Surprisingly enough, paediatricians have not been very eager to apply the same concept to the functional development of low birth-weight infants. There are two main reasons for this. Firstly, in low birth-weight infants many functions depend on conceptional age during the first days of life, but then develop in relation to age from birth under the influence of environmental factors. Temperature regulation (Brück, 1961) and bilirubin binding are more effective in preterm infants of 36 weeks' conceptional age born at 34 weeks than in fullterm infants of 40 weeks who have just been born. Secondly, since 1886, when Miller introduced the definition of prematurity by reference to birth weight, paediatricians have usually looked upon body weight as the main determining factor for maturity. However, the relation between functions and "maturity" thus determined was frequently found to be poor. Although the definition of prematurity by weight was opposed by some obstetricians and paediatricians—notably by von Pfaundler (1941)—during the entire first half

[1] This investigation was supported by grants from the Deutsche Forschungsgemeinschaft, Schwerpunktprogramm Nervensystem Schu 120.

[2] The authors express their gratitude to the Max Planck Institute Computing Facility, Göttingen, for computing assistance.

of the century, this definition was accepted by the World Health Organization in 1948 and revised in 1961.

Only more recently has it become obvious that the maturation of nervous activity in newborn infants proceeds with age from conception rather than with age from birth or with body weight. This had already been shown for some aspects of psychomotor development by Gesell and Amatruda (1964), and for behavioural phenomena in the newborn period by Saint-Anne Dargassies (1955, 1966), Robinson (1966), and Babson and McKinnon (1965). Age-dependent development of the EEG has been repeatedly stressed by Dreyfus-Brisac (Dreyfus-Brisac and Blanc, 1956; Dreyfus-Brisac, 1964), and quantitatively confirmed by Parmelee and associates (1968) by means of a pattern recognition programme and by ourselves when we applied Grey Walter computer analysis to the EEG of term, preterm, and small-for-dates infants (Nolte *et al.*, 1967, 1968). The purpose of the present study was to find out which neurophysiological functions proceed with conceptional age independently of abnormal environmental factors and are therefore suitable for estimation of age, and which are heavily influenced by pathological conditions during pregnancy and the neonatal period. These investigations are part of a longitudinal study with the ultimate goal of finding neurophysiological deviations characteristic of certain gestational abnormalities and determining their prognostic significance.

METHODS

General

Impulse conduction along nerve fibres and the computational process of impulse transmission at synapses are the two fundamental electrophysiological mechanisms of nervous activity. Impulse conduction speed proceeds with myelination (Erlanger and Gasser, 1924; Hursh, 1939) and this in turn with age from conception (Carpenter and Bergland, 1957; Skoglund, 1960b; Thomas and Lambert, 1960; Gamstorp, 1963; Raimbault and Laget, 1963; Dunn *et al.*, 1964). Therefore, peripheral motor nerve conduction velocity was selected as a parameter for the degree of maturation. The electromyographic technique for conduction velocity measurement, its limitations, and the results are fully described elsewhere (Schulte *et al.*, 1968b). The development of spinal synaptic connections, both excitatory and inhibitory, can be investigated by electromyographic evaluation of spinal reflexes. For this study we chose the monosynaptic so-called tendon reflexes and their subsequent silent period as well as the Moro reflex. A detailed description of our technical approach and the results regarding the Moro reflex are given in a recent paper (Schulte *et al.*, 1968a). We used needle electrodes in order to be able to pick up such minimal activity as single motoneurone discharges and, at the same time, to avoid interference by mass activity from adjacent muscles not under investigation.

Subjects

A total of 83 newborn infants were classified into five groups according to the following criteria.

Group 1 was a control group of 20 normal fullterm infants. The pregnancies were uneventful and terminated spontaneously. The deliveries and routine paediatric examinations were normal. The birth weights were between the 10th and 90th percentile according to both Hosemann (1948) and Lubchenco and associates (1963), and ranged from 2,970 to 4,120 g. The gestational age ranged from 39 to 41 weeks measured from the first day of the last menstrual period.

Group 2 consisted of 25 small-for-dates infants. The weight both at birth and at the time of conduction velocity measurement was more than two standard deviations below the mean for the age, that is, below the 5th percentile according to Hosemann (1948) and well below the 10th percentile according to Lubchenco and associates (1963). The gestational age ranged from 36 to 45 weeks (Fig. 1).

Group 3 consisted of 38 preterm infants of gestational age less than 38 weeks. In all cases the pregnancies were normal except for the premature delivery which occurred without complication spontaneously or by Caesarian section. Postnatal courses were uneventful with the exception of the most immature child (gestational age 25 weeks) who died after 8 days. The weight of all infants both at birth and at the time of electromyographic examination was between the 10th and 90th percentile according to Hosemann (1948) and Lubchenco and associates (1963).

Group 4 contained all preterm infants who fell into the same weight range as the small-for-dates infants.

Group 5 was made up of 14 pairs of twins and 1 set of triplets who were included whether or not their gestational age was known. The triplets were divided into pairs, the medium-sized in each case being treated as the reference infant. Twins whose gestational ages were known were also placed in groups 2 and 4 according to the specifications.

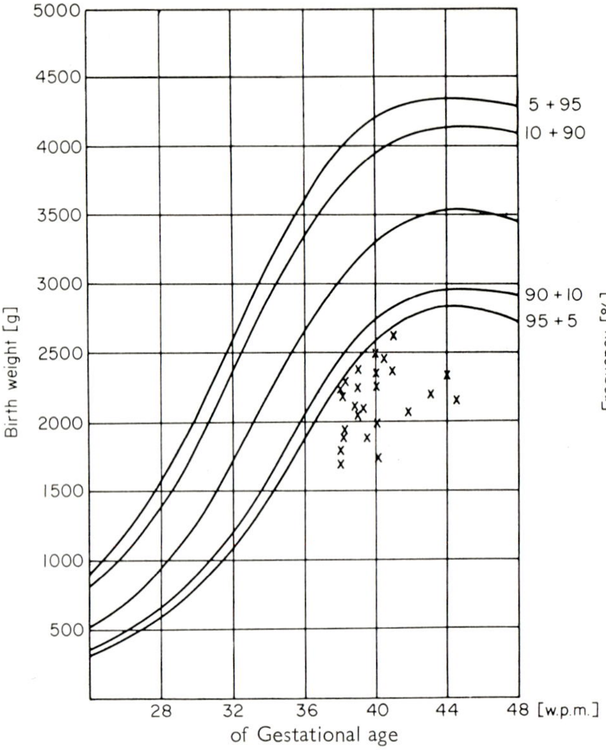

FIG. 1. Birth weights and gestational ages of the small-for-dates infants of this study indicated (x) in relation to the normal intra-uterine growth curves established at Göttingen by Hosemann (1948.)

The rectal temperatures of all infants studied were between 35·8 °C and 37·8 °C with only one exception: the youngest preterm infant had a rectal temperature of 35·0 °C. The five most immature and two small-for-dates infants were examined in their incubator. For technical reasons not all procedures were applied to each infant. The actual numbers of infants for each test can be seen from the tables and figures.

RESULTS AND DISCUSSION

Nerve Conduction

Impulse conduction along myelinated motor nerve fibres was found to be correlated with the infant's conceptional age but independent of his birth weight (Fig. 2). Small-for-dates infants had a higher conduction

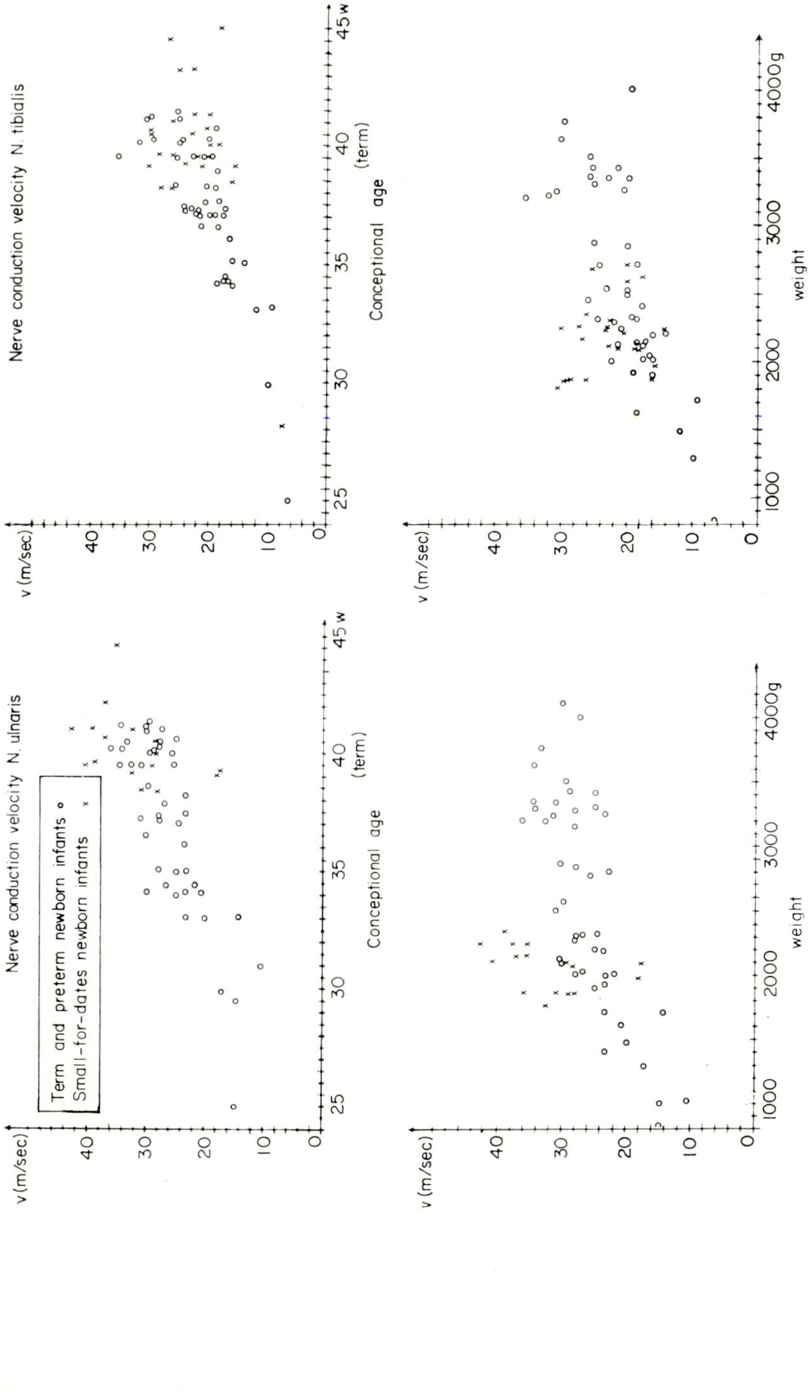

FIG. 2. Ulnar (left) and tibial (right) motor nerve conduction velocity in relation to conceptional age (above) and to body weight (below). Nerve-conduction velocity increases with age. Small-for-dates infants have a higher conduction velocity than preterm infants of comparable weight. [From Schulte *et al.* (1968b).]

TABLE I. STATISTICAL ANALYSIS (*t*-TEST) OF NERVE-CONDUCTION VELOCITY IN FULLTERM AND PRETERM INFANTS OF NORMAL WEIGHT AND IN SMALL-FOR-DATES INFANTS

	N. ulnaris					*N. tibialis*				
	n	*conceptional age* [*weeks*]	*weight* (*g*)	*conduction velocity* [*m/sec*]	*β* (*p*=0·05)	*n*	*conceptional age* [*weeks*]	*weight* (*g*)	*conduction velocity* [*m/sec*]	*β* (*p*=0·05)
term	19	40·6 ± 0·61	3345 ± 349	*30·4 ± 3·40	31·87 28·82	15	40·5 ± 0·20	3355 ± 316	*25·8 ± 2·0	26·85 24·82
small-for-dates	17	40·3 ± 1·58	2068 ± 183	°32·4 ± 7·25	35·95 28·85	20	40·7 ± 1·78	2139 ± 231	°23·68 ± 4·02	25·29 22·07
preterm	16	35·8 ± 1·64	2129 ± 243	*°25·9 ± 4·08	27·87 24·0	24	36·3 ± 1·56	2224 ± 219	*°18·6 ± 3·71	20·26 17·0
				*$t = 4{\cdot}520$ $p < 0{\cdot}001$ °$t = 3{\cdot}360$ $p < 0{\cdot}005$					*$t = 5{\cdot}934$ $p < 0{\cdot}001$ °$t = 6{\cdot}516$ $p < 0{\cdot}001$	

In each group the mean values and standard deviations are given for conceptional ages and body weights at the time of examination and for both ulnar and tibial nerve-conduction velocities. In addition, the confidence interval for the mean value of the conduction velocities is indicated (β) when the probability is 95% ($p = 0{\cdot}05$). Statistically significant differences in nerve-conduction velocities between the three groups of infants are indicated by * and ° with the corresponding t values and the level of probability (p). [From Schulte *et al.* (1968b).]

velocity than preterm infants of comparable weight (Table I). In twins of different body weight no correlation between weight and conduction velocity was found (Fig. 3). These findings indicate normal or near-normal myelination of peripheral nerve fibres in the majority of small-for-dates infants, which is in agreement with studies on brain weight.

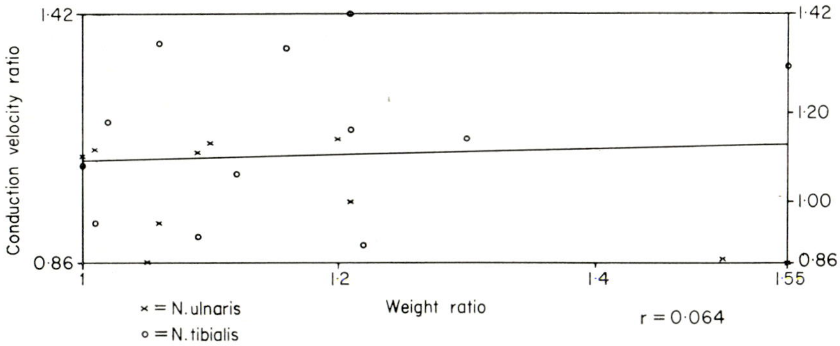

FIG. 3. Relationship between body weight ratio (Twin I: Twin II) and nerve conduction velocity ratio (Twin I: Twin II) in newborn twins. The heavier twin is always Twin I. No significant correlation could be found between the ratios for body weight and conduction velocity. The regression line is almost exactly horizontal, the Pearson correlation coefficient (r) being +0·06 [From Schulte *et al.* (1968b).]

A large proportion of brain weight is contributed by myelin, and in small-for-dates infants brain weight is less affected by intra-uterine malnutrition than is the weight of other organs or total body weight (Larroche, 1962; Gruenwald, 1963). In newborn rats nutritional deprivation led to a body weight 50 per cent that of control animals but reduced brain weight, total brain lipids, cholesterol, and phospholipids by only 20 per cent (Benton *et al.*, 1966). For those small-for-dates infants which had a lower conduction velocity than the fullterm control infants two explanations are possible: the dates given by the mothers might have been wrong; or, on the other hand, there is some evidence from animal experiments that intra-uterine malnutrition sometimes affects the myelination of only certain nerve fibres. Insufficient fetal nutrition which coincides with periods of rapid myelination in one particular group of axons will involve those axons but will not affect those whose myelination is already completed or has not yet started (Culley and Hertz, 1965; Dobbing, 1966). In general the fairly strong correlation between nerve conduction velocity and conceptional age is not surprising but one might expect a greater variability in other functions in which more complex nervous mechanisms are involved.

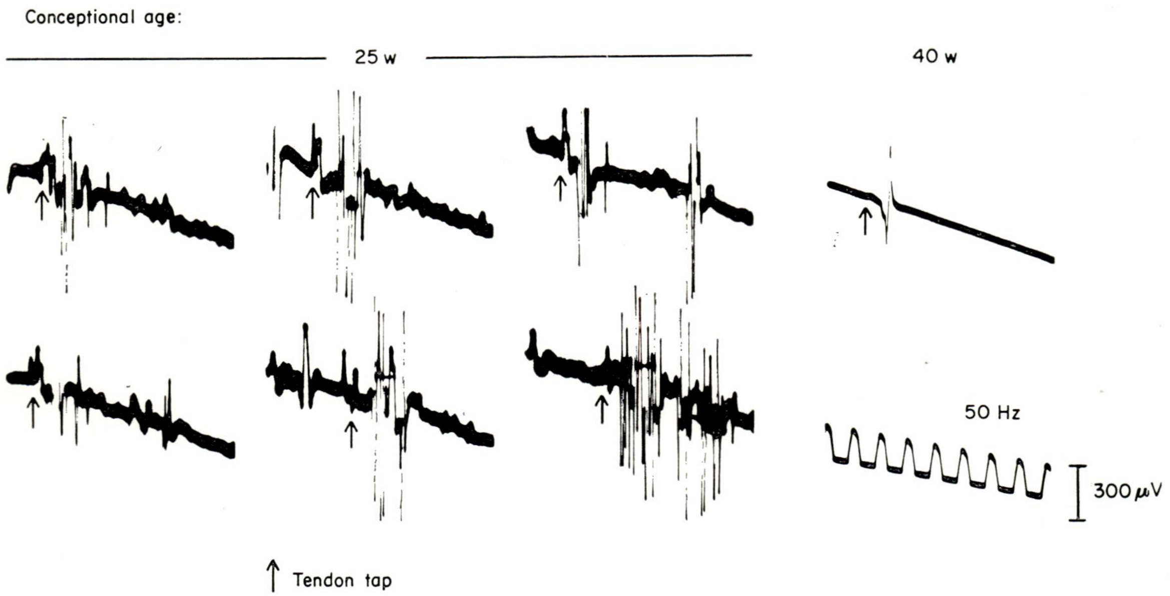

FIG. 4. The monosynaptic stretch reflex elicited by a tendon tap in a preterm infant of 25 weeks' conceptional age consisted of a burst of impulses rather than of one compound muscle action potential, such as was seen in the infant of 40 weeks' conceptional age.

Monosynaptic stretch reflex

The simplest test of synaptic transmission is the monosynaptic muscle stretch reflex elicited by a tendon tap or an electrical stimulus to the sensorimotor nerve. In all infants tested from 25 weeks' conceptional age up to term we never failed to evoke the monosynaptic reflex muscle action potential, although in some preterm infants the corresponding muscle contraction could not be seen. Its absence might have been due either to a low degree of synchronization of spinal motoneurones or to a lack of muscle power or both. In the youngest preterm infant of 25 weeks' conceptional age the low degree of motoneurone synchronization could be demonstrated electromyographically. The bioelectric reflex muscle activity evoked by a tendon tap consisted of a short train of impulses rather than of one compound muscle action potential as normally seen in older infants, children, and adults (Fig. 4). Various reasons could account for this asynchrony.

1. A wide variation of a comparatively low impulse conduction velocity in afferent and efferent nerve fibres would result in asynchronous activation of both spinal motoneurones and muscle fibres.
2. It is reasonable to assume that in very immature preterm infants the muscle stretch receptor activity evoked by a tendon tap is monosynaptically transmitted only to some spinal motoneurones and that, in addition, other motoneurones are activated after polysynaptic delays. Such a build-up of motoneurone depolarization pressure in excitatory spinal interneurones is by no means restricted to very immature preterm infants. However, in adults—both human and animal—the first synchronous reflex burst of spinal motoneurones creates strong inhibitory influences on themselves and on surrounding motoneurones, thus eliminating the possibility of immediate repetitive firing.

Spinal Inhibition

Inhibitory pathways. In older infants, children, and adults nerve cell inhibition following the discharge of spinal motoneurones is guaranteed by several mechanisms (Fig. 5).

1. Each spike potential is followed by membrane hyperpolarization due to a postexcitatory increase of membrane permeability to potassium. This membrane potential shift is called positive after-potential.
2. Each motoneurone action potential, before leaving the grey matter of the spinal cord, activates interneurones, called Renshaw cells, which in turn inhibit the surrounding motoneurones. This pathway represents an intraspinal inhibitory feedback mechanism.

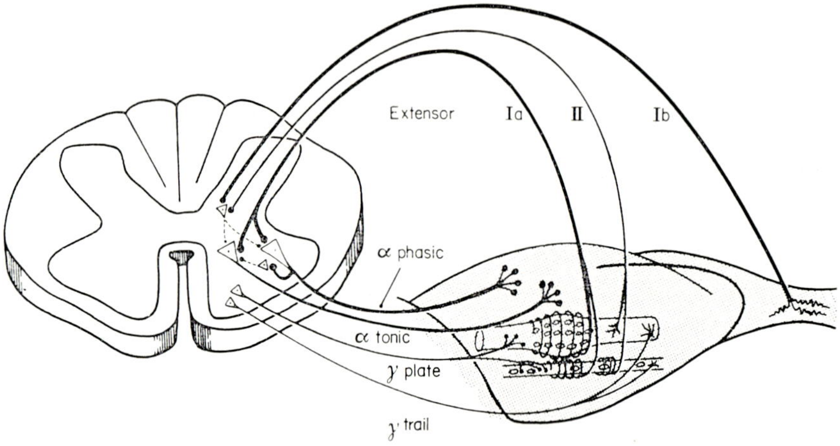

FIG. 5. Important pathways in the spinal motor system for extensor muscles. ——— excitatory connections; – – – – – inhibitory connections. α phasic: phasic α-motoneurones which activate the skeletal muscles and generally cause fast movements by means of short bursts of action potentials. α tonic: tonic α-motoneurones which activate the skeletal muscle for longer periods of contraction by means of a series of repetitive action potentials. While still within the grey matter, axon collaterals of the α-motoneurones activate Renshaw cells which act as inhibitors on the α-motoneurones. γ-plate, γ-trail: fusimotoneurones innervating muscle fibres within the muscle spindles (intrafusal muscle fibres).

Ia, II, Ib: Sensory afferent nerve fibres of muscle receptors activated by stretch.

Ia: Primary sensory muscle spindle ending of spiral formation located in the equatorial zone of the intrafusal muscle fibres. The impulses of these nerve fibres activate the motoneurones of the same muscle monosynaptically.

II: Secondary sensory muscle spindle endings of spiral or semi-spiral formations. The impulses of the secondary muscle spindle fibres via interneurones activate the motoneurones of flexors but inhibit the motoneurones of extensors.

Ib: Sensory nerve fibres from Golgi tendon organs which inhibit the motoneurones of the same muscle via interneurones. [From Schulte (1968).]

3. The reflex muscle twitch activates Golgi tendon organs, the afferent impulses of which inhibit spinal motoneurones via interneurones. This pathway represents a musculo-spinal inhibitory feedback mechanism.

4. Muscle spindle afferents are silenced by the reflex shortening of the muscle, thus part of the continuous afferent drive of spinal motoneurones from peripheral sources is eliminated for the short time while the muscle is contracting.

Silent period. The sum of spinal inhibitory mechanisms, activated by a synchronous burst of motoneurone discharges, can be demonstrated electromyographically. Each reflex compound action potential

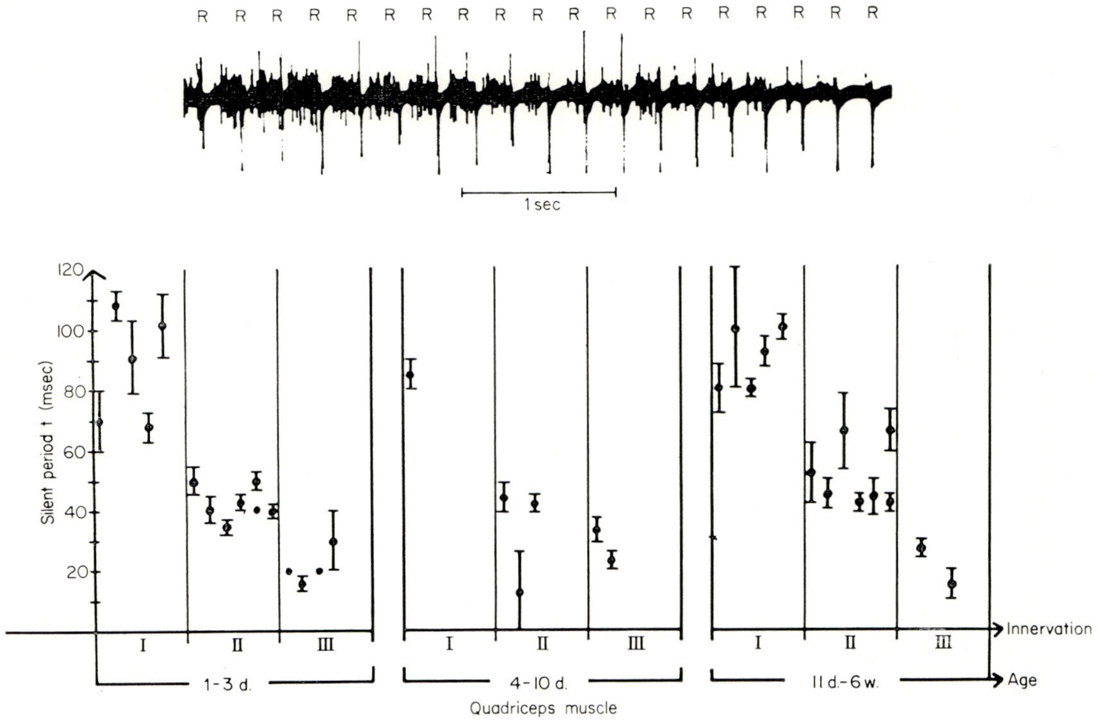

FIG. 6. Each reflex action potential evoked by tendon tap is followed by a silent period, the duration of which decreases with increasing background activity, the amount of which is indicated by I-III:

I (weak): sparse activity, only single action potentials.

II (moderate): background activity with one action potential immediately followed and sometimes even superimposed by another.

III (strong): maximum activity with the action potentials superimposed on each other.

The silent period is measured from the end of the reflex action potential to the recurrence of the background activity. Possible age-dependent changes in the duration of the silent period were not statistically evaluated for the time after birth at term. [From Joppich and Schulte (1968).]

is followed by the "*Innervationsstille*" (Hoffmann, 1922, 1934) or silent period in the ongoing background activity (Fig. 6). In newborn infants as well as in adults the duration of this silent period depends on the amount of background activity, that is, the supraspinal depolarization pressure on spinal motoneurones (Schulte and Schwenzel, 1965). The duration of the silent period decreases with increasing background activity: this shows that spinal inhibitory mechanisms can in part be outweighed by supraspinal excitatory drive (Paillard, 1955). The

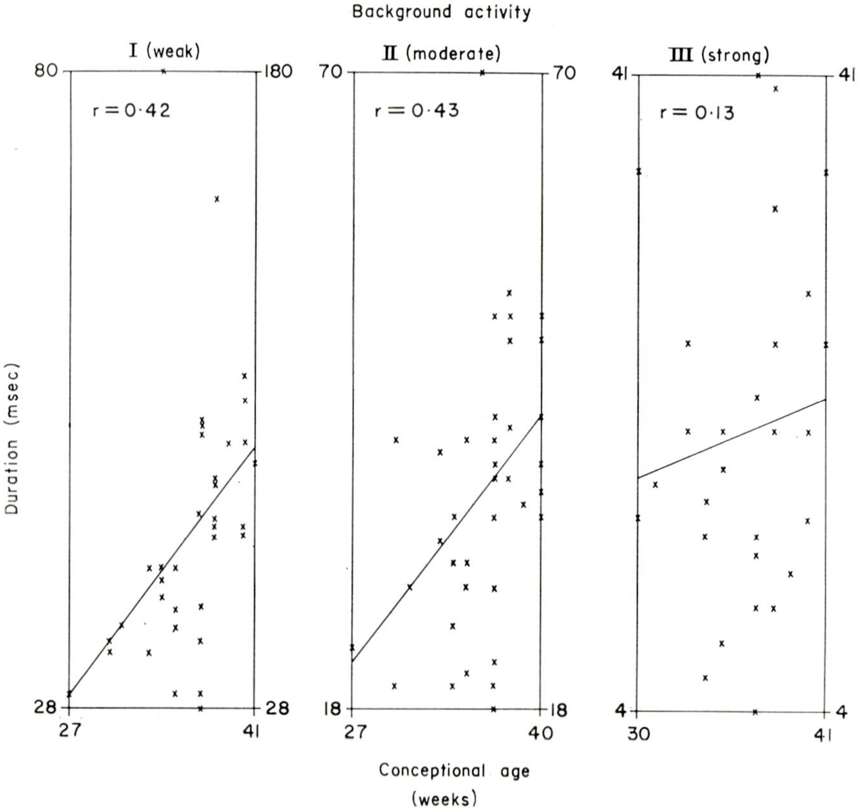

FIG. 7. The duration of the post-reflex silent period, being dependent upon background muscle activity (weak, moderate, strong) increases slightly with conceptional age, the Pearson correlation coefficient (r) being 0·42 during weak, and 0·43 during moderate, background activity. However, the duration of the silent period subsequent to a monosynaptic reflex elicited during strong muscle contraction shows only slight variation with age.

duration of the silent period—measuring the amount of inhibitory influences on spinal motoneurones subsequent to the monosynaptic stretch reflex—increases with conceptional age (Fig. 7). However, the minimum duration of the silent period after the monosynaptic reflex during the strongest supraspinal motoneurone excitation is almost equally maintained through all ages, including immature preterm infants. This result is consistent with the hypothesis that a minimum of postexcitatory inhibition, possibly due to basic membrane phenomena, is well developed in preterm infants of 30 weeks' conceptional age. However, surplus inhibition, due to more complex computational synaptic mechanisms in the spinal cord, proceeds with conceptional age.

Moro Response

Extensor: flexor ratio. More complex interactions of excitatory and inhibitory synaptic structures in the spinal cord of newborn infants can be examined by studying the Moro response pattern. It is well known that the Moro response pattern is dependent upon the infant's gestational age (Saint-Anne Dargassies, 1955, 1966; Babson and McKinnon, 1965; Brett, 1965). In preterm infants of less than 35 weeks' conceptional age the reaction consists of a brisk extension and abduction of the upper extremities. The subseqent flexion and adduction component is missing or incomplete (Fig. 8). After 35 weeks' conceptional age the infant develops the characteristic flexion posture of the fullterm neonate. In the Moro response, extension and abduction decrease at the same time as flexion and adduction become more prominent.

The purpose of this part of the study was to evaluate the age-dependent changes of the Moro reaction pattern by means of electromyography, and more specifically, to determine whether these changes in pattern are due to an increase in muscle mass or to a change in spinal motoneurone activity.

With increasing conceptional age the duration and the amount of biceps activity in the Moro response pattern significantly increased while the same values for the triceps activity remained almost constant (Fig. 9). A slight decrease in the amount of triceps activity with age was statistically insignificant. Thus electromyographic analysis indicates that the age-dependent flexor predominance is due to an increase of flexor, rather than to a decrease of extensor, activity.

The triceps-to-biceps Moro response activity ratios were below one in fullterm, and above one in preterm, newborn infants; the difference is statistically significant although the variance was very high in each

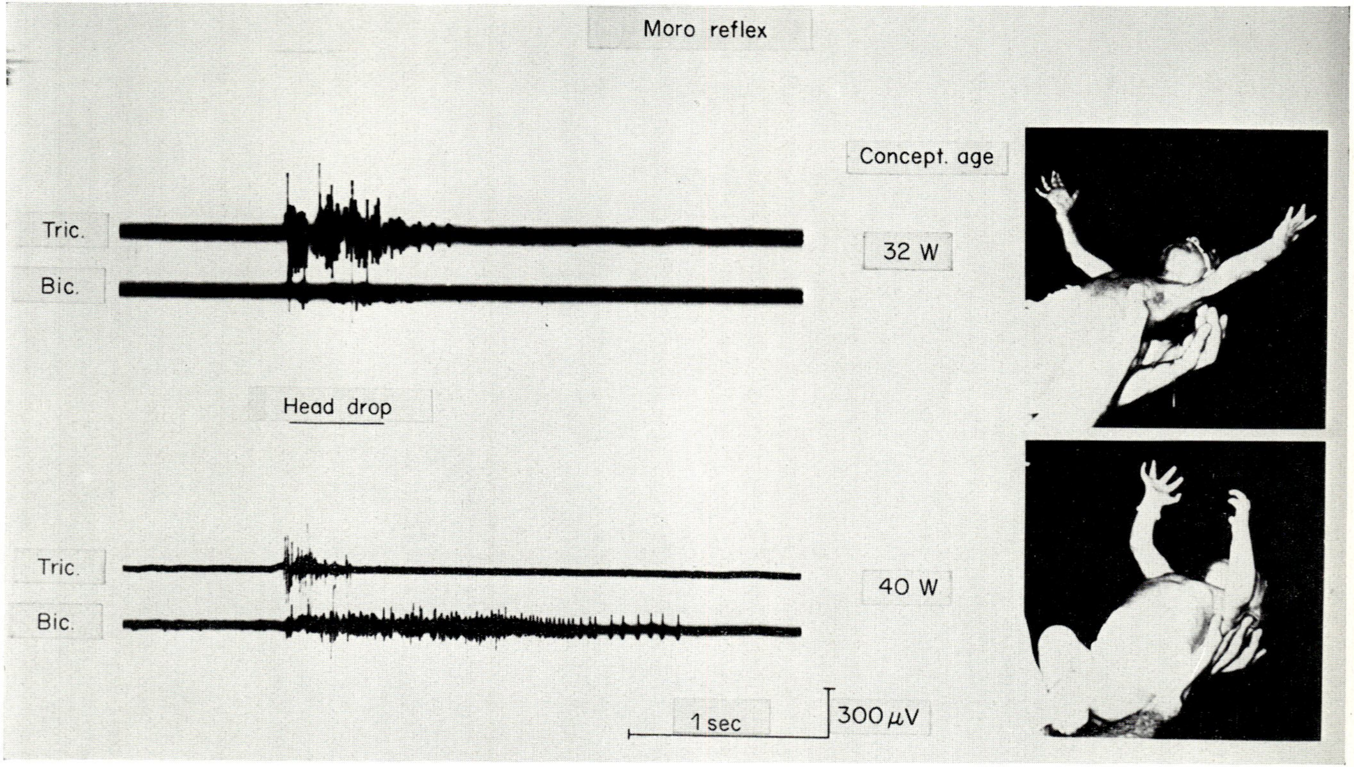

FIG. 8. At 32 weeks' conceptional age the Moro response consists of extension and abduction of the upper extremities. With increasing maturation both extension and abduction decrease whereas adduction and flexion become more prominent. Electromyographic activity subsequent to the head drop starts in the triceps muscle, being outlasted by activity in the biceps in fullterm newborn infants. [From Schulte *et al.* (1968a).]

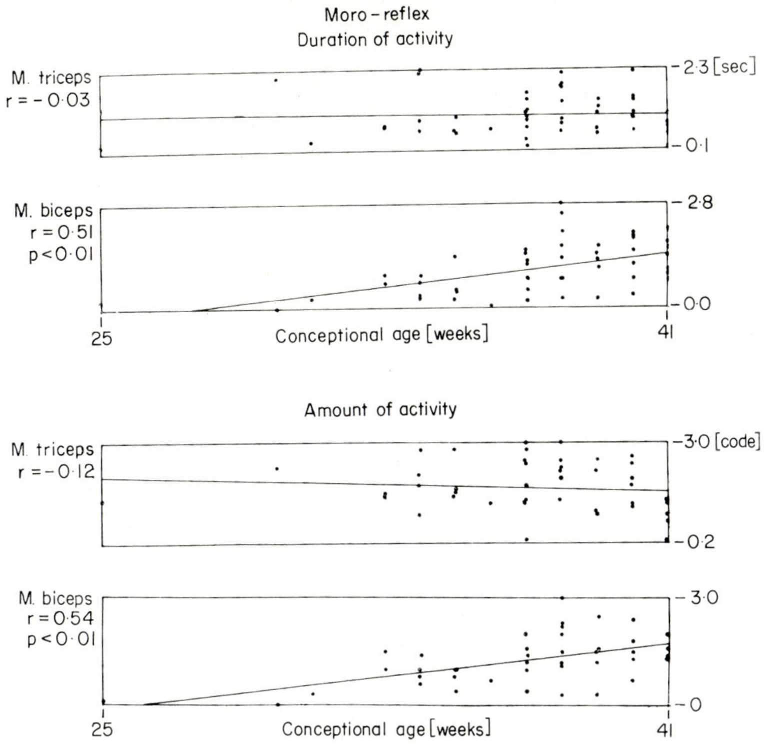

FIG. 9. Regression lines for the amount and the duration of biceps activity rise with conceptional age, the Pearson correlation coefficient (r) being significantly different from zero. Triceps activity is not related to conceptional age. [From Schulte *et al.* (1968a).]

group (Table II). Small-for-dates infants with a conceptional age comparable to that of the normal fullterm infants and a birth weight comparable to that of a group of preterm infants had a triceps-to-biceps activity ratio different from that of either the normal fullterm or the preterm infants. The variability of this triceps-to-biceps ratio in infants of equal conceptional age was considerable. The Moro reflex, therefore, was not suitable for an exact estimation of conceptional age. This might in part have been due to the fact that minimal pathology in the newborn period affected the Moro response more than age differences. In spite of this high variability of the Moro response pattern a statistically significant decrease of the triceps-to-biceps activity ratio with age could be demonstrated. So far, the electromyographic data confirmed the results of observational studies mentioned earlier.

TABLE. II STATISTICAL ANALYSIS (*t*-test) OF THE TRICEPS-TO-BICEPS ACTIVITY RATIO IN NORMAL FULLTERM, PRETERM, AND SMALL-FOR-DATES INFANTS

		Conceptional age [*weeks*]	Weight (*g*)	*MORO-REFLEX* $\frac{TRICEPS}{BICEPS}$ Duration of activity	β $p = 0{\cdot}05$	*MORO-REFLEX* $\frac{TRICEPS}{BICEPS}$ Amount of activity	β $p = 0{\cdot}05$
term	N = 18	40·17 ± 0·79	3344·74 ±348·94	▲*0·89 ± 0·66	1·20 0·58	▲*1·16 ± 0·94	1·59 0·72
small-for-dates	N = 23	40·61 ± 1·83	2118·70 ±244·64	▲1·25 ± 1·93	2·04 0·46	▲1·54 ± 1·31	2·08 1·00
preterm	N = 21	36·19 ± 1·63	2194·76 ±250·09	*1·93 ± 1·99	2·78 1·08	*2·21 ± 1·76	2·97 1·46
				*$t = 6{\cdot}14$; $p < 0{\cdot}001$ ▲$t = 2{\cdot}27$; $p < 0{\cdot}025$		*$t = 4{\cdot}18$; $p < 0{\cdot}001$ ▲$t = 2{\cdot}23$; $p < 0{\cdot}025$	

(From Schulte *et. al.*, 1968*a*). For symbols see Table I.

Delayed biceps response. In some infants the biceps activity started only after the triceps activity had already ceased (Fig. 10). This Moro response pattern with delayed biceps activity occurred more often in preterm, than in fullterm, newborn infants.

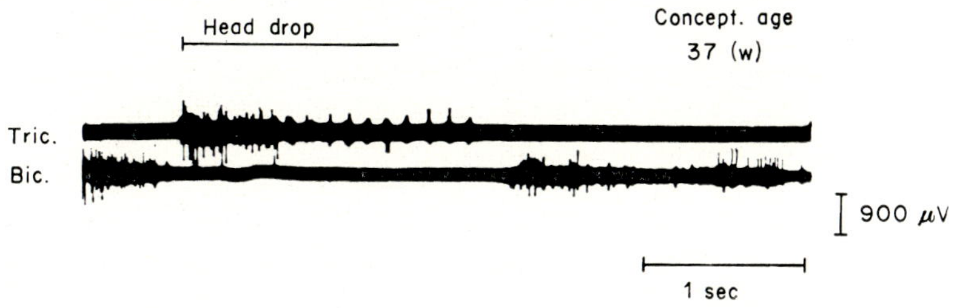

	N	*infants with delayed biceps activity*
preterm 25–33 w concept. age	9	4 (44·5%)
preterm 34–38 w concept. age	27	4 (14·8%)
term 39–41 w concept. age	37	4 (10·8%)

FIG. 10. In some infants, ongoing biceps activity abruptly ceases after eliciting the Moro response in the triceps muscle. Activity in the biceps starts again only when the triceps motoneurones are silent. This Moro response with delayed biceps activity occurs more often in preterm, than in term, infants, in the latter sometimes under abnormal conditions. [From Joppich and Schulte (1968).]

The delay in the biceps response demonstrates another aspect of the function of inhibitory spinal interneurones in preterm infants. The early immature Moro response consists of an immediate and strong activation of extensor motoneurones of the upper extremities. This reaction is already present in the 25-week-old preterm newborn infant and remains constant through all ages. As we know from animal experiments (Sherrington, 1889), a strong activation of extensor motoneurones very often implies a concomitant inhibition of flexors and vice versa. It is reasonable to assume that for flexor motoneurones in preterm infants the depolarization pressure, that is, the excitatory afferent inflow from central and peripheral origin, is too weak to overcome the hyperpolarization pressure which is raised in the inhibitory interneurones of the spinal cord by strong synchronous bursts of extensor motoneurone activity. The increasing flexor Moro response with conceptional age can be due to an increase in excitatory influences from either supraspinal or peripheral sources. Considering the results from animal experiments we think it very likely that proprioceptive influences enhance the Moro flexor reaction with increasing age. During the primary Moro extension response, flexor muscle spindles are stretched—thus eliciting a phasic or tonic myotatic reflex activity in spinal flexor motoneurones. In kittens the ability to sustain activity of muscle spindles develops in the first weeks after birth. In the immature animal only phasic, but no tonic myotatic reflexes can be elicited (Skoglund, 1960a,c). It is likely that the same developmental sequence occurs in the human fetus and newborn infant. Thus the brisk Moro extension creates a tonically sustained increase in flexor muscle spindle discharges—and therefore tonic myotatic reflex activity in spinal flexor motoneurones—only in more mature infants. In the immature preterm infant the spindle discharge frequency rapidly accommodates. Thus the proprioceptive depolarization pressure on the flexor motoneurones would be less in preterm, than in fullterm, newborn infants.

Rhythmic Moro response. In some infants of more than 34 weeks' conceptional age part of the Moro reaction pattern consisted of rhythmic, instead of tonic, motoneurone activity (Fig. 11). The rhythms represent burst-like discharges of spinal motoneurones. These bursts are separated from each other by periods of strong motoneurone inhibition due to negative feedback systems such as outlined earlier. These rhythms almost invariably occur in hyperexcitable infants, especially in infants of diabetic mothers. In addition, a rhythmic Moro response pattern is the most regular abnormal finding in the Moro response of small-for-dates infants, and that is particularly true of those who had an abnormal gestational period. We are at present investigating the reason for this tendency for rhythmic motoneurone discharges to occur. Hypoglycaemia, which sometimes occurs in small-for-dates infants and is the cause most usually suspected, has already been ruled out for the majority of our cases.

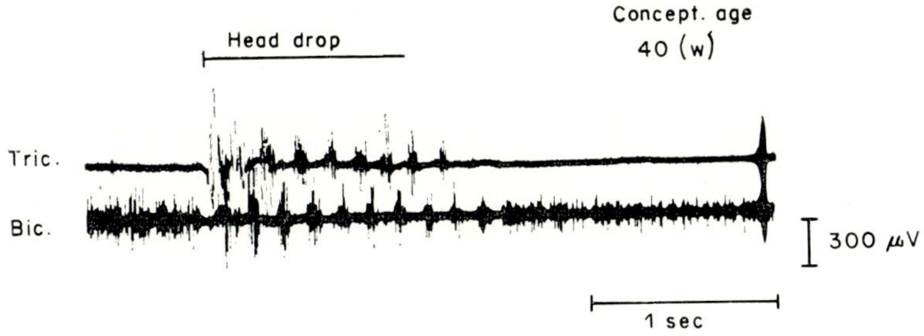

		infants with rhythmic Moro response	*% of rhythmic activity Triceps*	*Biceps*
preterm 34–38 w concept. age	27	9 (33%)	28	22
term 39–41 w concept. age	17	5 (28%)	23	10
hyperexcitable term	7	7 (100%)	65	85
small-for-dates abnormal gestation	15	8 (53·2%)	30	22·5

FIG. 11. In some neonates, particularly in hyperexcitable and in small-for-dates infants, the Moro response pattern consists of rhythmic rather than of tonic motoneurone activity. [From Joppich and Schulte (1968).]

CONCLUSION

In newborn infants of low birth weight neurophysiological and behavioural mechanisms develop with conceptional age and are independent from body weight. However, because of the frequent occurrence of abnormal environmental factors in the pre- and perinatal period the neurophysiological parameters fall into one of two categories (Fig. 12).

The first category comprises neurophysiological mechanisms which mainly depend on structural maturation. These phenomena are not greatly influenced by abnormal environmental factors and are therefore suitable for an estimation of conceptional age. According to our experi-

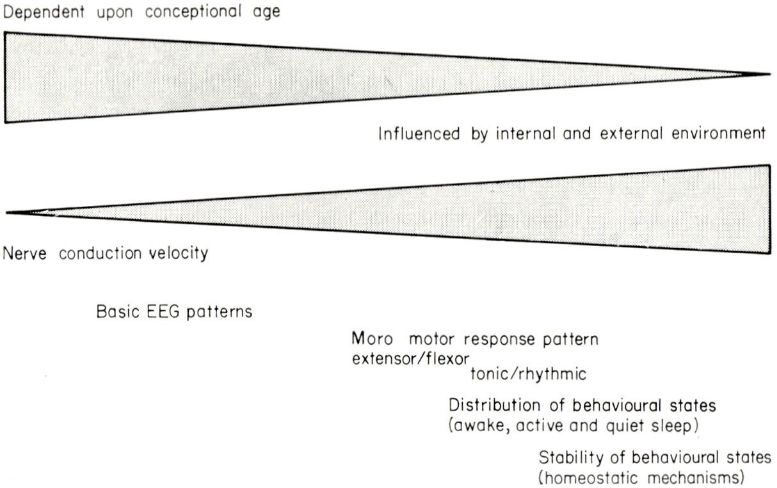

FIG. 12. Brain mechanisms are dependent upon both structural maturation and environmental influences. Complex synaptic functions and homeostasis of behavioural state are more easily altered by abnormal conditions and less suitable for an age estimate than comparatively simple neuronal activities like impulse conduction.

ence two phenomena belong to this group: nerve conduction velocity as an indicator of myelination, and basic EEG patterns probably as an indicator both of dendritic arborization and of formation of intracortical synaptic connections. Even these parameters can be influenced by certain abnormal circumstances, particularly when they are of severe degree.

The second category comprises neurophysiological mechanisms which vary considerably with the infant's external and internal environment. These phenomena seem to be most promising for the detection of neurological abnormalities but they are less suitable for an age estimate, particularly under abnormal conditions. Complex nervous activity belongs to this group, the Moro response pattern being one example. Another example, probably even more revealing because it is more complex, is the behavioural state stability. Basic EEG patterns, merely indicating the presence, the amount, and the sequence of bioelectric activity generators, are age-dependent but their circadian distribution and their coincidence with other parameters of respiration, heart rate, muscle activity and so on are heavily influenced by environmental factors (Monod *et al.*, 1967; Prechtl, 1968). All the second category phenomena also show various characteristics depending on conceptional age. This relation, however, is immediately masked when abnormal conditions like hypoxia, hypoglycaemia, electrolyte changes, polycythaemia, hyperbilirubinaemia and many other unknown factors influence nervous activity.

REFERENCES

BABSON, S. G. and MCKINNON, C. M. 1965. A preliminary report on the neuromuscular milestones in premature infant development, presented at 13th Annual Meeting, Western Society for Pediatric Research, Portland, Oregon.

BENTON, J. W., MOSER, H. W., DODGE, P. R. and CARR, S. 1966. Modification of the schedule of myelinisation in the rat by early nutritional deprivation. *Pediatrics, Springfield.* **38,** 801–807

BRETT, E. M. 1965. The estimation of foetal maturity by the neurological examination of the neonate. In M. Dawkins and W. G. MacGregor (Eds.), *Gestational age, size and maturity.* No. 19 in Spastics Society series Clinics in Developmental Medicine. Heinemann, London. Pp. 105–115.

BRÜCK, K. 1961. Temperature regulation in the newborn infant. *Biologia Neonat.* **3,** 65–119.

CARPENTER, F. G. and BERGLAND, R. M. 1957. Excitation and conduction in immature nerve fibres of the developing chick. *Am. J. Physiol.* **190,** 371–376.

CULLEY, W. J. and HERTZ, E. T. 1965. Effect of restricted food intake on growth and composition of preweanling rat brain. *Proc. Soc. exp. Biol. Med.* **118,** 233–234.

DOBBING, J. 1966. The effect of undernutrition on myelination in the central nervous system. *Biologia Neonat.* **9,** 132–147.

DREYFUS-BRISAC, C. 1964. The electroencephalogram of the premature infant and full-term newborn. In P. Kellaway and I. Petersén (Eds.), *Neurological and electroencephalographic correlative studies in infancy.* Grune & Stratton, New York. 186–707.

DREYFUS-BRISAC, C. and BLANC, C. 1956. Electro-encéphalogramme et maturation cérébrale. *Encéphale* **45,** 205–241.

DUNN, H. G., BUCKLER, W. ST. J., MORRISON, G. C. E. and EMERY, A. M. 1964. Conduction velocity of motor nerves in infants and children. *Pediatrics, Springfield.* **34,** 708–727.

ERLANGER, J. and GASSER, H. S. 1924. Compound nature of action current of nerves as disclosed by cathode ray oscillograph. *Am. J. Physiol.* **70,** 624–666.

GAMSTORP, J. 1963. Normal conduction velocity in ulnar, median and peroneal nerves in infancy, childhood and adolescence. *Acta. paediat., Stockh. Suppl.* **146,** 68–76.

GESELL, A. and AMATRUDA, C. S. 1964. *Developmental diagnosis.* 2nd ed. Harper & Row, New York.

GRUENWALD, P. 1963. Chronic fetal distress and placental insufficiency. *Biologia Neonat.* **5,** 215–265.

HOFFMANN, P. 1922, *Untersuchungen über Eigenreflexe (Sehnenreflexe) menschlicher Muskeln.* Springer, Berlin.

HOFFMANN, P. 1934. Die physiologischen Eigenschaften der Eigenreflexe. *Ergebn. Physiol.* **36,** 15–108.

HOSEMANN, H. 1948. Schwangerschaftsdauer und Neugeborenengewicht. *Arch. Gynäk.* **176,** 109–123.

HURSH, J. B. 1939. Conduction velocity and diameter of nerve fibres. *Am. J. Physiol.* **127,** 140–153.

JOPPICH, G. and SCHULTE, F. J. 1968. *Neurologie des Neugeborenen.* Springer: Berlin, Heidelberg, New York.

LARROCHE, J. C. 1962. Quelques aspects anatomiques du développement cérébral. *Biologia Neonat.* **4,** 126–153.

LUBCHENCO, L. O., HAUSMAN, C., DRESSLER, M. and BOYD, E. 1963. Intrauterine growth as estimated from liveborn birth weight data at 24 to 42 weeks of gestation. *Pediatrics, Springfield.* **32,** 793–800.

MILLER, N. T. 1886. Die Frühgeborenen und die Eigenthümlichkeiten ihrer Krankheiten. *Jb. Kinderheilk.* **25,** 179–192.

MONOD, N., ELIET-FLESCHER, J. and DREYFUS-BRISAC, C. 1967. Le sommeil du nouveau-né et du prématuré. *Biologia Neonat.* **11,** 216–247.

NOLTE, R., SCHULTE, F. J., MICHAELIS, R. and JÜRGENS, U. 1967. Power spectral analysis of the electroencephalogram of newborn twins in active and quiet sleep. In P. Kellaway and J. Petersén (Eds.), *Clinical electroencephalography of children.* Almqvist & Wiksell, Stockholm. Pp. 89–96.

NOLTE, R., SCHULTE, F. J., MICHAELIS, R., WEISSE, U. and GRUSON, R. 1968. Bioelectric brain maturation in small-for-dates infants. *Devl Med. Child Neurol.* **11,** 83–93.

PAILLARD, J. 1955. *Réflexes et régulations d'origine proprioceptive chez l'homme.* Arnette, Paris.

PARMELEE, A. H., SCHULTE, F. J., AKIYAMA, Y., WENNER, W. H., SCHULTZ, M. A. and STERN, E. 1968. Maturation of EEG activity during sleep in premature infants. *Electroenceph. clin. Neurophysiol.* **24,** 319–329.

PFAUNDLER, M. VON. 1941. Studien über Frühtod, Geschlechtsverhältnis und Selektion; zum perinatalen Sterben; die Neugeborenensterblichkeit. *Z. Kinderheilk.* **62,** 351–495.

PRECHTL, H. F. R. 1968. Polygraphic studies of the full-term new-born: II. Computer analysis of recorded data. In M. Bax and R. C. MacKeith (Eds.), *Studies in infancy.* No. 27 in Spastics Society series Clinics in Developmental Medicine. Heinemann, London. Pp. 22–27.

RAIMBAULT, J. and LAGET, P. 1963. Étude de la vitesse du conduction des fibres chez le jeune enfant. *Revue Neurol.* **108,** 204–208.

ROBINSON, R. J. 1966. Assessment of gestational age by neurological examination. *Archs Dis. Childh.* **41,** 437–447.

SAINT-ANNE DARGASSIES, S. 1955. Le maturation neurologique du prématuré. *Revue Neurol.* **93,** 331–346.

SAINT-ANNE DARGASSIES, S. 1966. Neurological maturation of the premature infant of 28–41 weeks gestational age. In F. Falkner (Ed.), *Human development.* Saunders, Philadelphia. Pp. 306–325

SCHULTE, F. J. 1968. Die Elektromyographie. In K. A. Bushe and P. Glees (Eds.), *Neurochirurgie des Gehirns und Rückenmarkes im Kindes- und Jugendalter.* Hippokrates Verlag, Stuttgart.

SCHULTE, F. J. and SCHWENZEL, W. 1965. Motor control and muscle tone in the newborn period. Electromyographic studies. *Biologia Neonat.* **8,** 198–215.

SCHULTE, F. J., LINKE, I., MICHAELIS, R. and NOLTE, R. 1968a. Electromyographic evaluation of the Moro reflex in preterm, term, and small-for-dates infants. *Devl Psychobiol.* **1,** 41–47.

SCHULTE, F. J., MICHAELIS, R., LINKE, I. and NOLTE, R. 1968b. Motor nerve conduction velocity in term, preterm, and small-for-dates newborn infants. *Pediatrics, Springfield.* **42,** 17–26.

SHERRINGTON, C. S. 1889. On nerve-tracts degenerating secondarily to lesions of the cortex cerebri. *J. Physiol., Lond.* **10,** 429–432.

SKOGLUND, S. 1960a. On the postnatal development of postural mechanisms as revealed by electromyography and myography in decerebrate kittens. *Acta physiol. scand.* **49,** 299–317.

SKOGLUND, S. 1960b. The spinal transmission of proprioceptive reflexes and the postnatal development of conduction velocity in different hindlimb nerves in the kitten. *Acta physiol. scand.* **49,** 318–329.

SKOGLUND, S. 1960c. The activity of muscle receptors in the kitten. *Acta physiol. scand.* **50,** 203–221.

THOMAS, J. E. and LAMBERT, E. H. 1960. Ulnar nerve conduction velocity and H-reflex in infants and children. *J. appl. Physiol.* **15,** 1–9.

Discussion

BERGSTRÖM: How is the EEG connected with the peripheral events?

SCHULTE: I put in the EEG only because it is part of the way we study these infants. We do polygraphic—electroencephalographic and electromyographic—studies in order to find out which neurophysiological parameters are influenced in abnormal infants and in what way. We now have a group of more than 30 abnormal newborn infants, on whom we have done a gestational age estimate from the nerve conduction velocity, from the electromyogram of the Moro reflex, from the neurological examination, and from the EEG. We found that conduction velocity provides the most accurate age estimate since, unlike any other parameter, it seems to be hardly influenced by pathology. This estimate is even more accurate than appeared in the slides I showed, which were of the first infants we examined. The variance for the conduction velocity is now smaller since we have eliminated some of the technical difficulties. The EEG seems to be not quite as independent from pathology. But from the basic EEG patterns one can estimate the gestational age with an error of about 2 weeks. This is influenced by abnormal circumstances, although to a surprisingly small extent. Even in some very abnormal infants, where the EEG has many abnormal potentials, the basic EEG patterns during active and quiet sleep are still visible. But in these infants other parameters of the polygraphic recording are very heavily disturbed, for instance, the regularity of respiration during quiet sleep. In fact in some very abnormal newborn infants there is hardly any regular respiration. The behavioural state stability or homoeostasis is very easily disturbed in abnormal newborn infants.

ROBINSON: Do pathological states have any effect on nerve conduction velocity?

SCHULTE: Not very often, apparently. We had one asphyxiated newborn infant who had hardly any heartbeat for 20 minutes after birth and who was artificially ventilated for 1 hour. This infant, who was almost decerebrate, had an ulnar nerve conduction velocity of 28 m/sec at 40 weeks' gestational age. This is less than one standard deviation below the normal mean. One can still do a fairly accurate age estimate from nerve conduction velocity in a case like this, whereas the EEG, the Moro response, and other neurological parameters are too abnormal to be useful for an age estimate.

ROBINSON: Have you any figures on hypocalcaemia?

SCHULTE: We know from animal studies that electrolyte changes do have some effect on conduction velocity but the effect is so slight that it does not show up in human neonatal pathology. It may be 5 per cent or so, but this is within the first standard deviation.

Significance of Nerve Conduction Time in Conditioning

LIPSITT: It is part of the lore of the infant-conditioning laboratory that nerve conduction velocity probably has something to do with the optimal circumstances for producing conditioning behaviour. The primary implication is that the CSUS interval, the interval between the conditioning stimulus and the unconditioned stimulus, may be affected to some extent by nerve conduction velocity, and with adults it seems as though 500 milliseconds is the optimal CSUS interval. There are some data on young organisms, for example Golubeva's work with newborn guinea-pigs (1939. *Psychol. Abstr.* **13,** No. 6113), indicating that the optimal CSUS may be considerably longer for the newborn. Have your findings any bearing on this?

SCHULTE: At a first guess I would say that compared with the length of the CSUS interval the differences in conduction time are extremely small if, indeed, they exist at all. We are now dealing with conduction times rather than velocities, and the distances involved are much smaller in newborn infants—which offsets the effect of slower conduction. I should think that synaptic delays are much more important here than delays in conduction.

Effect of Extra-uterine Experience

BRONSON: The nerve conduction rate increases very regularly with gestational age. In your prematures does it continue at about the same rate after birth when they are exposed to the external environment or is there evidence of acceleration?

SCHULTE: We have not completed this study yet, but we have compared three or four infants who reached term partly extra-uterinally with others born at term. From these preliminary results I am almost convinced that we shall find no great differences between these two groups of infants.

ROBINSON: R. S. Paine has some figures which show no significant difference in conduction velocities whether the baby had been maturing intra-uterinally or extra-uterinally (1966. *Clin. Proc. Child. Hosp. Wash.* **22,** 247).

BRONSON: Have you looked at the development of visual functions at all from this point of view?

SCHULTE: No, but we have done this for another parameter, the EEG. Together with Parmelee we compared extra-uterine and intra-uterine development of bioelectric brain activity. We coded every page of the EEG in a 3-hour polygraphic recording and then we counted the different codes for each infant. We found that premature infants reaching term, and fullterm infants born at term, have roughly the same distribution of codes. There were a few premature infants who at their expected term still had premature codes, but that might have been due to the fact that their mothers' dates were wrong, or that some of these infants were delayed in their development of the EEG patterns. This study—like all our others—was done blind, the examiner not knowing an infant's age, and it gives quantitative confirmation of Dreyfus-Brisac's position. Possibly with more sophisticated types of analysis one might find differences in the EEG between premature infants reaching term and fullterm infants born at term.

PRECHTL: What evidence have we of the effect of extra-uterine experience? We have learnt that accelerated maturation of nerve conduction velocity and of the EEG is not evident in preterm infants who have reached full term. We have also learnt that the state cycles are not influenced, and I should not expect conditioning to be influenced. Do we know anything at the moment which really is affected by extra-uterine experience?

WOLFF: Sucking frequencies are no different, but Benjamin and Metcalfe at Denver report that sleep spindles appear earlier in those who have had some time outside the uterus (J. D. Benjamin. 1961. In

A. W. Brosin (Ed.), *The Innate and the Experiential in Development*, p. 19. Univ. of Pittsburgh Press, Pittsburgh).

SCHULTE: I would be surprised.

ROBINSON: The critical thing is vision.

BRONSON: Which would make a nice distinction between neural systems which have intra-uterine input and those in which the input must await birth.

SCHULTE: Michaelis has found that social smiling appears earlier in relation to gestational age in infants born 5 weeks before term than in infants born at term (*see* also p. 165).

Significance of Myelination in CNS Development

PRECHTL: What are the effects of myelination and the change in synaptic time on the function of the developing nervous system? Does the CNS improve with myelination? Is the increase in nerve conduction velocity—at least to a large extent—wiped out by the increase in length of the nerves as Schulte has told us? Certainly, the synaptic time will be changing, but in the light of what we heard yesterday from Bergström could there be also a change in the synchronization of nerve-cell activities?

SCHULTE: To answer your first question first, about nerve conduction velocity and its meaning for development. In newborn infants the conduction time is even shorter than in adults. Because of the shorter distances, a lower conduction velocity in itself should not be a reason for functional incapacity. But myelination may not be so unimportant. With myelination many other parameters develop and they may be important. For instance, with an increasing thickness of the myelin sheath, the excitability, the maximum spike frequency, and the amplitude of the action potential increase. Motoneurones with high conduction velocity usually have a discharge pattern with a higher frequency than those with a lower conduction rate. Skoglund studied newborn kittens and found a conduction velocity of about 10 metres per second at term and these kittens had no tonically sustained discharges from their muscle spindles. He did find, however, tonic discharge patterns from the muscle spindle when the myelination had proceeded up to a conduction velocity of about 20 to 25 metres per second. Some weeks after term the muscle spindles could maintain high frequencies over a long period of time. Coming back to human infants—the term infant has a conduction velocity in the tibial nerve of about 25 metres per second. At about 36 weeks' gestational age (4 weeks preterm) conduction velocity is 20 metres per second, and it is just at this time that the baby develops the characteristic flexion posture. Surprisingly enough, this is very similar to the situation in kittens. Thus, I am quite convinced that myelination, indicated by a higher conduction velocity, and the tonic muscle spindle and motoneurone discharge patterns, have something to do with one another. If the myelin sheath reaches a certain thickness, whose value seems to be comparable in different species, there is the possibility of maintained, tonic discharge frequencies' originating at the first Ranvier node. Thus, conduction velocity is not the only parameter connected with the myelin sheath.

Another relation exists between myelination, amplitude of the action potential, and the amount of transmitter being released at interneuronal synapses. If the action potential is small, the amount of transmitter is small, and if the action potential is high the amount of transmitter is great. The amount of transmitter determines all excitatory and inhibitory synaptic activities, and hence is the main factor which determines the state of excitation and, finally, behaviour. Thus, I am reluctant to say that myelination has nothing to do with function.

BERGSTRÖM: There are many other factors involved here. First, the action potentials early in development, at least at the central level, are of very long duration. That would, of course, contribute to the amount of transmitter. It is possible that the long duration of immature spikes compensates for the small amplitude so that the electrical output, which determines the transmission in the immature synapse, remains constant. The second thing is that in early development, also at the central brain level, there appears to be some kind of giant action potential. This makes the problem even more complicated. Therefore, we just don't know what happens in the very beginning at the synaptical level.

What is the connection between excitation and myelination? We should remember that it is not the fibres which are excited; the excitation occurs in places where there isn't any myelin. It may just happen that the myelination occurs at the same time as the maturation of some other processes.

SCHULTE: I would partly agree with that. However, though excitation occurs in places where no myelin is present, the transformation of the generator potential into spikes at different frequencies occurs at the first Ranvier node, which means myelinated nerve fibre.

ROBINSON: Myelin really consists of a set of unit membranes, derived from Schwann cells, coiled in a spiral fashion. Do you think there is some critical number of unit membranes?

SCHULTE: It is really not the thickness of the myelin sheath which is important but the distance of the Ranvier nodes. The action potential jumps from one Ranvier node to the next, and the internodal distance rather than the thickness of the myelin sheath is what determines the conduction velocity. But the thickness of the myelin sheath and the internodal distance are correlated to each other.

ROBINSON: Does the internodal distance depend on the interval between the Schwann cells along the nerve?

SCHULTE: I do not know.

Brain and Behavioural Mechanisms in the Human Newborn Infant

H. F. R. PRECHTL

Department of Developmental Neurology,
University Hospital, Groningen.

INTRODUCTION

IN THE STUDY of patterns and cycles of sleep, physiological and behavioural research overlap widely. During the last few years investigations of behavioural states such as quiet sleep, rapid-eye-movement (REM) sleep, and various awake states have provided a powerful method for research on brain mechanisms and behavioural phenomena, not only in animals, but also in the human infant. Physiological methods and behavioural observation techniques have been used together very profitably, with deliberate disregard for the traditional borders of these fields. Complex phenomena such as the states require complex techniques of investigation. Many functions have to be recorded simultaneously and multidimensional automatic analysis of the data is required. Some of the techniques have even been borrowed from disciplines as far removed as engineering, geophysics, and meteorology.

I would like to present some of the results of studies in which we attempted to explore certain behaviours occurring in newborn infants during early extra-uterine life and their brain mechanisms. Neonates were chosen for two reasons: (1) their brain functions and their behavioural repertoire are still relatively simple as compared to those of the human adult; (2) we had encountered clinical problems in the early neurological assessment of brain damage which demanded further investigation.

APPROACH AND METHODS

We tried to attack the problem of behavioural states in the infant within the theoretical framework of a "black box" analysis. Baseline data are collected by observing or recording the various outputs such as head and limb movements, closing or opening of the eyes, eye movements, respiration, heart rate, EEG, and EMG from various muscle groups, while the infant is kept under constant and neutral environmental conditions: he is naked in a climate chamber whose ambient temperature is 32 °C and humidity 55 per cent. By keeping the ambient noise level at about 55dB, and the artificial light in the room at medium intensity, a constant auditory and visual input is ensured. The babies are investigated between two feeds or are bottle-fed every 3 hours during the recording.

Under these conditions a number of states consisting of characteristic constellations of certain functional patterns occur cyclically and can readily be recognized not only in any given baby, but in all babies. These states are stable over periods ranging from a few minutes up to 45 minutes. They are separated from each other by transitions in which the parameters change their properties; for example, regular respirations become irregular or phasic EMG activity becomes tonic, until a new stable constellation is reached. All these phenomena can also be observed in infants lying clothed in their cribs in a nursery. However, in the experimental conditions of the climate chamber the awake states occur less often and are of shorter duration.

The first task of our analysis was the investigation of the statistical properties of the various parameters and of their inter-relations in the different states. In a second series of studies we attempted to shed light on the internal organization of the underlying brain mechanisms by applying various inputs (tactile, proprioceptive, auditory, vestibular, and nociceptive stimulation) in the different states.

Details of the methods have been fully described previously (Prechtl, 1968; Prechtl *et al.*, 1968); only the main points will be mentioned here. In all our polygrams the following standard variables were recorded: respiration, electrocardiogram (ECG), heart rate (by cardiotachometer), electro-oculogram (EOG), electroencephalogram (EEG), and electromyogram (EMG). We employed an Offner Beckman Dynograph Type R with 16 recording channels. At the time of recording, the paper was run at a speed of 6 mm per second; during play-back it was run at various slower speeds down to 6 mm per minute. The recorded data were stored in analogue form on an instrumentation tape recorder (Ampex CP-100 or Ampex FR-1800). Computer analysis was carried out off-line on TMC special purpose computers (CORR-100; with amplitude discriminator, amplitude-time converter) and the results were printed, punched on paper tape (Tally), and plotted on an

X-Y-plotter (Mosely Autograph 2D-2). For further computation the 8-channel punch-tape output was fed into a Telefunken TR4 general-purpose computer of the University Computer Centre.

RESULTS

Polygraphic Recordings of States

The classification of states in young infants was originally based on behavioural criteria which could be observed (Wagner, 1939; Wolff, 1959, 1966; Escalona, 1962; Brown, 1964; Prechtl and Beintema, 1964).

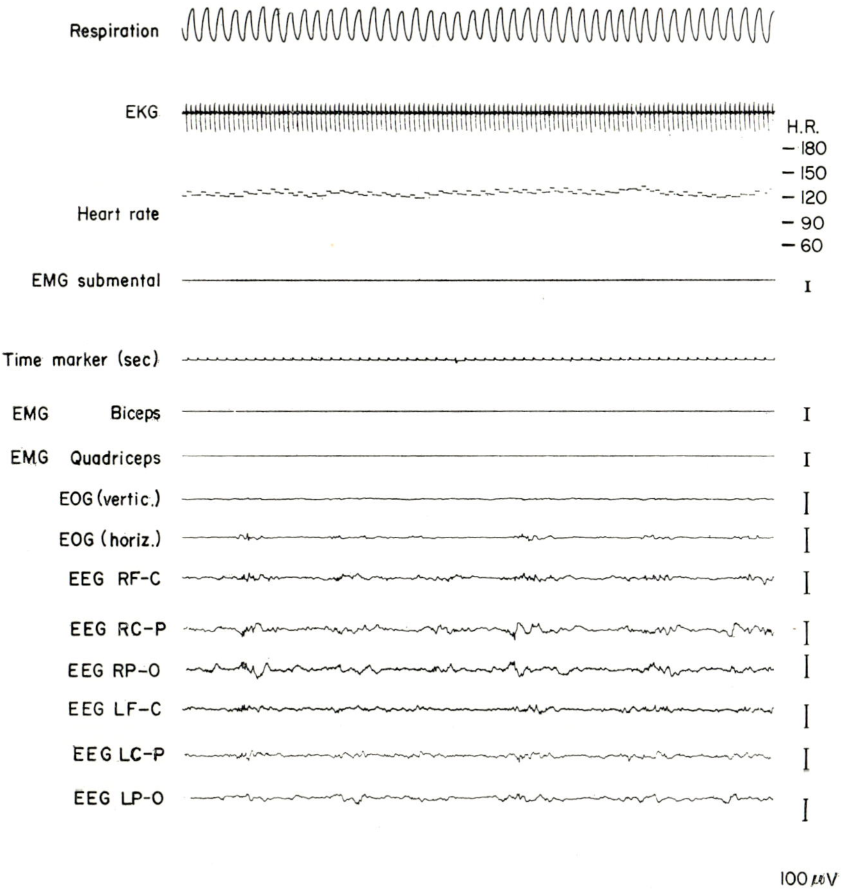

FIG. 1. Polygraphic record from an 8-day-old infant during a 1-minute period of regular sleep. A break through of the *tracé-alternant* bursts of the EEG can be seen in the EOG.

A varying number of items was included in the definitions and this resulted in different, often non-comparable, scales of classification. Independently from these efforts, EEG studies led to the recognition of particular states of sleep and wakefulness which have specific EEG patterns (Dreyfus-Brisac *et al.*, 1955; Dreyfus-Brisac, 1959; Dreyfus-Brisac and Monod, 1965; Delange *et al.*, 1962; Petre-Quadens, 1965, 1966).

Modern electronic recording devices make it possible to take many variables into account, some of which cannot be observed with the unaided eye. The assessment of these physiological concomitants of the behavioural states facilitates the analysis of the underlying regulating processes in the nervous system.

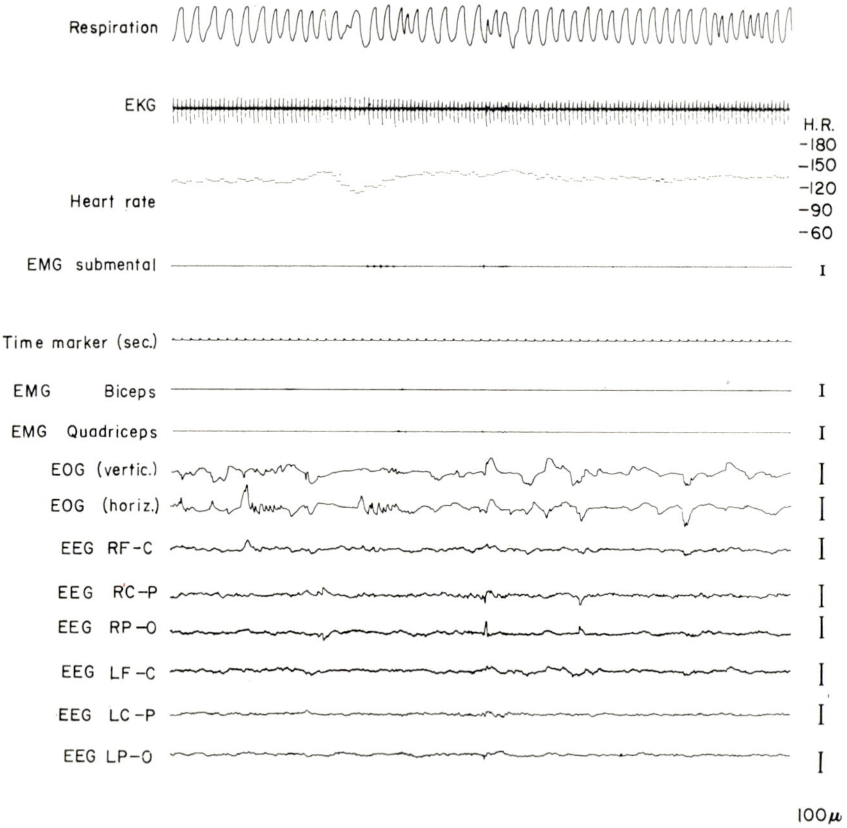

FIG. 2. Polygraphic record from an 8-day-old infant during a 1-minute period of irregular sleep.

A few examples of polygraphic recording may serve as illustrations. Figure 1 shows one minute of a regular-sleep state, when the baby's eyes remain closed, respiration is regular, and no body movements occur. The heart rate is stable and relatively slow, the EEG contains periodic bursts of waves with high amplitude (the *tracé alternant* pattern), and the absence of eye movements is expressed in the EOGs as a straight base-line. The irregular-sleep state is portrayed in Fig. 2. The irregular respiration is accompanied by irregular and fast heart rate, eye movements can be clearly observed in the vertical and horizontal EOG, the EEG is of a low amplitude, and phasic activity occurs irregularly in the EMG channels corresponding with small jerky movements. In the quietly-awake state (Fig. 3), the baby's eyes are open, the respiration is slightly irregular, the heart rate is fast, there is

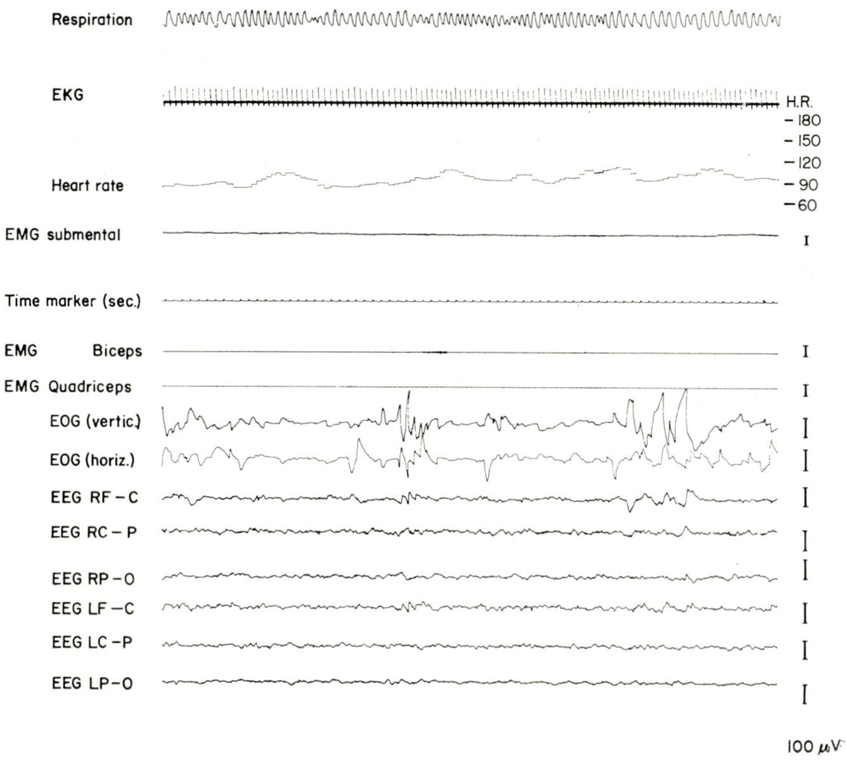

FIG. 3. Polygraphic record from an 8-day-old infant during a 1-minute period of quiet wakefulness.

little EMG activity, and fast-scanning eye movements and big phasic blink artefacts occur in the EOG.

A clear picture of the duration of states, of the transitions between the stable states, and of the inter-relationship between the various recorded parameters can be obtained from compressed records, which are made by playing the signals back from magnetic tape onto paper running at low speed. Figure 4 is such a record, beginning with the

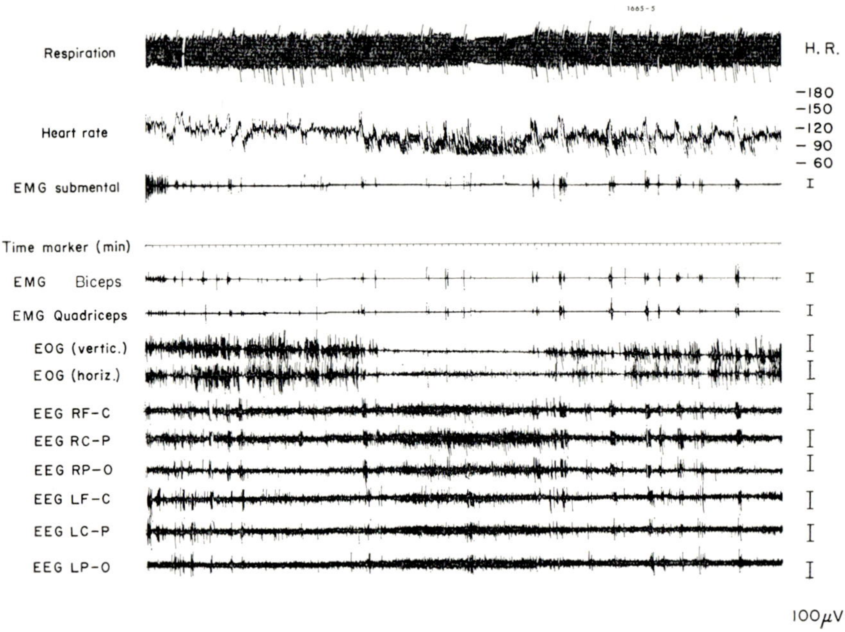

FIG. 4. Polygraphic record from a 5-day-old infant during a 90-minute period, compressed by running the paper at 6 min/min.

infant sucking on a bottle (EMG activity present in the submental muscle), followed by a transition into irregular sleep (irregular respiration, fast heart rate, eye movements, and low-voltage EEG). When this epoch is terminated the respiration becomes regular, the heart rate decreases, the eye movements cease and the EEG gradually develops a higher amplitude. The period of regular sleep which results lasts for about 23 minutes. From time to time, however, the stable pattern is interrupted by startles accompanied by a deep inspiration and expiration followed by apnoea of several seconds' duration. Simultaneously with the deep sigh there is a generalized phasic contraction of all muscles and a brief tachycardia. After the end of the regular-sleep epoch the baby passes into a new period of irregular sleep with the same characteristics as the one before.

Computer Analysis of the Polygraphic Data

Individual parameters. A polygraphic recording made over the course of several hours contains a huge amount of analogue data. Visual inspection of the records, as described in the previous paragraph, cannot provide more than a global and subjective evaluation, with all its shortcomings. Before the data can be analysed, it is essential both to quantify them and drastically to reduce them. Since methods of analysis by hand are extremely time-consuming and since the results obtained are nevertheless of only limited precision, modern techniques of automatic data processing are of great help. Applying such techniques of analysis we have been able to convert the polygrams into quantified data and finally to plot them as sequential diagrams to show the course of the various parameters.

In order to make these transformations, the separate signals are subjected to statistical treatment by the computer. The respiration signal, recorded with a thermistor across the nostrils, is analysed by an amplitude discriminator which measures the length of each breath-cycle. This is carried out for consecutive epochs each of 3 minutes, and for each epoch a non-sequential histogram of breath-to-breath intervals is obtained. This technique is superior to ordinary counting of the respiratory rate because it supplies not only the preference interval, which can easily be converted into rate, but also the variation of the signal, which is a measure of the regularity or irregularity of respiration. From these interval histograms, the median interval and the 25th percentiles and 75th percentiles (quartiles) are computed. These measurements are used because the distributions are often skewed and the means and standard deviations are therefore not proper descriptions of the data.

The analysis of the heart rate is based on the same principles, and the intervals between consecutive QRS complexes on the ECG are measured. From the distribution of beat-to-beat intervals the median and the quartiles are again computed for consecutive 3-minute epochs.

A quantitative analysis of the EEG amplitude can be made by hand-measurement of the peak-to-peak amplitudes of many waves in a given record. However, this technique is tedious and very inaccurate. Automatic sampling by the amplitude-time converter of the amplitudes at regular short intervals now makes it possible to analyse very exactly the distribution of the amplitudes and the mean-square voltage of a particular portion of an EEG record. By computing the mean, standard deviation, skewness and kurtosis of the amplitude distributions, information can be obtained as to whether a deviation from a Gaussian distribution can be rejected or not. In addition, squaring the voltages of the sample points and averaging the sum gives the mean square voltage in μV^2 which is an expression of the power of the EEG signal in the epoch analysed. The distribution of the power across the frequencies contained in the EEG can be obtained from the power density spectra.

Quantitative analysis of the rapid eye movements (REMs) in irregular sleep or when the baby is looking around with his eyes open in the quietly-awake state has been reported in detail in a previous paper (Prechtl and Lenard, 1967). Here I shall refer to the number of rapid eye movements which occur in each 3-minute epoch. Automation of this counting process is still very difficult and would require pattern discrimination programmes which for this type of signal are very elaborate and unsatisfactory. Hand analysis of the paper write-out of the EOG records seems to supply sufficiently accurate data.

The data which have been analysed separately are finally compiled in a plot diagram, of which an example is given in Fig. 5. Recordings were made from this 8-day-old baby continuously for 5 hours. He was fed 1 hour and 20 minutes after the beginning of the recording and again near the end. During the second half of the recording—3 hours and 15 minutes after the beginning—the baby was given a dummy (nipple) so that he performed non-nutritive sucking during a state of wakefulness. The first 20 minutes of the recording consisted of a regular-sleep epoch in which the respiratory rate (calculated from the median breath-to-breath interval) was about 40/min, the heart rate was about 110/min, the mean-square voltage of the EEG was between 100 and 140 μV^2, and there was a complete absence of eye movements. Respiration and heart rate were stable, as is shown by the small inter-quartile ranges.

Following the initial period of regular sleep there was a period of irregular sleep lasting about 50 minutes, with many rapid eye movements, fast and irregular respiration and heart rate, and with the mean square voltage of the EEG decreased to about 40–50 μV^2. This pattern of regular, followed by irregular, sleep repeated itself several times, and was interrupted only by brief states of wakefulness and sucking.

It is obvious that diagrams of this kind provide more information than any compressed record can supply. However, the more intimate

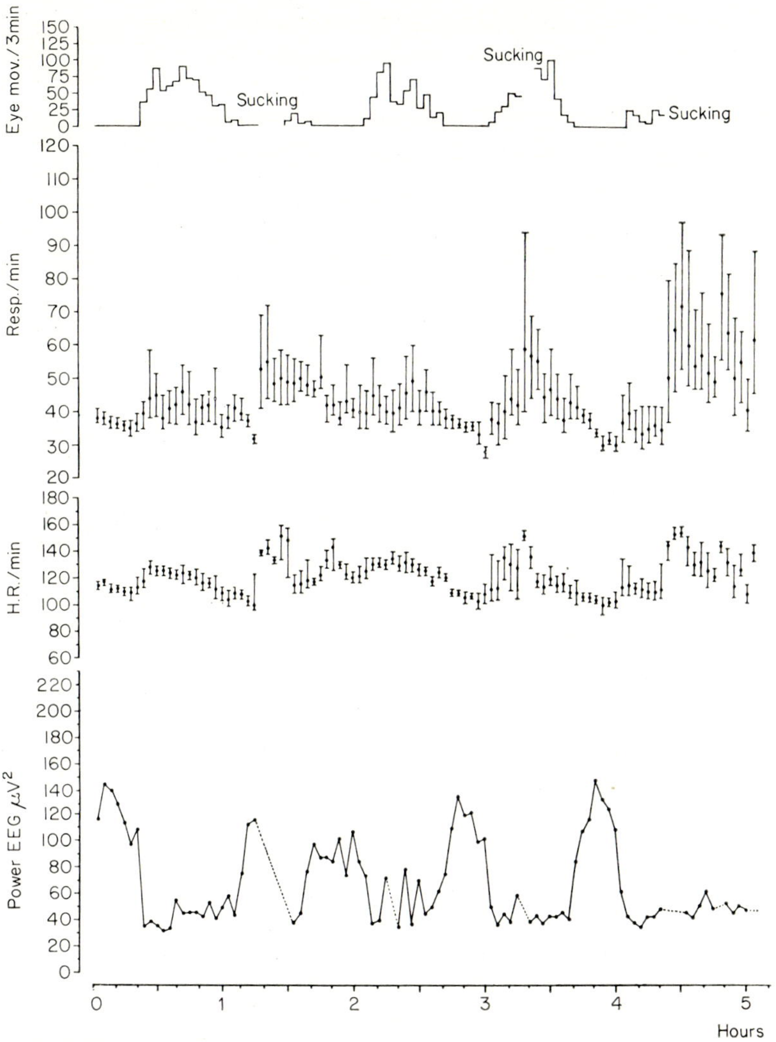

FIG. 5. Record compiled from the data on eye movements, respiration, heart rate, and EEG collected polygraphically in an 8-day-old infant over a 5-hour period. Each point represents the median value for the parameter over a 3-minute epoch; the range is the interquartile range.

relations between the statistics of the various parameters are still impossible to see. Further analyses are therefore required.

Relations between parameters. It is of great interest to see how, for instance, respiration and heart rate are correlated. For this purpose the ratio between the median intervals of respiration and the median intervals of the heart beats is computed. In general the ratio varies between 1 and 4, being high during regular sleep and during or shortly after sucking, and relatively low during irregular sleep. A positive correlation exists between respiratory rate and heart rate, as shown in Fig. 6.

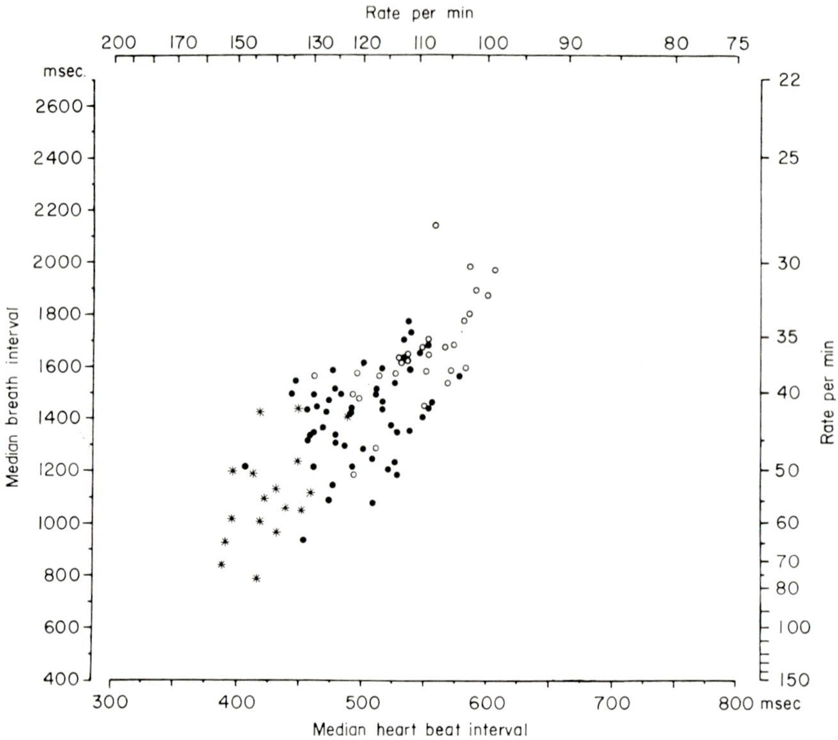

FIG. 6. Plot diagram of the correlation between median breath-to-breath intervals and median heart beat-to-beat interval. Circles = regular sleep; dots = irregular sleep; asterisks = awake.

The values cluster for each particular state. As proved by discriminatory analysis the clusters are significantly separated from each other. The interquartile ranges of respiration and heart beat also show a high correlation which means that the occurrence of irregularity in the one parameter is always accompanied by irregularity in the other parameter.

There is a close relationship between the median values of breath-to-breath intervals and the corresponding interquartile ranges (Fig. 7, upper part). During the regular-sleep state the median is high and the

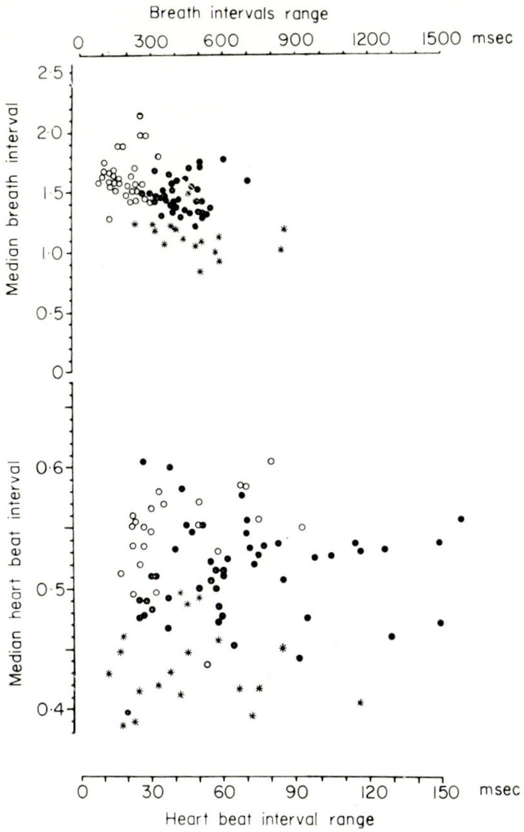

FIG. 7. Upper part: Plot diagram of the correlation between median breath-to-breath intervals and interquartile ranges of breath-to-breath intervals. Lower part: Plot diagram of the correlation between median heart beat-to-beat intervals and interquartile ranges of beat-to-beat intervals. Symbols as in Fig. 6.

interquartile range low; during irregular sleep the median intervals are shorter, but the interquartile range is larger. During the awake states the intervals are even shorter, but the range values are widely scattered. Disregarding the states, the data as a whole show a negative correlation between breath-to-breath intervals and the range of these intervals (Fig. 7, upper part). Discriminatory analysis shows a highly significant separation of the clusters belonging to the different states. Although these phenomena are evident for respiration, the statistics of the heart rate are less clear (Fig. 7, lower part). Another significant relationship exists between the median breath-to-breath intervals and the mean square voltages of the EEG. The correlation is positive and the separation of the clusters for the different states is highly significant. Finally I will mention the negative correlation which exists between the duration of EMG activity and the median beat-to-beat interval of the heart. Again there is a strictly state-specific patterning.

These relationships between the various parameters describe quantitatively the state-specific constellations. Regulating mechanisms within the "black box" are expressed in terms of the statistical properties of these constellations. The few examples given are no more than an outline illustration of this approach. In our current investigations both normative data and data from infants with neurological abnormalities are being collected. Striking differences have already been found in the statistics of polygraphic parameters recorded from neurologically abnormal newborns.

State and Responses to Stimulation

When the environmental conditions are kept as constant as possible, the parameters measured vary from time to time in accordance with the properties of the different states. These states are expressions of the internal regulating mechanisms within the "black box". To continue with this analogy, the analysis of these internal processes can also be achieved by changing the input parameters individually, and measuring the input-output relations.

The large variation of the responses to sensory stimulation is commonly considered to be one of the main difficulties in studies in young infants. However, in the light of the wide fluctuations of states, these variations are not surprising.

By exploring systematically the infant's responsiveness to stimulation through various input channels (that is, sensory modalities) we can obtain clues about the organization of the brain mechanisms which underline the regulation of state. While the state is continuously monitored, stimuli are presented at more or less regular intervals of suitable length.

The data collected so far are summarized in Table I. It will be seen that the extent to which responses depend on state is closely linked to the modality of the input. Proprioceptive stimulation such as an abrupt stretch of a muscle or a short vibration of the body elicits strong or even exaggerated responses in regular sleep. During irregular sleep, however, these responses are weak or even absent, and they are of moderate intensity during the quietly-awake state. Ankle clonus is the only response whose occurrence is restricted to periods of regular sleep. The briskness of reflexes in regular sleep and their tendency towards

TABLE I. EFFECT OF STATE ON THE INTENSITY OF RESPONSES TO SENSORY STIMULATION IN DIFFERENT MODALITIES

	Regular sleep	*Irregular sleep*	*Quiet awake*	*Reference*
Proprioceptive reflexes				
ankle clonus	+++	±	±	Lenard *et al.*, 1968
knee jerk	+++	±	++	Prechtl *et al.*, 1967b
biceps jerk	+++	±	++	Lenard *et al.*, 1968
lip jerk	+++	±	++	Prechtl *et al.*, 1967a
Moro response (hit)	++	±	++	Lenard *et al.*, 1968
Exteroceptive skin reflexes				
Tactile and pressure				
rooting	—	—	++	Lenard *et al.*, 1968
lip protrusion reflex	—	++	+	Prechtl *et al.*, 1967a
plantar grasp	—	+	++	Lenard *et al.*, 1968
Babkin	—	+	++	Lenard *et al.*, 1968
palmar grasp	—	++	++	Lenard *et al.*, 1968
palmo-mental	—	++	++	Lenard *et al.*, 1968
finger reflex	—	+	++	Vlach *et al.*, 1968
toe reflex	—	++	+++	Vlach *et al.*, 1968
tibial reflex	±	++	++	Vlach *et al.*, 1968
fibular reflex	±	++	++	Vlach *et al.*, 1968
axillary reflex	±	++	++	Vlach *et al.*, 1968
Nociceptive				
thigh reflex	++	++	++	Lenard *et al.*, 1968
Babinski reflex	++	+++	+++	Lenard *et al.*, 1968
abdominal reflex	++	+++	+++	Lenard *et al.*, 1968 Vlach *et al.*, 1968
pubic reflex	++	+++	+++	Vlach *et al.*, 1968
inguinal reflex	+++	+++	+++	Vlach *et al.*, 1968
Auditory response				
auditory orienting	±	++	+++	Hutt *et al.*, 1968
Vestibular response				
doll's eye response	±	++	+++	Von Bernuth and Prechtl, 1969

+++ very strong response; — absent response

clonic discharges may be attributed to a high sensitivity of the muscle spindles, due in turn to strong gamma activity during this state. The finding of tonic activity in antigravity muscles of the jaw supports this hypothesis.

The weakness or absence of proprioceptive reflexes during irregular sleep has not yet been explained for human infants. In cats it has been shown that presynaptic inhibition occurs in group Ia muscle afferents during REM sleep, especially when REM bursts occur (Gassel *et al.*, 1964). This relationship is also present in the human infant (Prechtl and Lenard, 1967). Thus, the greater the number of eye movements, the smaller the reflex discharge at that particular time (Fig. 8). However,

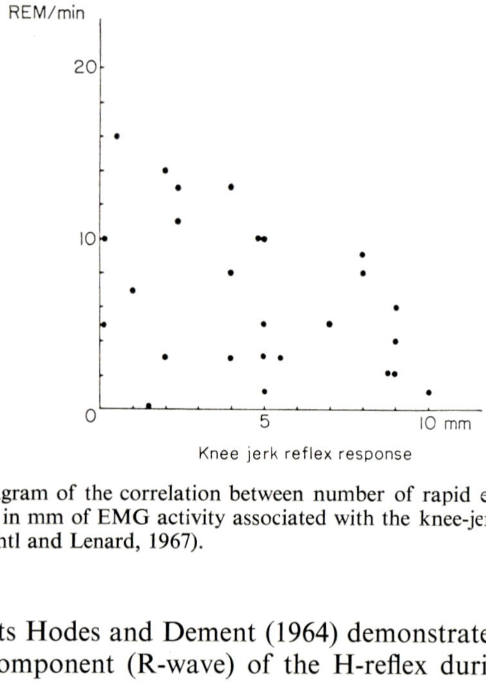

FIG. 8. Plot diagram of the correlation between number of rapid eye movements per minute and height in mm of EMG activity associated with the knee-jerk reflex during the same minute (Prechtl and Lenard, 1967).

in human adults Hodes and Dement (1964) demonstrated a depression of the reflex component (R-wave) of the H-reflex during REM-sleep and they believe that the phenomenon is mainly due to changes in the alpha motoneurones.

In sharp contrast to the responses to proprioceptive input, the exteroceptive skin reflexes elicited by tactile stimuli or pressure are absent during regular sleep, but are clearly present during irregular sleep and wakefulness. The stimuli have a gradual onset and last for several seconds, as do the responses. To find such strong responses during irregular sleep came as a surprise. Experiments with adult cats have shown that polysynaptic skin reflexes are diminished or abolished during REM-sleep (Pompeiano, 1967). It is not yet clear whether this discrepancy in the findings is due to species differences or to the difference in developmental stage, since neither young kittens nor human adults have yet been studied from this point of view.

Skin reflexes of the nociceptive type do not show any state dependency. Stroking the skin of the abdominal wall, of the inguinal area, of the thigh, and of the sole of the foot probably excites pain receptors; though, since the intensities of the stimuli are low, the nature of the stimulus is perhaps often a tickle. The biological significance of protective responses' being independent of state is evident.

In experiments on the auditory-orienting response in newborns, using EMG activity in the limb muscles as an index of response, a very low responsiveness has been demonstrated during regular sleep. Responses during irregular sleep are only slightly weaker than during the awake state. Similar behaviour is seen with the vestibulo-ocular response. The doll's eye response, which consists of compensatory eye movements in response to side-to-side rocking of the baby along its longitudinal axis and which we measured from the electro-oculographic recording, is weak or absent during regular sleep and present during irregular sleep and the awake state. For obvious reasons it is difficult to study visual responses (such as the optokinetic nystagmus) during sleep.

The abolition of non-nociceptive skin reflexes, auditory-orienting, and vestibular responses during regular sleep is still unexplained. Since motor units are readily activated by nociceptive and proprioceptive stimuli during this state, inhibitory processes—which act primarily on the afferent side but do not block the efferent side—may be involved.

CONCLUSION

In the analysis of states in the newborn infant, "black box" theory has been applied as a theoretical framework. The heuristic value of this approach is obvious. Experiments and techniques can be designed which are adapted to the methodological restrictions encountered in work with human subjects. Without penetrating the baby's skin, or disturbing the infant's well-being in any way, it is possible to record a spectrum of outputs over comparatively long periods of time. Often of course, these measurements are not direct assessments of particular functions but rather of derivations of them or even of epiphenomena. The EEG reflects only in a limited way the neuronal activity in the cortex and subcortical structures, and respiratory rate is only one aspect of gaseous metabolism, as is the heart rate of circulation. Despite these shortcomings in the recording techniques, to which there is no alternative at present, it seems possible to investigate underlying regulating brain mechanisms if—but only if—multidimensional data analysis is employed. Modern mathematical techniques, developed in the areas of probability theory, random-noise theory, and control-system theory are invaluable. Stochastic analysis of polygraphic data is a comprehensive approach which could be called "brain engineering". We are still at the very beginning but it seems reasonable to assume that along these lines we shall achieve further progress in research on normal and impaired brain mechanisms and behaviour in the human infant.

REFERENCES

Brown, J. L. 1964. States in newborn infants. *Merrill-Palmer Quart.* **10,** 313–327.

Delange, M. M., Castan, P., Cadilhac, J. and Passouant, P. 1962. Les divers stades du sommeil chez le nouveau-né et le nourrisson. *Revue neurol.* **107,** 271–276.

Dreyfus-brisac, C. 1959. Electroencephalography in infancy. In F. Linneweh (Ed.), *Die physiologische Entwicklung des Kindes.* Springer; Berlin, Göttingen, Heidelberg, Pp. 29–40.

Dreyfus-brisac, C. and Monod, N. 1965. Sleep of premature and full-term neonates —a polygraphic study. *Proc. R. Soc. Med.* **58,** 6–7.

Dreyfus-brisac, C., Samson-Dolfus, D. and Fischgold, H. 1955. L'activité électrique cérébrale du prématuré et du nouveau-né. *Semaine des Hôpitaux, Paris.* **31,** 135–142.

Escalona, S. K. 1962. The study of individual differences and the problem of state. *J. Am. Acad. Child Psychiat.* **1,** 11–37.

Gassel, M. M., Marchiafava, P. L. and Pompeiano, O. 1964. Tonic and phasic inhibition of spinal reflexes during deep desynchronized sleep in unrestrained cats. *Archs ital. Biol.* **102,** 471–499.

Hodes, R. and Dement, W. C. 1964. Depression of electrically induced reflexes ("H-reflexes") in man during low voltage EEG sleep. *Electroenceph. clin. Neurophysiol.* **17,** 617–629.

Hutt, S. J., Hutt, C., Lenard, H. G., Von Bernuth, H. and Muntjewerff, W. J. 1968. Auditory responsivity in the human neonate. *Nature, Lond.* **218,** 888–890.

Lenard, H. G., Von Bernuth, H. and Prechtl, H. F. R. 1968. Reflexes and their relationship to behavioural state in the newborn. *Acta paediat., Stockh.* **57,** 177–185.

Petre-quadens, O. 1965. Étude du sommeil chez le nouveau-né normal. In *Le sommeil de nuit normal et pathologique.* Electroencéphalographie et Neurophysiologie-Clinique, Nouvelle Série, Vol. 2. Masson, Paris. Pp. 149–155.

PETRE-QUADENS, O. 1966. On the different phases of the sleep of the newborn with special reference to the activated phase, or phase d. *J. neurol. Sci.* **3,** 151–161.

POMPEIANO, O. 1967. The neurophysiological mechanisms of the postural and motor events during desynchronized sleep. In S. S. Kety, E. V. Evarts, and H. L. Williams (Eds.), *Sleep and altered states of consciousness.* Williams & Wilkins, Baltimore, Md. Pp. 351–423.

PRECHTL, H. F. R. 1968. Polygraphic studies of the full-term newborn infant. II. Computer analysis of recorded data. In M. C. O. Bax and R. C. MacKeith (Eds.), *Studies in Infancy.* Clinics in Developmental Medicine No. 27. Heinemann, London. Pp. 26–40.

PRECHTL, H. F. R. and BEINTEMA, D. J. 1964. *The neurological examination of the full-term newborn infant.* Clinics in Developmental Medicine No. 12. Heinemann, London.

PRECHTL, H. F. R. and LENARD, H. G. 1967. A study of eye-movements in sleeping newborn infants. *Brain Res.* **5,** 477–493.

PRECHTL, H. F. R., AKIYAMA, Y., ZINKIN, P. and KERR GRANT, D. 1968. Polygraphic studies of the full-term newborn infant. I. Technical aspects and qualitative analysis. In M. C. O. Bax and R. C. MacKeith (Eds.), *Studies in infancy.* Clinics in Developmental Medicine No. 27. Heinemann, London. Pp. 1–25.

PRECHTL, H. F. R., KERR GRANT, D., LENARD, H. G., and HRBEK, A. 1967a. The lip-tap-reflex in the awake and sleeping newborn infant. A polygraphic study. *Expl Brain Res.* **3,** 184–194.

PRECHTL, H. F. R., VLACH, V., LENARD, H. G. and KERR GRANT, D. 1967b. Exteroceptive and tendon reflexes in various behavioural states in the newborn infant. *Biologia Neonat.* **11,** 159–175.

VLACH, V., VON BERNUTH, H. and PRECHTL, H. F. R. 1969. State dependency of extroceptive skin reflexes in newborn infants. *Devl Med. Child. Neurol.* **11,** 353–362.

VON BERNUTH, H. and PRECHTL, H. F. R. 1969. Vestibulo-ocular response and its state dependency in newborn infants. *Neuropädiatrie* **1,** 11–24.

WAGNER, I. F. 1939. Curves of sleep depth in newborn infants. *J. genet. Psychol.* **55,** 121–135.

WOLFF, P. H. 1959. Observations on newborn infants. *Psychosom. Med.* **21,** 110–118.

WOLFF, P. H. 1966. The causes, controls, and organization of behaviour in the neonate. *Psychological Issues.* Vol. 5, No. 1, Monogr. 17. International Univ. Press, New York.

Discussion

BERGSTRÖM: Is there any connection between the different states and such concepts as consciousness or arousal?

PRECHTL: I stopped using the term arousal because I found it to be related to particular modalities of stimulation—there is no such general thing as arousal. In regular sleep the baby does not respond to tactile stimulation: in REM sleep it does. This suggests that REM sleep is the lighter. But, taking the monosynaptic reflexes as a criterion, the response is exaggerated in regular sleep, and absent in REM sleep—so now REM sleep is the deeper sleep. Studies on cats confused those working on infants. Most cat responses disappear in REM sleep, and in slow-wave sleep they have some responses; not so in the baby. There are no satisfactory criteria for defining consciousness.

BERGSTRÖM: Can these states be found only in very young children?

PRECHTL: No, there are two types of sleep which occur at all ages—regular and irregular.

BERGSTRÖM: Can you relate consciousness to these states in older subjects?

PRECHTL: I doubt that REM sleep is always dream sleep. The most immature prematures have the most REM sleep. Do they dream the most, and if so what about?

PETRE-QUADENS: Foulkes has shown that 58 per cent of dreaming occurs outside REM sleep. It must be related to something else apart from dreaming.

PRECHTL: That was why we compared the rapid eye movements in sleep with scanning movements. We first believed that they were associated with visual scanning in dreams, but found that the interval distribution in rapid eye movements is quite different from that in scanning eye movements (H. F. R. Prechtl and H. G. Lenard, 1967. *Brain Res.* **5**, 477–493.)

BRONSON: Presumably the different pattern of eye movements which you found in state 2 (as compared with the quietly-awake state with the eyes open), is due to the infant's responding to the external environment. But there remains a possibility that it has to do with the internal state rather than to opening the eyes and seeing the outside. Have you looked at awake infants either staring at a homogeneous field or in a very dim light to see if the patterns then go back more towards those seen in REM sleep (state 2)?

PRECHTL: No, not yet. The view our newborns have is not homogeneous; they look around. There are no slow eye movements as in state 2—this is a very characteristic difference.

BERGSTRÖM: Have you tried to analyse more exactly the types of those different distributions of respiration and the other parameters? It would perhaps tell us something about the basic process.

PRECHTL: We are now doing that. We also want to introduce measures of the stationarity of the process—we want to see when a particular signal changes or loses its stationarity.

Significance of the EEG

PLOOG: Is there any way to show a power spectrum of an EEG which takes into account not only the amplitude but also the frequency? Or don't you think that is important in this context?

PRECHTL: I was very interested in the frequency changes within and between the various states, but they are in fact minimal. In adults, where all-night sleep records have been made and power-density spectra constructed, there are quite dramatic shifts in the frequency. Surprisingly this is not the case with the newborn. State 1 differs dramatically from the other states only in that there is a sharp peak of frequency around 1 to 1·2 cycles per second, and this is exactly the frequency of the bursts of *tracé alternant*, visible to the naked eye.

BRONSON: I have been assuming that increased amplitude of the EEG meant greater synchrony in the pattern of neural activity, and therefore that it was correlated with the presence of slow rhythmic activity. The recorded amplitude would therefore begin to fall when you began to get what in an adult would be Beta rhythm.

PRECHTL: No. High amplitude-slow wave EEGs are often differentiated from low amplitude-high frequency EEGs. If you amplify this low amplitude EEG in the newborn, it is very hard to differentiate it from the high amplitude EEG. When we look at EEGs we usually ignore the slow waves of relatively low amplitude. This has something to do with our Gestalt perception.

BRONSON: What is the cause of greater voltage if it is not a matter of greater synchrony, in newborns anyhow? It is surely not due to greater action potentials; is it more neurones firing?

SCHULTE: What we record from the scalp are not action potentials of cortical nerve cells, probably they are postsynaptic potentials. The EEG is the sum of all postsynaptic potentials. In addition, the glia may contribute to the EEG, particularly to the slow and ultra slow waves of the neonatal EEG. Most electroencephalographers refuse now to imply stronger synchronization solely on the basis of higher EEG amplitude.

PLOOG: I disagree. I think there is a certain definite relationship between the EEG waves and the firing cortical units underneath, which cannot all be explained by postsynaptic dendritic potentials.

SCHULTE: Nobody would deny such a relationship. But this power might not be due to spike potentials and it does not necessarily imply stronger synchronization. Under certain conditions you might have a lot of postsynaptic potentials in one area of the brain and you are very likely to have many spike potentials too. But it is possible to think of other conditions, where you have no—or only very few—spike potentials, but where there is still much activity going on in the form of slow potentials. Under normal circumstances it is very unlikely that spikes contribute significantly to the EEG.

Transition Between States

DITTRICHOVÁ: It is important to recognize that a behavioural state is not necessarily a stable state. This is true not only of state 2 which is characterized by great variations, but also of state 1, because we can see that even during that state there are changes in various parameters. For example, the frequency of respiration decreased from the beginning to the end in a period of state 1; and there are also changes in the EEG from the beginning to the end of such a period. So state 1 is a stable state when you compare it with state 2, but nevertheless there are changes during it.

PRECHTL: I agree. There are microfluctuations within a stable state, and then, of course, it is just a matter of degree of resolution whether you call it stable or not. However, the changes within one of the defined states are much smaller than the changes between states.

WOLFF: Similarly, during sucking on a pacifier throughout a period of about 20 minutes of regular sleep, gauged by regular respiration, there is a gradual diminution in the amplitude—not in the frequency, which remains constant—until you reach a point where you get no sucking whatsoever, perhaps 15 minutes after the start of regular sleep. After 20 minutes the reverse of this happens. Just before the deep sigh which marks the change from regular to irregular respiration, the amplitude of sucking is again as high as initially. This is not a matter of habituation, because if you wait until somewhere in the middle of the period of regular sleep to insert the pacifier, then the amplitude of sucking is immediately rather low and sucking stops fairly soon. This is a property of what we call regular sleep or state 1—it has different levels.

PRECHTL: With the knee jerk response we didn't see much difference in intensity during state 1. However, eye movements in response to rocking show differences during state 1. So we have to refine our state concept.

WOLFF: I think refine is the wrong word because you can then refine to an infinite regress. We have to agree on the most suitable arbitrary definitions of state and then keep to them.

AMBROSE: Does the nature of the respiratory change during transition between states depend on which states are involved?

PRECHTL: In Fig. 5 you have the impression that in the transition from regular to irregular sleep, the change in respiration is very abrupt, in rate and especially in scatter. The transition from irregular into regular sleep is very often a much more smooth and gradual change, as if the organism had difficulty in building up all these regular activities. It takes more time to develop this more stable, homeostatic state of regular sleep than to break it up. The same is true of the heart rate and of the EEG. In fact the changes in EEG correspond remarkably with those in respiration.

Asynchrony of Cerebral Measures in Normal Babies

PRECHTL: Figure 9 shows a 5-hour record on an abnormal baby. He was hyperexcitable in the neurological examination. The record was made when he was 8 days old, the same age as the normal baby (Fig. 5). For the first 9 minutes there was fairly acceptable regular sleep —no eye movements, slow stable respiratory rate, slow stable heart rate and a high average-power of the EEG. But after that the record shows dissociation: there are periods of very high and stable heart rate and epochs of slow and stable heart rate but with a very high and very irregular respiration and relatively high EEG amplitude. If we compute the correlation between the EEG power and the median respiration interval, the correlation coefficient is close to zero. In the normal baby this correlation is highly positive.

BRONSON: When would an infant like this begin to fall into the regular pattern of the normal infant?

PRECHTL: Our follow-up studies show that they are likely to be abnormal after 4 years. A hyperexcitable infant like this would be likely to show mild dyskinesia in the form of choreiform movements at 4 years.

KAUFMAN: Is there anything you can do to synchronize this baby's activities?

PRECHTL: Yes. Just in the last few weeks we found more or less accidentally that if you rock these babies across the transverse axis, you move the diaphragm up and down and that puts them into regular respiration. Of course you have to be careful to choose the speed of the rocking at around 30 to 40 per minute. This appears to suppress to a certain extent irregular sleep and even the eye movements by mechanically imposing relatively regular respiration. If you then stop rocking, an explosion of rapid eye movements and irregular respiration may occur.

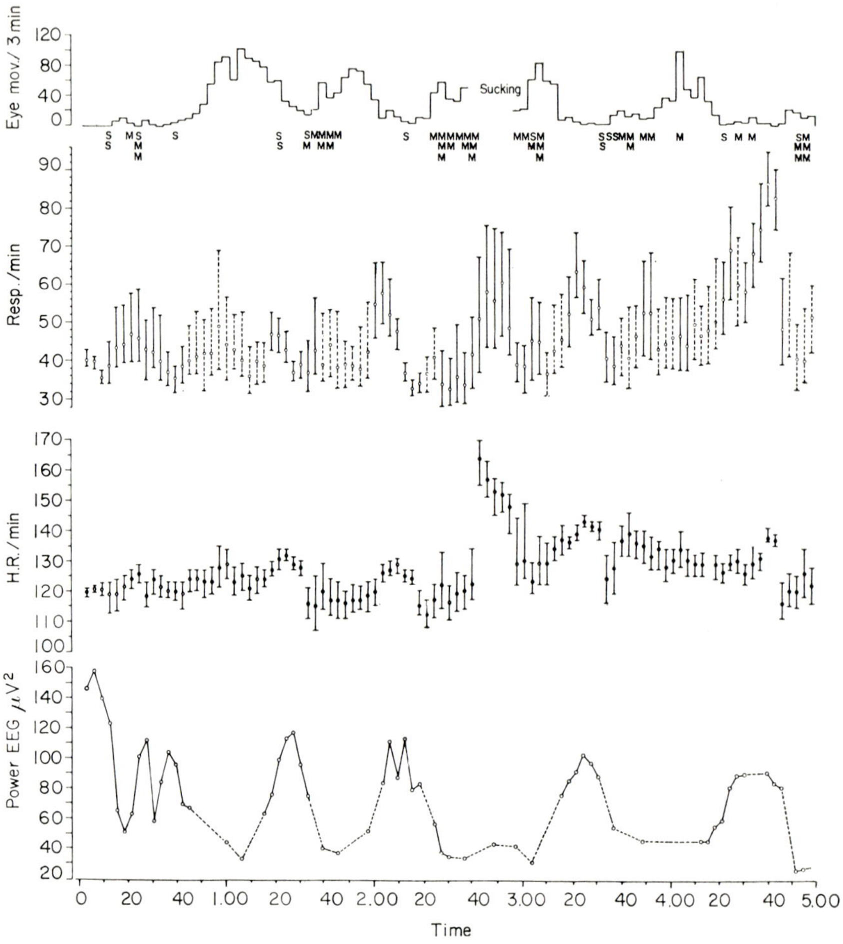

FIG. 9. Compiled polygram of an 8-day-old infant with hyperexcitability syndrome. Very short epochs of regular sleep, and dissociation of the pattern of intercorrelation, are seen. Dotted lines in the quartile ranges of respiration indicate periodic respiration.

AMBROSE: Certainly the vertical rhythmic rocking tends to facilitate regular respiration for as long as it is applied. We found that this is especially so at a rocking rate of 60 per minute, but I doubt if the rocking directly—mechanically—steadies respiration.

Habituation and State

LIPSITT: Prechtl implied that the habituation process is possibly, at least in some cases, a change in state rather than a change in cognitive capacity. Would the response recovery to a novel stimulus following habituation to a repetitive stimulus alter the argument? Let us say you habituated to an 85-dB tone, 200 cycles per second, and you then presented a novel stimulus of the same intensity but of a different frequency, with recovery of response resulting.

PRECHTL: Recently the Hutts (Hutt *et al.*, 1968. *Nature* **220,** 618) have demonstrated in human newborns that the intensity of the auditory orienting response (EMG activity in the limb muscles, heart-rate changes) depends on the state of the infant. While the responses to sound stimulation were consistent in the quietly awake state, somewhat fewer responses were seen during REM sleep, and hardly any response occurred in regular sleep. After repeated presentation of the stimuli (2 seconds' duration every 30 seconds) there was no systematic or progressive response decrement (habituation) during one stable state. A decrement of the responses was observed to be associated with changes from the quietly awake state to REM sleep or REM sleep to regular sleep. On the other hand, a recovery of the response occurred at state transitions in the other direction.

LIPSITT: Several studies of human newborns have claimed to show habituation. They have demonstrated response diminution, whatever the explanation or mechanism involved. Then in some studies novel stimuli have been introduced following the habituation trials, with recovery of response. Assuming these studies are replicable does that recovery to a novel stimulus destroy your argument concerning the contamination of the habituation or decrement by some state change?

PRECHTL: You have to show first that the response pattern would be the same to the stimulus type A and the stimulus type B.

LIPSITT: Many of these studies have involved counter-balance design whereby A is the habituating stimulus for some subjects and B is the habituating stimulus for some other subjects, with the alternative stimulus being the recovery stimulus. Those doing habituation work obviously assume that they are affecting the organism, that is, that the response diminution is coming from somewhere. Presumably all effects of stimuli are mediated by the nervous system or else we must believe in ghosts. Is the argument as to whether there are changes in state concomitant with response diminution effects pertinent to the question of whether there is or is not habituation in the newborn?

PRECHTL: What you are asking is: if you give repetitive stimulation and the response declines, does it matter whether there is a central inhibitory mechanism which reduces the response or whether the baby changes the state due to the stimulation? The whole point is that you need baseline data first, because there are state changes without stimulation. In our case the state cycles during stimulation were not different from those without stimulation.

PAPOUŠEK: That is an exquisite analysis of this problem but only from one side; you stress the effect of the state upon the response to stimulus too much. You should pay more attention to the effect of stimulation upon state—because what you say, that habituation can be an effect of change in the state, could also be put in another way, that repeated stimulation changes the state simultaneously with the decrease of the response.

PRECHTL: We did not find any evidence that repetitive stimulation using rocking, sound, knee jerk, or lip tap had any effect on the cycling of state. We did it on the very same baby; we did recordings for hours first without stimulation and then with stimulation to be able to compare the two situations.

PAPOUŠEK: This can be a question of what behavioural patterns you choose, and what methods of study. But the problem is a very old one. We have been studying behavioural states since 1954, and some of our results correspond with work done by Krasnogoski at the beginning of the century. He was always stressing that there is a bilateral relation between the effects of stimulation and state. I anticipate that you will come to small oscillations of the states which are superimposed on your main cycles. I disagree with your statement that there are cycles which are independent of stimulation. At any moment, the infant is stimulated by hundreds of stimuli but you don't record them. "No experimental stimulation" does not mean no stimulation at all. Very frequently, our experimental stimulation is just a superimposing of one kind of stimulation on a basic constellation of stimuli which influence the child's behaviour.

PRECHTL: I agree, but I did not say there was no stimulation—I said the conditions were constant.

WOLFF: One has to distinguish between changes in state which have nothing to do with what you do to the baby and the fact that by repetitive stimulation you can quite clearly alter the state of the baby. Did Lipsitt use 30-second intervals between each stimulation?

LIPSITT: Yes.

WOLFF: Certainly with rapid, flashing lights you can very easily convert state 2 to state 1 sleep; change the frequency of stimulation and the baby reverts to state 2. It is not so much the flashing light as the monotony of the stimulation which does the trick, and any number of things, such as rapid repeated sounds, can do exactly the same.

Motor Development and Holotelencephaly[1]

PETER H. WOLFF[2]
Harvard Medical School

INTRODUCTION

THIS PAPER DESCRIBES the clinical course and motor development of an infant with a major congenital brain malformation. The clinical diagnosis of *arrhinencephaly*, made at birth, was confirmed at autopsy 4½ months later, when a *holotelencephaly* or failure in hemispheration of the frontal lobes was specifically identified (Yakovlev, 1959).

Previous clinical and neuroanatomical reports on such infants have agreed about the gross morphological and pathophysiological features: these infants are microcephalic, have marked orbital hypotelorism, flattened nasal bridges, and bilateral hare-lips. Their EEGs are invariably abnormal; they frequently have uncontrollable seizures, a marked instability of body temperature, and great difficulty in swallowing.

Within the general category of children with holotelencephaly two groups can be distinguished. One includes those with various extracephalic malformations of the skeletal, cardiovascular, and renal systems, as well as the characteristic brain malformation; these children

[1] During this study the author was supported by a Career Development Grant of the U.S.P.H.S.—N.I.M.H., KMH 3461, and a Research Grant of the U.S.P.H.S.—N.I.M.H., 06034.

[2] From the Children's Hospital Medical Center and Department of Psychiatry, Harvard Medical School, Boston, Massachusetts. The generous help of colleagues at the Children's Hospital Medical Center made this study possible. In particular I would like to thank Dr. John F. Crigler who directs the Clinical Research Center where this infant was studied (Clinical Research Center Grant S-R 00128); Dr. Cesare Lombrose, whose department carried out the electroencephalographic studies; and Dr. Floyd Gillis, who made the gross anatomical studies of the brain. I am much indebted to Dr. Paul Yakovlev, Director of the Warren Museum of Anatomy, who made the serial sections of the brain and provided invaluable guidance in the interpretation of the neuropathological findings.

have a specific chromosome abnormality (trisomy 13–15). Children in the other group show very few, if any, extracephalic malformations and their chromosome complement is normal, although the brain malformations are as severe as, or more severe than, those in the first group (Yakovlev, 1959; Bishop *et al.*, 1964; DeMyer *et al.*, 1964; Hintz *et al.*, 1968).

No systematic observations correlating the anatomical findings of such "experiments in nature" with relevant behavioural data have so far been carried out. The focus of this report will therefore be on observations of motor activity and the development of reflexes, which were made in conjunction with laboratory studies and a detailed examination of the brain after the infant's death.

CASE REPORT

Family History

The mother was a 27-year-old severely malnourished Cuban woman who had taken no special medications during her pregnancy. Two of her five previous pregnancies issued in normal children: a boy who is now 9 years old, and a girl of 5. Two other pregnancies resulted in microcephalic still-births with bulging eyes and "flat heads". One pregnancy ended as a spontaneous abortion in the first trimester. Neither parent recalls hearing about similarly abnormal infants on either side of the family.

Physical Examination

The patient was a female infant born at term weighing 6 lb 8 oz. Labour and delivery were uneventful, but the infant's Agpar score was only 2 at 1, 3, and 5 minutes after birth. Physical examination revealed an infant of normal size, well-formed below the neck. The microcephalic-scaphocephalic cranium measured 31 cm in the occipito-frontal circumference, the eyes were very protuberant, and there was a marked orbital hypotelorism. The skull did not transilluminate. The nasal septum was absent, and the common nares communicated anteriorly with the mouth as one chamber. The upper lip and gingivae were centrally cleft to the inferior border of the nasal cavity, but the rest of the palate was intact, and the uvula was a single midline structure. The eyebrows were prominent, and the eyelashes were very long. The low-set ears were elfin shaped; no antihelix was noted.

Although a grade 1 systolic murmur was occasionally heard, the electrocardiogram was normal. There was no webbing of the neck or

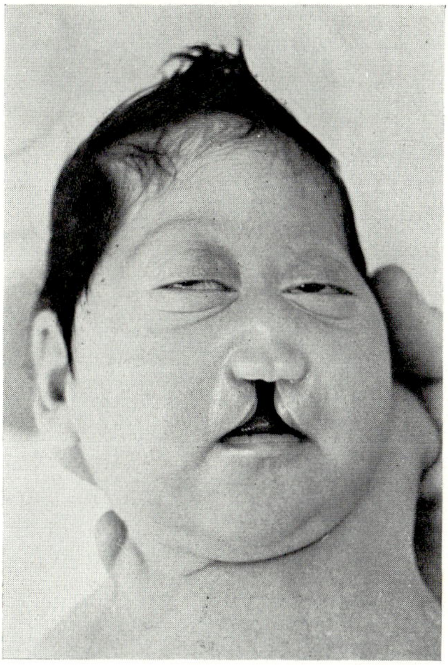

FIG. 1. Frontal view of patient at 3 weeks.

polydactyly, and no other extracephalic abnormalities were noted. Neurological examination revealed a lethargic infant who responded readily to loud noises but moved her extremities slowly. In sleep her extremities were flaccid but they became rigid and resisted passive movement whenever she was awake. The face was symmetrical.

During the first week after birth it was difficult to elicit the deep tendon reflexes. The grasp and rooting reflexes were absent, the Galant and Moro reflexes were weak, and the Babinski reflex was positive. It was impossible to elicit any eye movements in response to a moving light because the infant was usually asleep or having a mild clinical seizure. Routine laboratory examinations in the first week were within normal limits.

Special Investigations

Five days after birth the child was transferred to the Children's Hospital Medical Center for detailed behavioural and other studies. The results of these studies will be summarized overleaf in logical, rather than chronological, sequence so that they can be surveyed more easily. Wherever necessary, the relevant chronological ages are given.

Laboratory findings. The haematogram was normal until the end of the third month, when a hypochromic anaemia appeared. Fasting blood sugar levels, serum calcium, phosphorus, and potassium values were normal for this age. There was a persistent hypernatraemia (sodium: 165 m Eq./l., 164 m Eq./l.; chloride: 121 m Eq./l.) but the infant was never oedematous. Glucose tolerance tests on two occasions, and repeated assays of PBI and BEI were normal, but the capacity to concentrate the urine was abnormal. (Maximum urine concentration: 232 milliosmoles/l.)

One month after delivery the eyes followed a moving light for a few seconds at a time and the optokinetic reflex could be elicited on both sides. Iced water to the middle ear provoked a normal caloric response bilaterally.

X-ray examination. Roentgenograms of the skull showed that the vault was small but that the cranial sutures were normally patent. There was marked orbital hypotelorism and a midline cleft of the maxilla, but the very small nasal bones were visible on X-ray. Pneumo-encephalographic studies revealed a moderate ventricular dilatation with grossly enlarged cisterns. The fourth ventricle was enlarged but of normal shape, the third ventricle was difficult to delineate, and the lateral ventricles were joined as a single chamber anteriorly. The cortex above the ventricles was of reasonable thickness although asymmetrical on the two sides. The greatly enlarged cisterna magna suggested that the cerebellum might be deformed or absent (Fig. 2).

EEG studies. Routine EEGs at 12 days after birth revealed continuous periodic spike-and-wave discharges at a frequency of 1—2 cycles/second, which were synchronous over both hemispheres. High voltage 6—7 cycles/second rhythms were seen between seizures and were better represented over the left, than the right, hemisphere (Fig. 3). Two weeks later continuous seizure activity was again noted. In addition, several electrical and clinical seizures with a right-sided predominance of clonic movements were recorded. Electrical activity at those times was characterized by polyspikes followed by general flattening changing to high voltage delta slowing, gradually replaced by spikes until the cycle repeated itself. A month later, the EEG showed almost continuous ictal status similar to that already described, although the rhythmical spikes and waves were now replaced by general polyspikes followed by slow waves. Intravenous Diazepam (Valium) had no effect on the EEG pattern or on the clinical seizures, even when given in doses large enough to depress respiration.

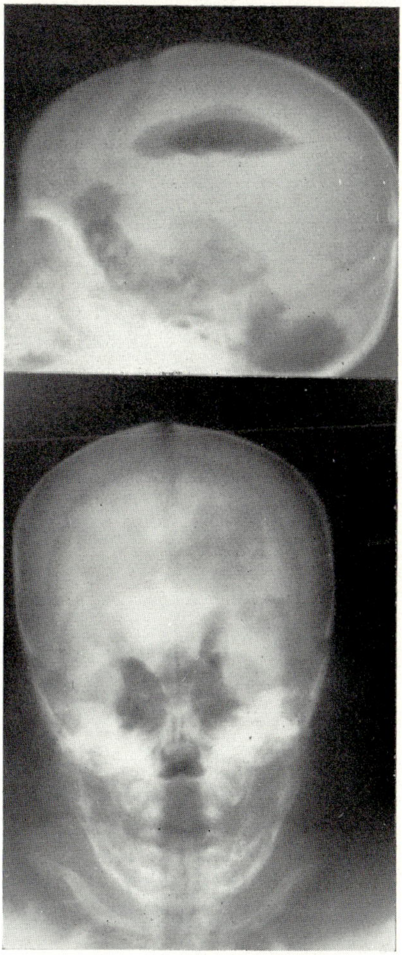

a

b

FIG. 2. Pneumoencephalogram. (a) Lateral view: Note thickness of cortex; greatly enlarged cisterns; presence of nasal bones. (b) A-P view: Note orbital hypotelorism; absent nasal septum; common space of the lateral ventricles.

Because the incidence of clinical seizures was directly related to body temperature, serial EEGs were taken as the infant's temperature was experimentally lowered from 102° to 94° F, and then allowed to rise again. At 94° electrical activity was only slightly altered. The least amount of electrical discharge occurred while the infant was warming up from 94° to 98° F. Once the body temperature had risen to 98° the seizure pattern was exactly the same as before.

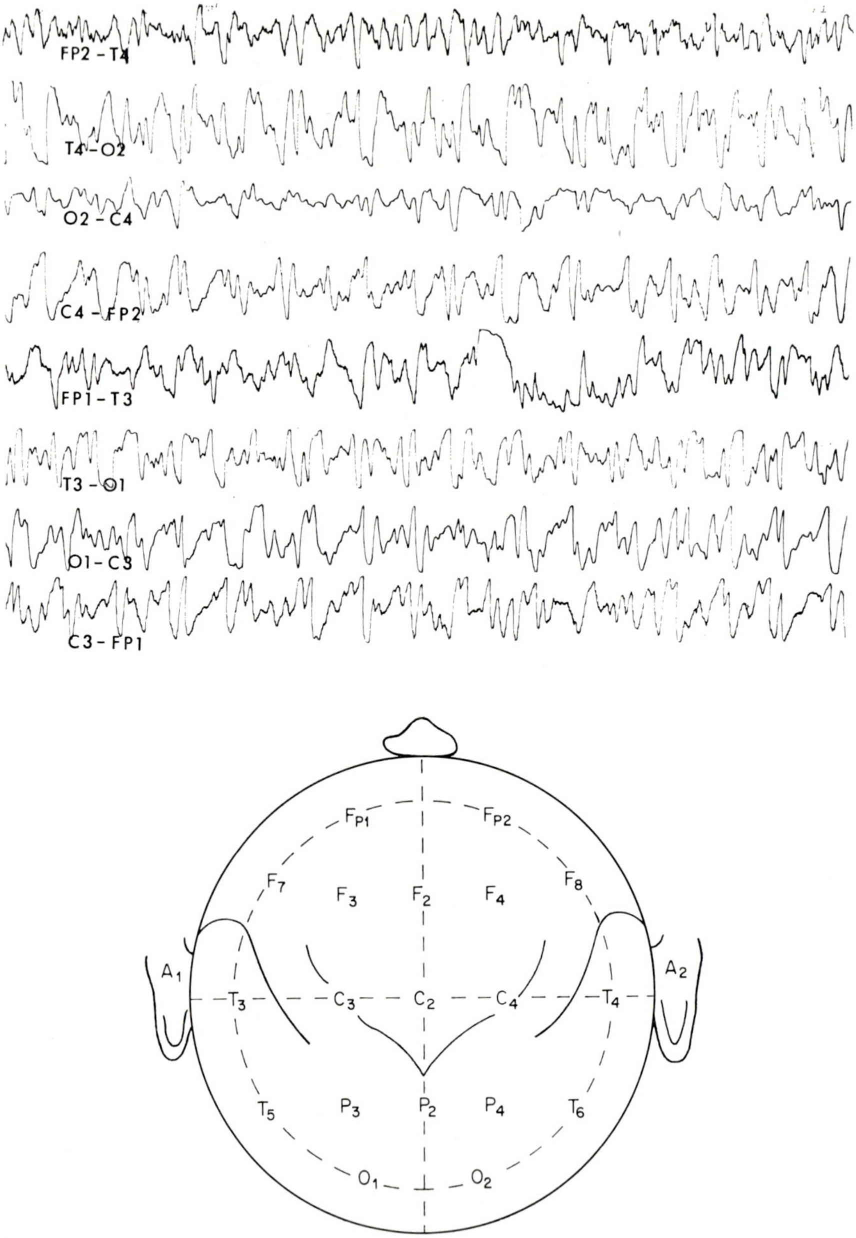

FIG. 3. Electroencephalographic sleep tracing at 2 weeks of age.

Definite evoked potentials to light were seen on the left side, but the response on the right could not be distinguished from background activity. There were no evoked potentials to sound.

Chromosome studies. Chromosome studies of the patient's peripheral blood on two occasions revealed a normal female complement; the chromosome patterns of the parents were also normal.

Observations of Behaviour

Because of the wide range of temperature fluctuations without signs of infection, it was considered useful to explore the relation of body temperature to (1) the incidence of seizures; (2) diurnal rhythms; and (3) the basic rates of rhythmical motor reflexes (in this case non-nutritive sucking; Wolff, 1968).

1. Direct observations on the one hand, and the nursing notes on the other, indicated a close correlation between high body temperature and frequent clinical seizures; and between low body temperature and few seizures (Table I). During a phase when the infant had an elevated temperature and frequent seizures, the temperature was experimentally

TABLE I. RELATION OF BODY TEMPERATURE TO SEIZURES

Age in days	*Low temperature*		*High temperature*	
	°F	*Comments*	*°F*	*Comments*
13	94·6	sleeps more		
16			101–104	convulsions every 5 min. lasting 1 min.
27	98·6	as usual		
32			102	more seizures after meals
44	95·3	sleeping no seizures		
46	94·6	no seizures except on stimulation		
50	95·6	sleeping no seizures		
55	94·8	quiet, awake		
71			100·2	continuous seizures
			99·8	continuous seizures
94	94·7	no seizures		
99			104·4	constant seizures
114			103·6	constant seizures

depressed to 92—93° F for a 12-hour period, after the mean rate of seizures at the higher temperature had been tabulated. Cooling reduced the rate of convulsions from one every 3—5 minutes at 98—99° F, to two per hour at 93°.

The incidence of seizures was also affected by the infant's arousal state. When she was awakened during a period which, by clinical criteria, could be identified as restful, seizure-free sleep she often began to have massive seizures which might last until she fell asleep again. On being reawakened, she repeated the whole cycle. The incidence of seizures was therefore directly related to body temperature and arousal state.

2. No obvious diurnal fluctuations in temperature were demonstrated either by continuous rectal temperature recording or by temperature readings taken every 2 hours. Fever spikes and episodes of hypothermia were randomly distributed over a 24-hour day. Furthermore, since there was no systematic relationship between the infant's sleep-waking cycle as inferred from detailed 24-hour recordings of crying and waking on the one hand, and the diurnal cycle or hospital feeding schedule on the other, it was impossible to determine whether these "macro-rhythms" were temperature-sensitive.

3. Although the infant had difficulty in swallowing formula, even from a Breck feeder, her nutritive and non-nutritive sucking patterns were remarkably similar to those of normal infants when tested on a *blind* nipple. While her body temperature was in the median range (98—99° F) the mean rate of sucks per second increased over the 4-month period in about the same way as that of normal infants (Wolff, 1968).

Despite great difficulties in nutritive "sucking" on the Breck feeder the infant gained half a kilo in the first 2 months (from 2·9 to 3·4 kilos). However, by 4½ months she still weighed less than 4 kilos and was by then below the third percentile for weight and height.

All efforts to control the seizures by medication failed. Phenobarbitone in doses up to 2 mg three times a day reduced their number somewhat but produced a respiratory depression which at times reached alarming proportions. Phenytoin given in 2-mg doses four times a day had an initially beneficial effect, but after 3 days the incidence and severity of clinical seizures returned to the pre-medication level. Only cooling the infant to 92—93° F controlled the seizures to a significant degree, and on a long-term basis this was not a feasible therapeutic measure.

At 1 month of age, the patient began to swallow a great deal of air without being able to expel it. Consequently her abdomen was often so distended as to create respiratory distress and apnoea. Her abdomen could, however, be deflated by gastric and rectal tubes, and she was intubated at least once a week to avoid further respiratory distress.

Despite virtually continuous electrical seizure patterns on the EEG and innumerable clinical seizures (during an average day, one every 3—5 minutes), and despite the absence of cortico-spinal tracts (see below), the child showed some improvement in overall motor performance. Until the end of the first month she was either asleep or having seizures that were followed by post-ictal periods of somnolence. No sustained periods of waking that might be considered analogous to the alert-inactive state of the normal infant were recorded at that time (Wolff, 1966). By the end of the second week the diffuse twitches of the face and limbs were organized as full myoclonic seizures starting in the face, spreading to all four limbs, and ending as a hyper-extension of the head and neck.

By the end of the first month, the Moro reflex was well developed and symmetrical. The traction reflex became stronger and for the first time she rooted well when awake or drowsy. The limbs had developed greater muscle strength; the deep tendon reflexes were now brisk, with some variable asymmetry between the left and right sides. Initially, vocalizations had been limited to weak whimpers. Now they sounded like the usual cries of fullterm infants and could no longer be distinguished from the latter by spectrographic analysis. The hunger cry was clearly differentiated from the pain cry that was given in response to a pin prick (Wolff, 1969). During occasional periods of "alert-inactivity" lasting 3—4 minutes, she fixated and pursued a moving light (Tables II and III). These changes probably reflected a stabilization or late emergence of congenital reflexes usually present in the normal fullterm infant.

Other changes in motor performance observed in the infant might be classified as developmental advances, since they are not observed in the fullterm infant and normally do not appear until the end of the first month. By 6 weeks the patient showed some differentiation in the patterns of emotional expression. She began to cry, waved her arms before her face as if to bring them to her mouth, and gave the impression of general agitation whenever the Breck feeder was taken from her mouth in the early part of the feeding. This affective response to the interruption of feeding stopped whenever the feeder was reinserted.

Two months after birth the infant began to kick her legs and wave her arms in a rhythmical fashion during periods when she was awake and not convulsing. Although this activity was not goal-directed in the

TABLE II. REFLEXES THAT DID NOT CHANGE WITH TIME

Reflex	*State*			
	4	*3*	*2*	*1*
Glabella	+	+	+	+
Pupillary reaction to light	+	+		
Acoustic blink		+	+	?
Corneal	+	+		
Plantar grasp	+	+	?	○
Babinski	+	+	+	+
Galant	+	+	+	+

State refers to the infant's condition at the time of testing:

1 Quiet restful sleep (regular sleep)
2 Restless sleep—eyes closed (irregular sleep)
3 Drowsiness
4 Awake inactive ("alert")

TABLE III. DEVELOPMENTAL CHANGES OF REFLEXES

Reflex	*Age in days*					
	16	26	33	66	85	112
Abdominal	○	+	+	+	○	○
Biceps tendon	+	R > L	+	L > R	+	L > R
Patellar tendon	○	+	+	L > R	+	L > R
Palmar grasp	○	+	L > R	+	+	+
Rooting	○	○	+	+	+	+
Head holding	○	○		+	+	+
Elbow support	○	○	?	+	+	+
Stepping	○	○	○	?	○	○
Moro	?	○	+	+	+	
Gamper's	○		○	?	○	?

usual sense, it represented a major change from the unpatterned movements of the first month. At 3 months while in the prone position she held her head up for 2—3 minutes at a time and could lift her upper trunk from the bed by supporting herself on her elbows. She also had athetoid movements for the first time, which were similar in form to those of normal neonates. She made vigorous efforts to turn from prone to supine, and her reflex crawling became efficient enough for her to move the length of the crib in 3—4 minutes. Periods of "alert-inactivity" were now longer than they had been at the beginning. She was hypersensitive to touch and pressure, and acted as if she were trying to avoid all skin contact.

A week later she suffered a series of prolonged, violent seizures for several days which brought her apparent motor progress to a halt. Soon thereafter she died after aspirating her vomitus during a seizure.

Post-mortem Findings

General. At autopsy the infant was below the third percentile for weight and for all growth parameters. The left lobe of the thyroid gland was relatively hypertrophied and there was a slight asymmetry of the adrenal glands but there were no other organ defects below the neck.

The appearance of the head and skull have been described in detail above. The brain weighed 190 grams. There was no hemispheration of the frontal lobes. From the tip of the frontal lobe a longitudinal fissure diverged posteriorly, which was the only gyration found in the frontal or parietal lobe. The temporal lobes were quite well formed with early Sylvian fissure formation (Fig. 4). Except for their blunted appearance the occipital lobes were well developed but without gyral formation.

The olfactory nerves, bulbs, and tracts were totally absent; the optic nerves were firm and completely juxtaposed; no optic chiasm could be seen. In the region of the hypothalamus there was a firm white fibrous mass measuring 2·5 cm in diameter, and behind it were two tiny bumps suggesting mamillary bodies. The cerebral peduncles were almost invisible (Fig. 5). The medulla appeared as two parallel bars (presumably the inferior olives) but there were no pyramids. The cerebellum was well formed with remarkably normal folial and fissure formation. As the cerebrum was small the cerebellar/cerebral ratio was 1/2·5.

Gross examination of the brain thus revealed a holotelencephaly, lack of hemispheration in the frontal lobes, anolfactoria, immature gyration of the other lobes, agenesis of the pyramidal system, and a firm fibrous mass in the region of the hypothalamus.

Neuropathological. The brain was sectioned in the frontal plane. Since I am not competent to give a detailed neuropathological description I have relied on Dr. Yakovlev's preliminary analysis of the slides, but I accept full responsibility for any errors there may be in the interpretation.

The topography of the brain was compatible with the X-ray findings and external gross appearance. The frontal lobes were fused as a single

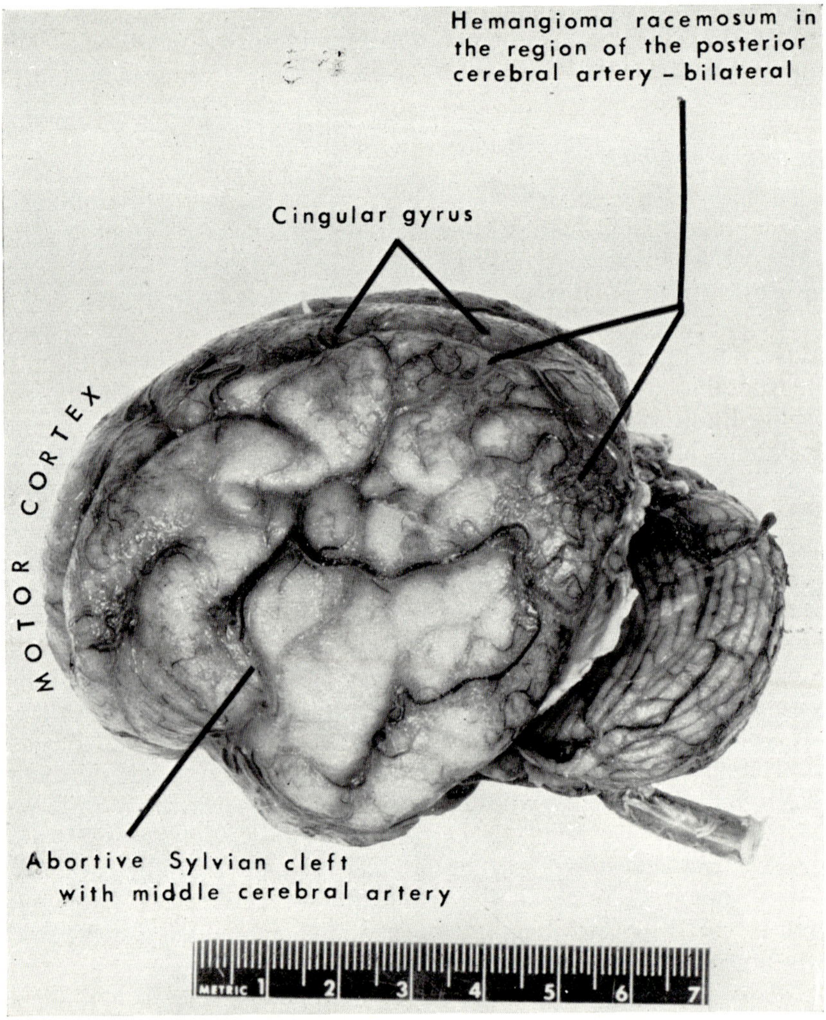

FIG. 4. Lateral view of brain before fixation. Failure of opercularization of the island of Reil.

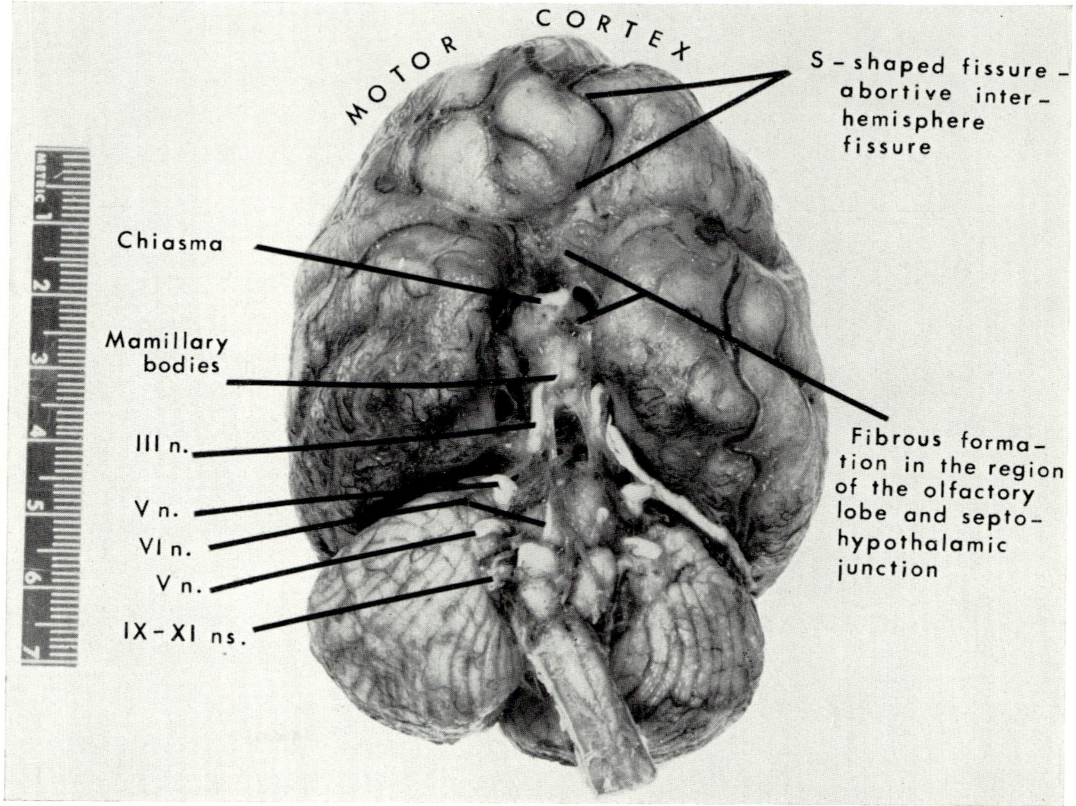

FIG. 5. Ventral view of brain before fixation. Holospheric hemispheres; failure of cleavage of the frontal lobes; failure of cleavage and evagination of the olfactory buds.

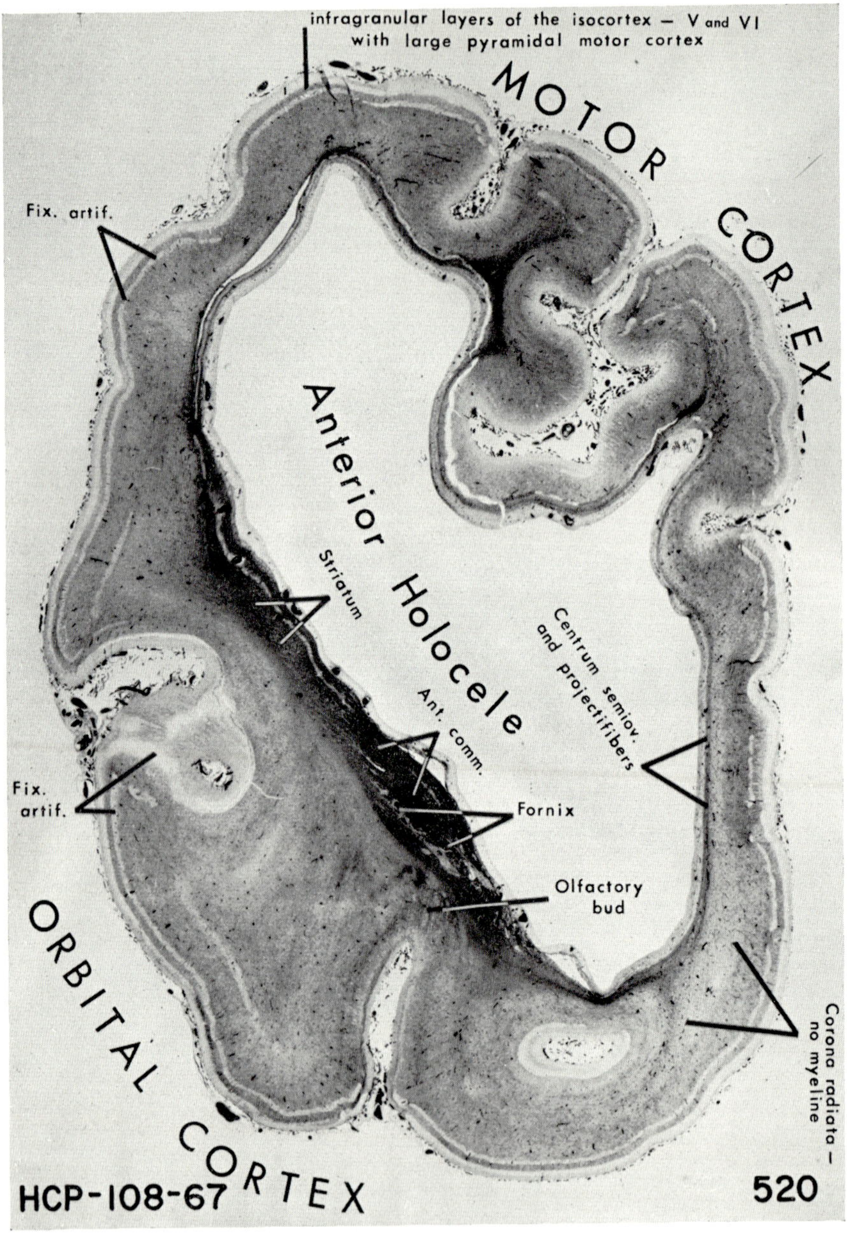

FIG. 6. Frontal section through frontal cortex and anterior holocele. Fix. Artif.—Fixation artifact, seen in all the brain sections.

structure which surrounded a single lateral ventricle. The corpus callosum and other dorsal midline structures were absent (Fig. 6).

The cortical plate was poorly differentiated. The superficial layers were indistinguishable and acellular, but the deeper layers were clearly delineated. In the frontal region the deeper layers still contained a number of large pyramidal cells (Fig. 7 and 8). The corpus striatum

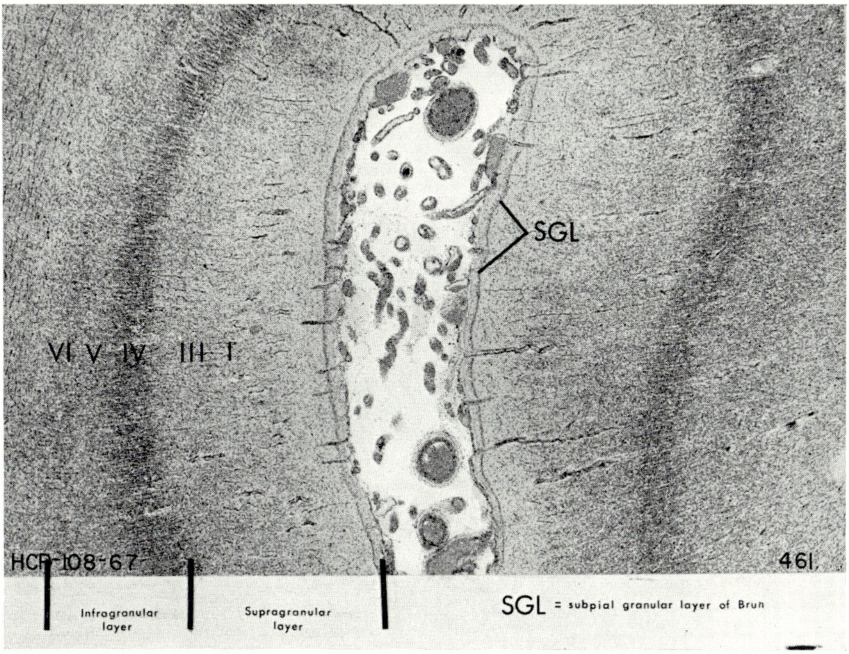

FIG. 7. Photomicrograph of frontal cortex, through portions of two gyri. Note diffuse arrangement of cell layers and unresolved subpial granular layer of Brun.

was represented by an undifferentiated midline structure separated into dorsal and ventral portions by a primitive internal capsule which probably carried only thalamic projections. Caudally the corpus striatum fused with the thalamus, which was also undifferentiated (Fig. 9). The lateral geniculate bodies were well formed but had not shifted from their dorsal position. The cerebral peduncles were entirely absent.

At the level of the red nucleus the brain topography was normal except that the pyramidal tracts were totally absent. The red nuclei

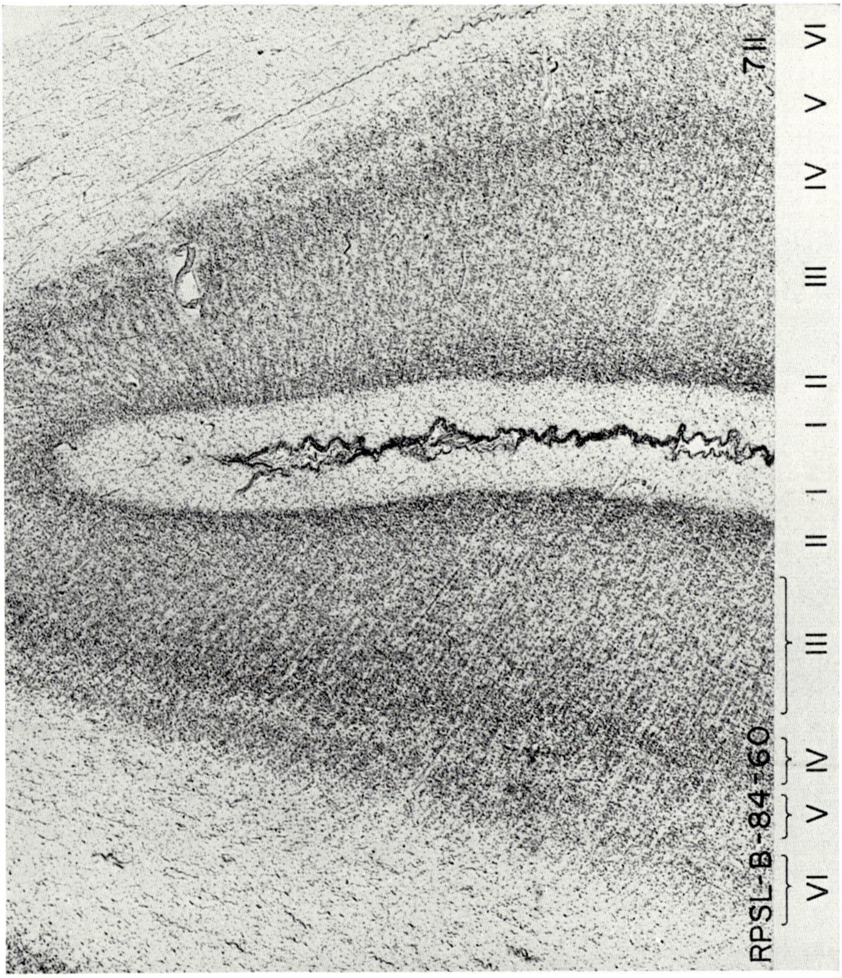

FIG. 8. Normal control. Photomicrograph of frontal cortex through portions of two gyri from a 44-week-old post-mature neonate. Note orderly arrangement of cell layers and total resolution of subpial granular layer of Brun.

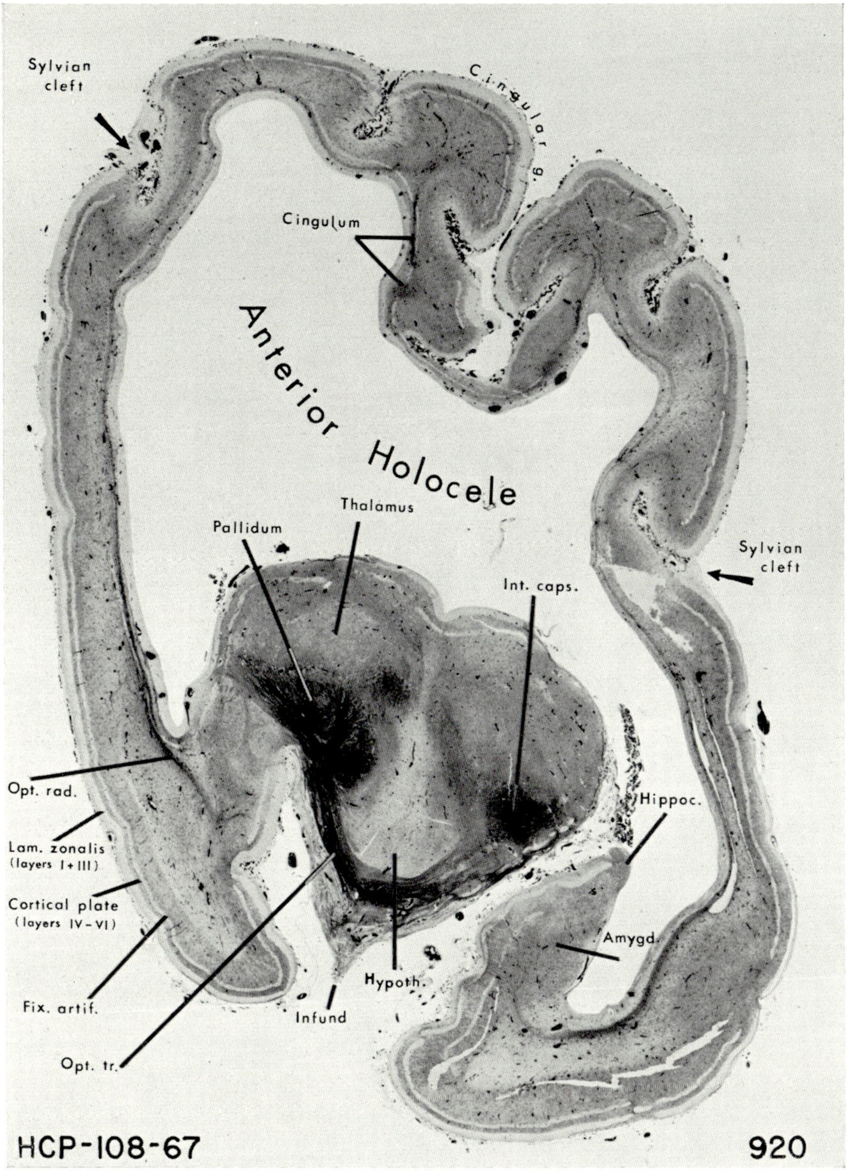

FIG. 9. Frontal section through brain at the level of the thalamus and hypothalamus.

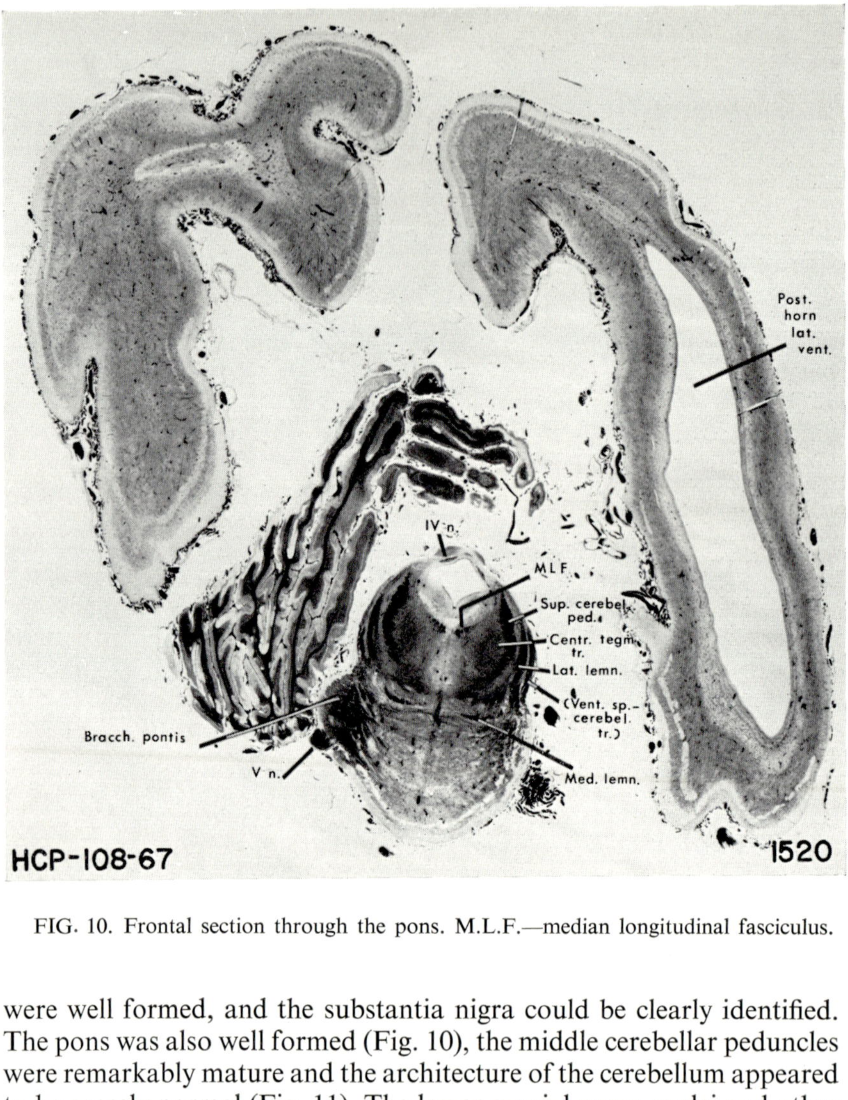

FIG. 10. Frontal section through the pons. M.L.F.—median longitudinal fasciculus.

were well formed, and the substantia nigra could be clearly identified. The pons was also well formed (Fig. 10), the middle cerebellar peduncles were remarkably mature and the architecture of the cerebellum appeared to be grossly normal (Fig. 11). The lower cranial nerve nuclei and other brain-stem structures including the cuneate and gracilis nuclei were easily identified; the medial lemniscus was present but stunted in its development.

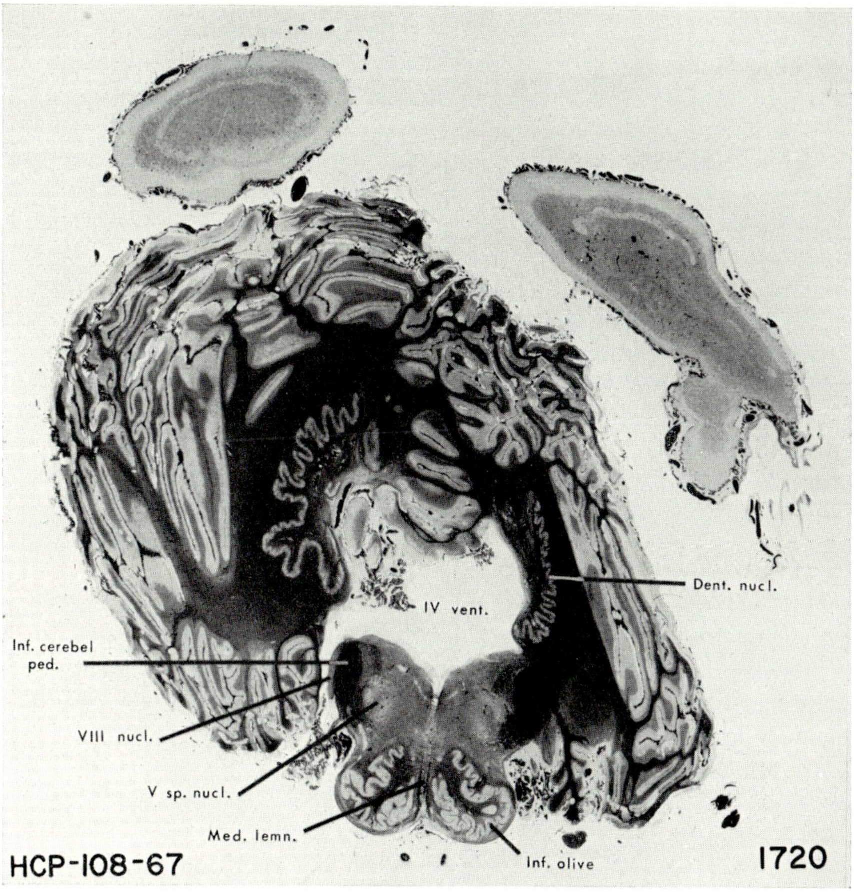

FIG. 11. Frontal section through cerebellum and medulla. Note complete absence of bulbar pyramids and cortico-spinal tracts.

DISCUSSION

The types and degrees of congenital brain malformation included under the term arrhinencephaly have been adequately reviewed in the past. For the purposes of this report it will therefore suffice to summarize the patient's outstanding anatomical and clinical features in terms of categories established in the literature (Yakovlev, 1959; DeMyer *et al.*, 1964).

Like the cases reviewed by Yakovlev (1959), DeMyer and associates (1964), and Bishop and associates (1964), this infant had the typical facial appearance and brain malformations embryologically related to a faulty induction by the prechordial mesoderm.

The extent of the brain malformation with almost no extracephalic abnormalities is compatible with the finding that the chromosome complement was normal (DeMyer *et al.*, 1964). Nevertheless, in view of the parents' tendency to produce offspring with arrhinencephalic malformations, they were advised to have no more children. Unlike the cases of familial holotelencephaly reported by Hintz and associates (1968), this infant had no major endocrine disturbances except in her ability to concentrate urine (but investigation of the endocrine system was not as thorough as it ought to have been). The disturbance in temperature regulation suggested that there must have been a structural defect in the hypothalamic region; yet the pituitary-hypothalamic axis was at least partly functional. The patient's glucose-regulating mechanisms were presumably adequate, and her pituitary secreted thyrotrophic hormone. Unfortunately the assay of her plasma growth hormone was unsatisfactory.

The significant clinical finding from a behavioural perspective was a slow but definite "progress" in motor performance despite the frequent clinical seizures and incessant electrical seizure activity. The changes in motor behaviour that might be designated as developmental acquisitions included the infant's ability to hold up her head at 2 months and to support the upper trunk on her elbows when in the prone position; the onset of rhythmical tandem movements of the limbs similar to the "exercise activity" of normal infants, even though the upper and lower limbs moved as pairs or in tandem rather than in alternating sequences; some integration of organismic states with an increase in periods of alert-inactivity (Wolff, 1969); and perhaps the early differentiation of affect-expressive movements in response to the interruption of feeding. To be sure, these were minor achievements and they required 4 months to develop. Although these acquisitions do not require the presence of a functional cerebral cortex, the fact that the changes did occur raises questions which are directly pertinent to the focus of this symposium. Given the child's clinical condition and structural defects, where and how did the changes towards greater organization occur? What, for example, were the relative contributions of the cerebellum and other non-cortical structures to the observed changes in posture and motility? To what extent did the motor patterns which were not observed until the second or third month represent a late-appearing, pre-functional organization of behaviour, and to what extent did they reflect the influence of exercise and experience? In other words, was the infant able to "learn"?

Most of our systematic information about the anatomical correlates of primitive motor functions in human infants is based either on analogies from animal experiments or on isolated reports of infants with various congenital malformations (Peiper, 1963). Clearly, analysis of a single case of this kind, even if it includes references—inevitably fragmentary—to the behaviour of similar infants and children in other reports, cannot produce conclusive evidence about the relation between functional competence and anatomical structure of the brain. Equally clearly, it is very difficult to obtain systematic information, based on concrete pathophysiological and anatomical correlations, about brain-behaviour relationships in human infants. Laboratory experiments have to wait on clinical opportunities. Systematic studies of the effects of destructive brain lesions in small infants to parallel the studies of brain function in adults with missile injuries will, it is hoped, remain impossible, unless the wars which affect civilian populations become a constant aspect of the human condition (Goldstein, 1942; Teuber, 1959).

The systematic collation of behavioural data on infants with congenital brain malformations is therefore of great importance. It may offer only partial solutions but may, nevertheless, raise and refine significant questions about brain structure and behavioural development. This is especially true of the general group of infants with holotelencephaly, which, by the methods of clinical genetics, can be divided into two large classes before death. Infants with a holotelencephaly that is associated with a 13—15 trisomy syndrome have a less profound disturbance of brain architecture than the group without chromosome abnormalities (their pyramidal tracts, for example, are intact) and the nature of the brain malformation is usually homogeneous. In contrast, children with holotelencephaly and no chromosome defect generally have a very extensive brain malformation. A systematic comparison of holotelencephalic children with and without chromosome lesions would thus permit us to compare neurological function and behaviour in children who have structural defects that are anatomically related but distinguishable.

Such comparative studies should include investigations of the following problems.

1. The anatomical locus of the observed developmental integration. Which gross structures are essential, and which are inessential, to the observed motor acquisitions? What difference does the presence or

absence of the pyramidal tracts make in the development of early postural reflexes and motility?

Since children with holotelencephaly usually die within the first year, the correlation of brain structure and behaviour also becomes a feasible undertaking.

2. The dynamic factors contributing to the observed changes in behaviour of such children who live beyond the first few months, or beyond the "reflex" stage of sensori-motor development (Piaget, 1952). What, for instance, is the role of experience and practice? How much would such children profit from systematically programmed experiences if they survived for a long enough training period?

3. The effects of continuous electrical seizures on the acquisition of experience, and on the neural integration which, we must assume, is responsible for the observed progressive coordination of motor patterns. Current views about the effects of convulsions on acquired behaviour are based on experiments in which normal animals are trained to perform specific tasks before or during electro-shock treatments, and on clinical impressions about the retention of memories in adult patients subjected to electro-shock therapy (Gerard, 1961; McGaugh, 1965). The results of such studies are not immediately relevant to us since they usually deal with the fate of discrete acquired habits and memories, and presuppose an intact cerebral cortex. Clinical evidence suggests that children with many seizures a day can develop and learn despite the seizures. So far we have no systematic information about the effects of electro-shock or seizure activity on the sub-cortical fixation of experience in humans, and we have no reason to assume that the phenomena recorded as seizures in this infant who had no functional cerebral cortex can be compared to the effects of electro-convulsive shocks in anatomically intact individuals. Indeed one might ask whether the recorded seizure activity was an irritative phenomenon at all, or simply the "natural" electrical activity of sub-cortical structures.

Learning experiments at various levels of complexity might help us to decide whether these children are capable of learning, and a comparison of the results of such experiments in children with and without seizures but in both cases suffering from holotelencephaly would help to answer the question of whether electrical seizure activity has any effect on primitive learning capacities.

Since many infants with the congenital malformations described above show a wide fluctuation in body temperature they also offer us a clinical opportunity for studying the relationship between body temperature and biological rhythms of various frequencies. In this patient the relation of body temperature to "high frequency rhythms" was explored. The effects of temperature fluctuation on other micro- and macro-rhythms of behaviour which are known to be partially sensitive to temperature fluctuations could be explored by more refined methods, especially in those infants who, unlike this one, are not subject to the incessant seizures which interfered with a systematic description of the temperature-dependent changes of sleep-waking cycles and the like (Solberger, 1965; Richter, 1965).

SUMMARY

The clinical course and post-mortem findings on an infant with holotelencephaly but with no chromosome abnormality have been described. Changes in behaviour over the course of the infant's 4-month life span were emphasized. It was suggested that some of the observed changes could be classified as developmental, and the question was raised as to what physiological conditions and anatomical substrates were required to account for them. Specifically it was proposed that a systematic comparison of arrhinencephalic children with and without the 13—15 trisomy syndrome might clarify some aspects of the structural-functional relationship between brain and behaviour, a clarification that could not be achieved by studying normal infants or isolated cases of gross congenital malformations.

REFERENCES

Bishop, K., Connoly, J. M., Carter, C. H. and Carpenter, D. G. 1964. Holoprosencephaly. *J. Pediat.* **65,** 406–414.

DeMyer, W., Zeman, W. and Palmer, C. G. 1964. The face predicts the brain: diagnostic significance of median facial anomalies for holoprosencephaly (arhinencephaly). *Pediatrics, Springfield* **34,** 256–263.

Gerard, R. W. 1961. The fixation of experience. In A. Fessard, R. W. Gerard, J. Konorski and J. F. Delafresnaye (Eds.), *Brain mechanisms and learning.* Thomas, Springfield, Ill. Pp. 21–36.

Goldstein, K. 1942. *After effects of brain injuries in war.* Grune & Stratton, New York.

Hintz, R. L., Menkin, G. M. and Sotos, J. F. 1968. Familial holoprosencephaly with endocrine dysgenesis. *J. Pediat.* **72,** 81–87.

McGaugh, J. C. 1965. Facilitation and impairment of memory storage processes. In D. P. Kimble (Ed.), *The anatomy of memory.* Vol. I. Science and Behavior Books, Palo Alto, Calif.

Peiper, A. 1963. *Cerebral function in infancy and childhood.* Consultants Bureau, New York.

Piaget, J. 1952. *The origins of intelligence in children.* 2nd. ed. International Univ. Press, New York.

Richter, C. P. 1965. *Biological clocks in medicine and psychiatry.* Thomas, Springfield, Ill.

Solberger, A. 1965. *Biological rhythm research.* Elsevier, New York.

Teuber, H. L. 1959. Some alterations in behavior after cerebral lesions in man. In A. D. Bass (Ed.), *Evolution of nervous control.* Am. Ass. Adv. of Sci., Washington, D.C. Pp. 157–194.

Wolff, P. H. 1966. The causes, controls and organization of behavior in the neonate. *Psychological Issues Monograph Series.* Vol. 5, No. 1, Monogr. 17. International Univ. Press, New York.

Wolff, P. H. 1968. The serial organization of sucking in the young infant. *Pediatrics, Springfield,* **42,** 943–956.

Wolff, P. H. 1969. The natural history of crying and other vocalizations in early infancy. In B. M. Foss (Ed.), *Determinants of infant behaviour IV.* Methuen, London. Pp. 81–109.

Yakovlev, P. I. 1959. Pathoarchitectonic studies of cerebral malformations: III. Arrhinencephalies (holotelencephalies). *J. Neuropath. exp. Neurol.* **18,** 22–55.

Discussion

Visual Behaviour and Role of Cerebral Cortex

Humphrey: The baby had optokinetic movements. They are cortical in origin and depend on areas 18 and 19 of the occipital and pre-occipital areas. That would explain your electrical findings from the cortex.

Wolff: Optokinetic movements are not cortically-dependent.

Humphrey: You can stimulate the cortex in the Rhesus monkey and secure them. I would think if that were true for the monkey it would be true for man, because man has a greater degree of corticalization.

Wolff: The fact that you can get something by stimulating a higher region doesn't necessarily mean that its presence requires that higher region.

Humphrey: Not necessarily, only after the brain is normally developed. Experimental work on monkeys shows that in the normal unoperated monkey optokinetic eye movements can be obtained by stimulating any point in the pathway as well as from the cortex. When you remove the cortical areas concerned, optokinetic movements are absent, but can be elicited from lower levels. Fixation is also cortical. Did the infant fixate?

Wolff: Yes, there were fleeting moments between seizures when one had the impression not only of visual fixation but also that the eyes moved in response to a moving object.

ROBINSON: There is a difficulty here, not only in translating from one species to another, but also in translating from the newborn to the adult. For instance it is generally thought that the blink response to light in adults depends on the cerebral cortex, but in the newborn this certainly can't be so because newborn babies with no cerebral hemispheres, like hydranencephalics, show a blink reflex (K. Hill *et al.*, 1961. *Am. J. Ophthal.* **51,** 267).

HUMPHREY: The blink reflex is subcortical, but fixation of the eyes—in the normal newborn infant or later—and optokinetic movements depend on areas 18 and 19 of the cortex.

BRONSON: I suggest that the visual phenomena you see at birth are subcortically mediated, and that only after a month do you begin to get capacities both for voluntary movements of the eyes and for the perception and memory of patterns—and that before this age the various visual phenomena are not primarily, and perhaps not at all, neocortically mediated.

HUMPHREY: In this baby there was another factor which indicates that the cortex was at least sending fibre tracts down: the good development of the cerebellar hemispheres. Their development is dependent on the cortico-ponto-cerebellar system. When there is a real agenesis of the cortex you have agenesis of the cerebellar hemispheres too.

Effect of Seizures on Development

PLOOG: One of the original questions Peter Wolff asked was to what extent seizure activity interrupts development, and he brought up this term "pure maturation". What evidence is there that seizure activity interrupts something? In conditioning studies, it was first believed that seizure activity would interrupt the pure Pavlovian conditioned reflex, and that is not true. You can establish a conditioned reflex and even train an animal while it has seizures. This means that something can be "encoded" while a seizure is going on.

KAUFMAN: The evidence is very confusing. Patients have been observed with continuous 3-per-second spike-and-wave activity in the EEG, who were not constantly having petit mal attacks. They were able a good deal of the time to function and carry on all kinds of activity during spike-and-wave electrical activity. So the EEG patterns do not tell you whether the patient is having a clinical seizure. On the other hand, R. S. Schwab (1941. *Am. J. Psychiat.* **97,** 1301) indicated that when patients do in fact have a seizure with 3-per-second spike-and-wave activity, their reaction time is prolonged and they very characteristically underestimate the passage of time, which would indicate that they are out of contact for a much longer time than they themselves realize, recognize, and recall. Conditioning during a seizure may depend on whether the pathway for the conditioning involved the parts of the brain in which the seizure was going on.

PLOOG: But in this infant I think we can neglect that factor because I think there was seizure activity all over.

PRECHTL: Recently J. Hutt and C. O. Ounsted tried to analyse information processing in children with petit mal. They used a simple sorting task in which it was known how many bits (binary units) had to be processed. The 0- or 1-bit task could be carried out during generalized spike-and-wave; with 2 bits there was partial impairment and with 3 bits total impairment. So the amount of information which has to be dealt with as well as the type of seizure and its localization are important.

BRONSON: The EEG abnormality in Wolff's child was a continuous state, not a periodic disruption. It was really the background pattern against which development proceeded.

SCHULTE: This problem can easily be studied in infants with hypsarrhythmia. The overall clinical experience with these children is that development greatly slows but by no means stops entirely. Some of these children make some progress, in motor development at least.

UNIDENTIFIED MEMBER: There is regression in some functions; it is not just a matter of stopping development.

SCHULTE: During clinical work with these children I never thought of them as providing a good opportunity to study the extent to which seizures and EEG abnormalities disturb learning and other developing functions. Some of these infants with hypsarrhythmia, about 10 per cent, subsequently develop normally—at least they are not grossly handicapped—whereas 90 per cent become severely mentally retarded.

MACKEITH: But had the 90 per cent been severely dulled before they started the seizures?

SCHULTE: You can have different histories. Some infants with hypsarrhythmia make good progress in the first 6 months of their life, then they start having infantile spasms and progress stops.

Cause of Temperature Fluctuation

PLOOG: Is the temperature fluctuating phenomenon you saw an exaggeration of a normally occurring phenomenon? Regulation of temperature is a very unstable function in prematures.

ROBINSON: Even in term babies the ability to withstand cold stress is much poorer than in older subjects.

WOLFF: This baby's temperature fluctuations were something different, because its body temperature didn't depend on the ambient temperature. Even in a constant ambient temperature the body temperature fluctuated. I think the premature baby is very much dependent on the ambient temperature. We checked every possible source of infection within reason and there was no sign. Many of these arrhinencephalic infants have these enormous fluctuations in temperature. Perhaps there is a direct relationship.

SCHULTE: We have to see this in connection with the hypernatraemia. There was some disturbance of electrolyte metabolism as well as of the temperature control system in that area of the hypothalamus.

Effects of Temperature on the EEG

PLOOG: How do you explain that the EEG became normal when the body temperature decreased?

SCHULTE: Maybe the EEG was not normal but some of the big waves disappeared. If the temperature drops to 32° C or 31° C then the EEG slowly decreases in amplitude, until at about 28° C it is almost inactive.

KAUFMAN: H. Hoagland plotted the frequency of dominant EEG rhythms against body temperature and found that it followed the Arrhenius equation according to which the velocity of chemical reactions is a function of temperature (1936. *Am. J. Physiol.* **116,** 604). Has this ever been repeated? Did you try the Arrhenius equation?

WOLFF: Just one EEG will show you that it's impossible to get anything out of that.

Social Smiling

GENERAL DISCUSSION

DITTRICHOVÁ: We observed children born 10 weeks prematurely for 6 months, and compared them with fullterm children. In social smiling we could not find any difference between them and the fullterm babies if we assessed their corrected age. They all started smiling at the same conceptional age, of about 45 weeks.

BOWER: Some people in Boston are claiming that prematures will smile socially in the thirty-second week.

SCHULTE: Do you mean that if you present stimuli, they will smile?

BOWER: They will smile at a human face.

SCHULTE: How do you look after the premature infant? Were they kept in your premature nursery, Dr. Dittrichová, or were they exposed to their parents?

DITTRICHOVÁ: They were in an environment similar to home. We have special nurses as mother substitutes, and it is also possible for the mothers to remain with their children. So the conditions are roughly the same in fullterm as in premature children, except that the premature infants are kept in incubators for approximately the first 4 weeks.

HUMPHREY: What is the stimulus for social smiling, so-called?

DITTRICHOVÁ: In our examination it was the adult, who was near the child and spoke to the child: visual *and* voice stimuli.

AMBROSE: It is important to define and standardize stimulus and conditions under which smiling is elicited. For instance, it is easier to elicit smiling in a 6-week-old baby (born at term) if you combine visual presentation of the face, auditory stimulation, and rhythmic movement stimulation, than if you use auditory or visual stimulation alone. I think most of the disagreements about the age at which smiling begins to occur have to do with the different conditions under which it is elicited.

WOLFF: A human stimulus that should provoke the so-called social smile may also function as a physical stimulus. Perhaps you can get a smile which seems to be a response to the social stimulus but which is really triggered by some other (internal or external) event. Then it becomes a matter of establishing the regularity with which the purported stimulus elicits a smile.

PLOOG: Why is it so important to make this distinction between the social smile and any other smiling? Wolff has published pictures of infants of 28 and 30 weeks' gestation which clearly demonstrated that these prematures smiled (P. H. Wolff. 1963. In B. M. Foss (Ed.), *Determinants of infant behaviour II*, p. 113. London, Methuen). This was not social smiling, but what is the difference? Eibl-Eibesfeldt (I. Eibl-Eibesfeldt. 1967. *Grundiss der vergleichenden Verhaltensforschung*. Piper, Munich) photographed a blind and a blind-and-deaf child, who not only smiled but also directed its eyes towards the vocal source or to the warmth of the face, which was close to it. Why discuss whether this is a response smile or just a spontaneous smile?

WOLFF: The smiles in the premature infants were elicited by clicking a pencil against the glass pane—not a social stimulus. Some may say this is not a real smile because it is not a "social" smile. The argument becomes ludicrous.

LIPSITT: The term "social smile" should not necessarily be dropped unless there is substituted for it some stimulus specification that will substitute for the word "social". It is possible to stimulate a smile in the newborn by doing certain things to him. One of them is to take the nipple out of his mouth very rapidly when he is sucking intensely; his lips then retract and his cheeks go up, and he looks as though he is smiling. It is very important to know that the "smile" was so induced rather than by a tap on the window or by a face.

PLOOG: Or by no stimulus at all.

AMBROSE: "Social smile" should be dropped: it confuses a number of different issues. That term is primarily relevant to the fact that from the second month on, the smile of the baby comes to perform an extremely important social function in the mother/infant relationship. But functional considerations in the second month must not be allowed to conceal other important matters concerning the ontogeny of the motor pattern of smiling and the way it is organized. Major changes take place in the causation of this from birth on and throughout the early weeks. Issues of causation should not be confused with issues of function. Various kinds of stimulation—not only external but presumably internal, also, because smiling can take place spontaneously—can elicit smiling, and I think this shouldn't be overlooked.

SCHULTE: There is a type of smiling in the premature infant which we see very often in active sleep, and which is nothing more than "rapid eye movements" in the facial muscles. This looks like smiling but it is not "social smiling". Yet Ambrose says that we should not distinguish these any more.

AMBROSE: Undoubtedly the internal stimuli that elicit the lip retraction motor pattern during sleep should be distinguished from the external stimuli that can also elicit the response, but I think it is unwise to make a distinction between different kinds of lip-retraction on the basis of differences in eliciting stimulation. Certainly you can get unilateral lip-retraction in sleep, as well as bilateral, but this motor pattern can be activated by a variety of different stimuli.

HUMPHREY: Does the term "social smiling" mean that emotional expression is involved?

WOLFF: There are morphological changes in the configuration of the smile, but not a radical change from one day to the next. Electromyography of the smile demonstrates that there are changes in the muscles used in smiling which continue until the child is 12 years old.

(M. Hanada, unpublished.) And I think the same thing is true of the set of stimuli which are adequate to elicit the smile. There is a gradation and it isn't that one day you have a social provocation. The term "social smile" has obscured this kind of progression.

KAUFMAN: From the evolutionary point of view the smile is basically a social signal, and there is no more reason to call it a social smile than there is to talk about a social threat in the monkey.

WOLFF: And a social cry in a baby.

SCHULTE: Surely, smiling in active sleep is something different from what Dr. Dittrichová has studied—the smile that you can evoke in an awake baby. There is an asleep smiling and an awake smiling. We get a "social smile" in an awake baby at about 44 to 45 weeks' gestation. The activity in the facial muscles which looks like smiling occurs in active sleep in a 28 weeks' gestation baby, without any stimulus. Is this something different?

WOLFF: Yes, in some dimensions obviously it is different, in other dimensions it is not. The smile of a 3-week-old is different from the smile of the adult.

AMBROSE: The younger the baby the less co-ordinated is this particular motor pattern.

SCHULTE: I am not talking about the motor pattern, but about the brain mechanism.

MACKEITH: Is there an analogy with speech? Perhaps as with early attempts at speech the baby is practising smiling.

BRONSON: At some point in development, smiling gets tied up with a feeling of pleasure—and probably quite early.

PLOOG: Are we discussing maturation? Kaufman said we are confronted with a social signal and here we use the word "social" and we mean that such a signal has a time in life to develop. This is true for other functions. If a male suckling develops an erection no one would deny that it is an erection, and no one would call another erection a social erection—that takes maybe 15 years until it becomes social, that is to say, partner-directed. It takes time for certain functions to ripen; smiling, language, and other functions. The point is not whether it is a stimulus-bound response; it can become such a response, but it is a signal.

BERGSTRÖM: If the observer thinks a smile is a social smile, he is himself responding to the smile.

LIPSITT: Much of the confusion in connection with the smiling response could probably be cleared up by making a distinction between respondent and operant behaviour—a respondent being an elicited response and an operant response being something that the child or the baby does in order to receive something else. Thus a "social smile" apparently spontaneous and designed to elicit a certain kind of reaction from some other person would be classified as an operant as opposed to an elicited response. A response to tapping on the window or to pulling a nipple out of the baby's mouth very rapidly is an elicited response.

AMBROSE: Much more observation of, and research into, the development of smiling, is needed. There has been quite a number of reports on smiling in the newborn, but much of the research on smiling starts only at the age at which the human face can begin to elicit smiling, namely in the second month. Wolff is one of the few people who have reported smiling in the newborn-to-six-week period; there is a need for a lot more work in that period.

The Infant:
development of sleep

Nomenclature of the Stages of Sleep

EDITOR'S NOTE

DURING THE SESSIONS of the study group it was evident—as it has for some time been evident from the literature—that there is confusion in the terminology used to describe the different stages, phases, or states of sleep in early infancy. I think there are two reasons for this confusion.

1. In the last decade there has been great interest in the nature, stages, and significance of sleep, in adults as well as in infants and children. Several research groups have independently observed that sleep in early infancy is not a uniform state, but that it consists of different stages or types which are easy to distinguish clinically—by observation of respiration and of eye and body movements, or by electroencephalography or electromyography. Having made these observations independently but more or less simultaneously, each research group devised a different set of names to describe its observations.

2. Though there are two major types or stages of sleep in early infancy, as set out in Table I, more detailed studies have shown that sleep in early infancy sometimes fails to fulfil all the criteria for either of the major stages of sleep. Consequently, regardless of differences in nomenclature, not all workers would classify some particular portions of sleep in the same way. They have adopted one of three possible approaches to this problem. The first is to regard one particular criterion, for example, regularity of respiration or the presence of eye movements, as being of overriding importance. If only one criterion is used it is obviously possible to classify the whole of sleep within the two major categories, but some portions of sleep would be put in a different major category if another overriding criterion was used. The second approach is to subdivide the major categories of sleep; and the third, which closely resembles the second, is to abide by strict and

TABLE I. NOMENCLATURE USED BY DIFFERENT AUTHORS TO DESCRIBE THE TWO MAJOR TYPES OF SLEEP OBSERVED IN THE NEWBORN AND IN EARLY INFANCY

Author	*Term for sleep characterized by:*	*Term for sleep characterized by:*
	Regular respiration No body movement or occasional startles No eye movements EMG activity at chin *Tracé alternant* (episodic sleep activity) on EEG	Irregular respiration Frequent small body movement Eye movements, rapid or otherwise No EMG activity at chin No *tracé alternant* on EEG
Prechtl, 1965	State 1	State 2
Aserinsky and Kleitman, 1955	No eye movement period	Interval of ocular and body activity, or active segment of motility cycle
Wolff, 1959	Regular sleep	Irregular sleep
Parmelee *et al.*, 1967 Dreyfus-Brisac and Monod, 1965 Dittrichová, 1969	Quiet sleep	Active sleep
Dreyfus-Brisac, 1964	Deep sleep	Light sleep
Dittrichová, 1962	State 1	States 2 and 3
Goldie and Van Velzer, 1965	Phase II	Phase I
Petre-Quadens, 1966	Stages (b) and (c) (distinguished by EEG)	Stages (a) and (d) (distinguished by frequency of eye movements)
Jouvet, 1961	Telencephalic sleep	Rhombencephalic, hind-brain, or paradoxical sleep
Other terms used	Synchronized sleep	Rapid eye movement (REM) sleep

exclusive definitions of the major categories of sleep but to recognize that there are transitional states between them.

It is clear that, of these two reasons for confusion in terminology, the first is a straightforward problem of nomenclature which, were it the only problem, should be readily resolved by agreement and goodwill. The second poses problems concerning the nature and the physiology of sleep states which make such a simple solution impossible. However, in order to understand the literature on this subject, it is essential for a start to know the terms which different authors use for the major categories of sleep. I have set out these terms in Table I, which I hope will prove a useful guide to the rest of this section. The table does not, and is not intended to, provide a comprehensive review of the literature on sleep in infancy; nor is the order in which the references are given meant to be a statement of priority—Prechtl's terms are given first because they were the ones most frequently used in the study group. The table is simply meant to show which terms can be regarded as more or less synonymous. All the studies cited refer to sleep in early human infancy except that by Jouvet (1961) which is concerned with adult cats. Strictly, this work is irrelevant to the present discussion: it has been included because Jouvet's work and nomenclature are frequently quoted with reference to sleep in infancy.

The table reveals just how confused and confusing the present terminology is. For example, a reader unfamiliar with this field of investigation might suppose, not unreasonably, that Prechtl's states 1 and 2 were equivalent to Goldie's and Van Velzer's Phases I and II or to Petre-Quadens' stages (a) and (b). In each case he would be totally wrong.

The most practical suggestion would be to ask authors to follow Aserinsky and Kleitman (1955) in using terms which are directly related to the observations they make: for example, "eye-movement sleep" or "no-eye-movement sleep". The result, though cumbersome, would at least be comprehensible. This method of nomenclature could also be adapted to include the extra or transitional states. I shall not elaborate on these transitional states and the physiological problems they pose, since the subject is extensively discussed in the papers by Prechtl, Petre-Quadens, and Dittrichová.

RJR

REFERENCES

Aserinsky, E. and Kleitman, N. 1955. A motility cycle in sleeping infants as manifested by ocular and gross bodily activity. *J. appl. Physiol.* **8**, 11–18.

Dreyfus-brisac, C. 1964. The electroencephalogram of the premature infant and full-term newborn. Normal and abnormal development of waking and sleeping patterns. In P. Kellaway and I. Peterson (Eds.), *Neurological and electroencephalographic correlative studies in infancy.* Grune & Stratton, New York. Pp. 186–207.

Dreyfus-brisac, C. and Monod, N. 1965. Sleep of premature and full-term neonates—a polygraphic study. *Proc. R. Soc. Med.* **58**, 6–7.

Dittrichová, J. 1962. Nature of sleep in young infants. *J. appl. Physiol.* **17**, 543–546.

Dittrichová, J. 1969. This volume. Pp. 193–201.
Goldie, L. and Van Velzer, C. 1965. Innate sleep rhythms. *Brain* **88,** 1043–1056.
Jouvet, M. 1961. Telencephalic and rhombencephalic sleep in the cat. In G. E. W. Wolstenholme and M. O'Connor (Eds.), *The nature of sleep.* Ciba Foundation Symposium. Churchill, London. Pp. 188–206.
Parmelee, A. H., Wenner, W. H., Akiyama, Y., Schultz, M., and Stern, E. 1967. Sleep states in premature infants. *Devl Med. Child Neurol.* **9,** 70–77.
Petre-Quadens, O. 1966. On the different phases of the sleep of the newborn with special reference to the activated phase or phase d. *J. Neurol. Sci.* **3,** 151–161.
Prechtl, H. F. R. 1965. Problems of behavioral studies in the newborn infant. In D. S. Lehrman, R. A. Hinde, and E. Shaw (Eds.), *Advances in the study of behavior*. Vol. 1. Academic Press, New York and London. Pp. 75–98.
Wolff, P. H. 1959. Observations on newborn infants. *Psychosom. Med.* **21,** 110–118.

Comparative Study of Sleep in Pregnancy and in the Newborn[1]

O. PETRE-QUADENS, J. L. HARDY, AND C. DE LEE

Born-Bunge Foundation,
and Hôpital St. Pierre, University of Brussels

INTRODUCTION

THE STUDY OF sleep is of interest because it allows the functional activity of the central nervous system to be measured. The electroencephalographic, electromyographic, and electrooculographic sleep patterns reveal phases which vary periodically during the night. Since the work of Aserinsky and Kleitman (1955), one of these phases, called paradoxical sleep (PS) or REM sleep and characterized by bursts of rapid eye movements (Dement and Kleitman, 1957), has been the object of numerous investigations. Neurophysiological data suggest that some of the cerebral circuits responsible for this phase interfere with the limbic midbrain circuit, described by Nauta (1958). It has been established that the total amount of sleep and the amount of PS vary according to the serotonin concentrations in the medial raphe of the pontine tegmentum (Jouvet *et al.*, 1967).

In the rabbit the proportion of PS varies with oestrus periods and with sex-hormone levels (Sawyer and Kawakami, 1959; Sawyer *et al.*, 1966). It has been suggested that the hormonal changes of the human menstrual cycle produce an increase in PS (Hartmann, 1966). In a previous study one of us demonstrated that the proportion of PS in the pregnant woman increases towards the end of gestation, and that the qualitative and quantitative variations of the other stages recall the sleep characteristics of the premature and the newborn at a corresponding gestational age (Petre-Quadens *et al.*, 1967). The sleep

[1] This research was sponsored in part by the Air Force Office of Scientific Research through the European Office of Aerospace Research, U.S. Air Forces, under Contract AF 61 (052) 949 and F6-1052-67 C 0066.

similarities of mother and newborn suggest that a common humoral mechanism might be responsible for the characteristics of both.

Since it is impossible to record the electroencephalogram (EEG) of the fetus through the abdominal wall, we wondered whether a study of the movements of the fetus would not reveal some correlations with his mother's sleep and throw some light on the many problems connected with sleep in the premature and newborn infant.

Furthermore, in order to quantify the qualitative changes observed in the rapid-eye-movement patterns themselves, we measured the intervals which separate the eye movements of PS in pregnancy and compared these measurements with those of non-pregnant subjects. We also compared the interval measurements of mentally normal, non-pregnant subjects with those of oligophrenics in whom Reiss (1961) suspected that endocrine deficiencies occurred.

MATERIAL AND METHODS

1. One hundred and twenty-one polygraphic all-night sleep recordings were made on 40 women, aged 21 to 28, at different periods of their gestation and postpartum. In some instances recordings took place at intervals over the whole period of pregnancy and postpartum; in others they were made for several successive nights at a given stage of pregnancy. Most subjects underwent at least two recordings on successive nights in order to prevent the first-night effect. Single recordings were made only from subjects from whom a previous recording had been made. For each subject at each period we used the averages of the data of successive nights, whatever their number.

2. The polygraphic recordings comprise the EEG; the electromyogram (EMG); and the electrooculogram (EOG) in horizontal and vertical bipolar shunts. For the EEG and EOG the time constants were 0·3 sec, and the amplitude 6 mm for 50 μV. The EMG was recorded with a time-constant of 0·1 sec and an amplitude of 10 mm for 50 μV. The paper speed was 15 mm/sec. The recording started at 10.00 or 11.00 p.m. and ended in the morning with the spontaneous awakening of the subject. In one subject at 33 weeks of pregnancy the fetal movements were recorded during four consecutive nights by means of a tocograph. The signals were integrated and transmitted to the polygraph with a time-constant of 0·3 sec.

3. Sleep recordings were made on 95 premature, fullterm newborn, and post-mature, normal babies; also on 4 mongols, 1 microcephalic, and 5 who had suffered from placental insufficiency. In order to avoid

the changes in the sequences of states, which are more numerous during the first 3 days of life, the recordings were made between the third and fifth days after birth (Prechtl, 1965). The technique was the same as described above. The duration of recordings varied from 2 to 3 hours so that a complete sleep cycle was obtained (Aserinsky and Kleitman, 1955; Dittrichová, 1962; Parmelee *et al.*, 1962).

4. The intervals separating the eye movements of PS were measured in fractions of seconds in the total night-sleep recordings of three women who were 33 weeks pregnant; the recording speed was 15 mm per second. A total of 12,662 eye-movement intervals was thus measured and converted into percentages with respect to a conventional duration of 100 seconds' PS, in order to render them independent of the duration of each PS epoch. The intervals between the horizontal and vertical eye movements were measured independently of each other. This method allowed us to compare them with those of two non-pregnant women of the same age.

5. By the same method 29,657 eye-movement intervals were measured in 13 mentally retarded, and 7 normal, subjects. The subjects were grouped according to age. The mentally retarded subjects had metabolic diseases—there were 5 cases of phenylketonuria, 2 of glycinuria, 2 of Prader's disease (Prader-Willi-Fanconi), 3 of unknown aetiology with albinism, and one of leucodytrophy with severe oligophrenia. They were grouped without reference to aetiology, for a previous study had shown that there is little correlation between sleep-stage percentages and aetiology.

Polygraphic night-sleep recordings were also made on 45 mentally retarded patients of all ages. Quantitative analysis of the different sleep stages was made according to the classification of Dement and Kleitman (1957). The results, classified by age, were compared to those of 25 normal subjects.

RESULTS AND DISCUSSION

Pregnancy and Postpartum

Between 33 and 36 weeks of pregnancy there is a marked increase on the amount of PS (Fig. 1). Changes in the EEG, EMG, and EOG are already apparent earlier in pregnancy.

1. *EEG*. The spindles increase considerably from the 20th week of pregnancy not only in amount but also in amplitude. This increase is accompanied by an increase of stage 2.[1] Moreover, this stage is over-

[1] For an explanation of sleep stages in the adult, see p. 190.

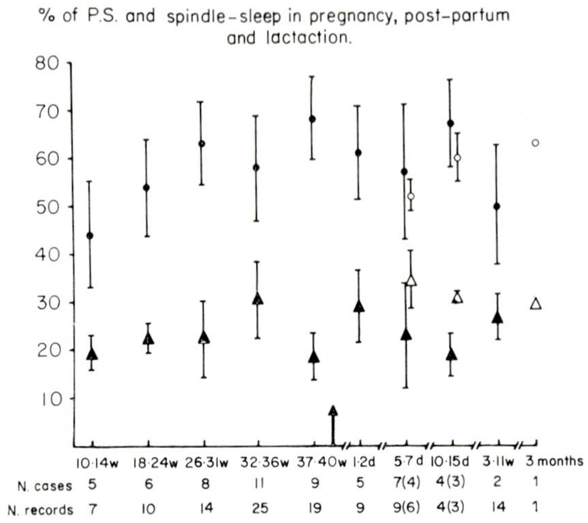

FIG. 1. Paradoxical sleep and spindle sleep as percentages of night sleep in pregnancy, postpartum and during lactation. ▲ Average percentage of PS in pregnant and non-breastfeeding women; ● Average percentage of spindle sleep in pregnant and non-breastfeeding women; △ Average percentage of PS in breastfeeding women; ○ Average percentage of spindle sleep in breastfeeding women. I One standard deviation above and below the mean value; distribution of the individual values is Gaussian; ↑ Time of delivery.

Abscissae: Gestational age in weeks (on the left of the arrow). Time elapsed since delivery (on the right of the arrow).

N. cases: Number of cases; the number of breastfeeding women is shown in brackets and is additional to the numbers not bracketed.

N. records: Number of recordings.

charged with spikes disseminated or grouped in polyspikes and waves, sometimes resembling epileptic discharges. The increase in spindles between 10 and 31 weeks is significant ($p < 0{\cdot}05$) and precedes the increase in PS. The spindles decrease slightly between 32 and 36 weeks, during which time a significant increase ($p < 0{\cdot}05$) of PS occurs. The correlation between EEG and EOG is less constant in pregnant, than in control, subjects. Bursts of rapid eye movements may be seen at the same time as spindles or alpha waves in the EEG. Spindles in PS are also found in the newborn (Petre-Quadens, 1965).

2. *EMG.* At the level of the chin muscles, EMG activity is present in all the sleep stages except that of paradoxical sleep, during which EMG activity is abolished in the normal healthy adult. In pregnant women as well as in the newborn the abolition of muscular tone during paradoxical sleep is inconstant and the EMG is often abolished during the other sleep stages.

3. *EOG.* From the 20th week of gestation, isolated eye movements, especially vertical, appear during all sleep stages. The isolated eye movements occur irregularly and reach their definitive proportion towards 20 weeks. They increase slightly between 33 and 36 weeks, that is, when PS reaches its highest proportion. The early appearance of isolated eye movements during pregnancy and certain other characteristics differentiate them from the grouped eye movements of PS. It is very likely a more primitive phenomenon, less organized than the eye movements of true PS.

Between 37 and 40 weeks, PS decreases ($p < 0{\cdot}01$). This decrease is accompanied by a significant increase of the spindling activity ($p < 0{\cdot}05$). After delivery, the percentage of PS decreases in the women who are not breastfeeding, as do the amounts of spindles and of isolated eye movements. In the breastfeeding women the proportion of PS remains high. The differences in PS between the two groups are significant ($p < 0{\cdot}05$). The marked decrease in the amount of PS between the 10th and 15th day after delivery in the women not breastfeeding looks similar to that occurring at the very end of pregnancy, and it is accompanied by a parallel increase of sleep spindles ($p < 0{\cdot}025$). In the breastfeeding woman the higher percentage of PS is accompanied, as during pregnancy, by a higher proportion of spindles and isolated eye movements.

The Newborn

PS characterized by rapid eye movements is very rare in the young premature (Fig. 2). It reaches its highest proportion at 37 weeks of gestational age, the increase occurring shortly after the increase of PS in the pregnant women. We recorded four newborn mongols and one microcephalic infant, and all had a low PS percentage. This decrease in eye movement time is also seen, though less constantly, in babies who have suffered from placental insufficiency.

Fetal Movements

From one pregnant woman during four consecutive nights, 26,245 fetal movements (FM) were recorded (Fig. 3). Their frequency was highest during sleep with isolated eye movements: 40·29 per minute, standard deviation (SD) = 17·3. Fetal movements were less frequent during PS (20·71, SD = 10·23) and awakening (FM 16·31, SD = 9·28). They were infrequent in stages 1, 2, and 3 without eye movements. (These are phases of quiet sleep in the adult which are distinguished from each other by their EEG characteristics.) The values were 4·71

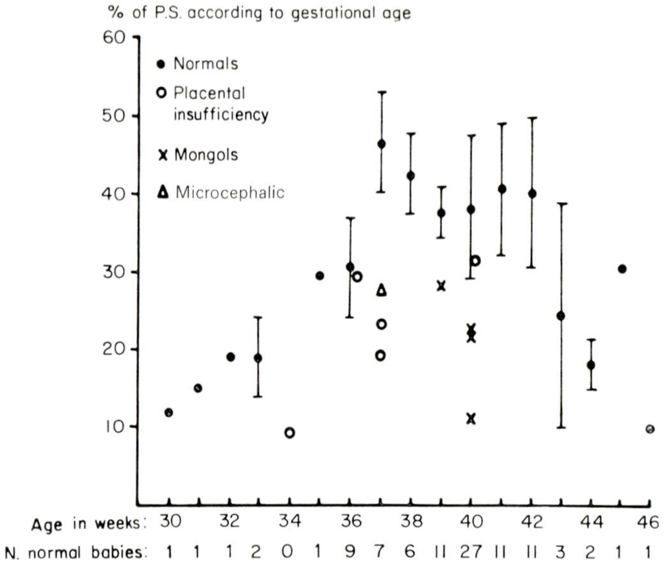

FIG. 2. Percentage of paradoxical sleep according to gestational age. The black circles indicate the average percentage of PS in 95 normal infants, born at different gestational ages, 3 to 5 days after birth. The lines above and below the symbols indicate the standard errors; the distribution of individual data is Gaussian. The other symbols refer to 4 mongols, 5 infants who had suffered from placental insufficiency, and 1 microcephalic infant.

(SD = 2·48) in stage 1; 3·75 (SD = 1·66) in stage 2, and 1·98 (SD = 0·86) in stage 3. The differences in the amount of FM were not significant ($p < 0{\cdot}1$) between stage 2 with isolated eye movement (IEM) and PS. They were significant ($p < 0{\cdot}05$) between wakefulness or PS and stages 1, 2, and 3. The frequency of fetal movements increased slightly as the EEG tracing desynchronized, but it was only when eye movements appeared that fetal movements increased significantly. The greatest frequency of fetal movements during stage 2 with isolated eye movements indicates that in this stage more fetal motor discharges took place than in PS. Interestingly enough in the premature and the newborn, stage *a* with its isolated eye movements (which is a phase of active sleep differing from true paradoxical sleep) is also characterized by more intensive motor discharges than occur in genuine PS (Petre-Quadens, 1966).

It may be suggested that in this fetus of 33 weeks, stage *a* occurred when his mother showed spindle sleep with isolated eye movements. But we do not know. In fact, an extra-uterine premature of 33 weeks shows not only the four sleep stages, but also awakens. We do not know

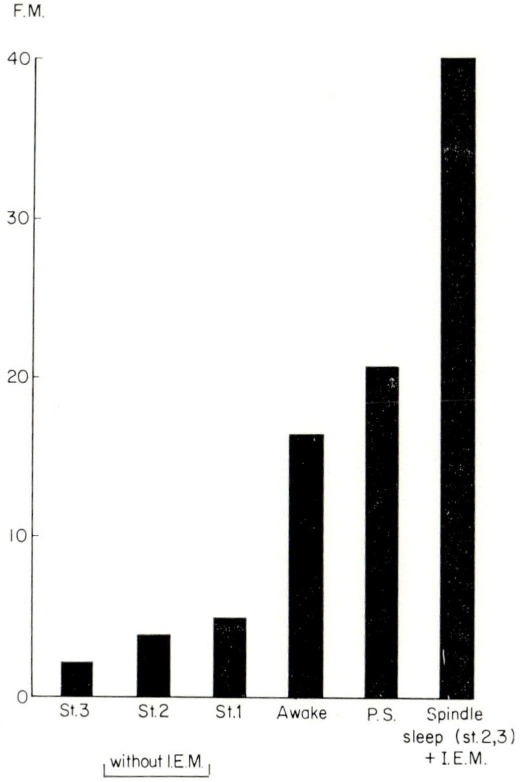

FIG. 3. Amount of fetal movement during sleep. Ordinates: the average number of fetal movements during each sleep stage of the mother. Abscissae: the mother's sleep stages. The differences between the number of fetal movements during stages 1, 2, and 3 without isolated eye movements is not significant. The same holds true during awakening and PS. On the other hand, the difference between the first group of fetal movements (stages 3, 2, and 1) and the second group (awakening and PS) is statistically significant at $p<0 \cdot 05$. The difference between the number of fetal movements during PS and that during spindle sleep + isolated eye movements (IEM) is significant only at $p<0 \cdot 1$.

what is the intra-uterine equivalent of awakening. In 1966 it was simultaneously demonstrated by Parmelee and associates in Los Angeles (Parmelee *et al.*, 1967), and by ourselves, that the young premature shows a preponderance of stage *a*. The amount of fetal movement when the mother is in PS may possibly suggest that PS in the fetus occurs at the same time as it does in the mother. This hypothesis was proposed by Sterman and Jeannerod (1967).

There is good evidence that, in the premature baby, stage *a* predominates because cortical maturation is not sufficiently advanced to allow the subcortical discharges to be inhibited. It is tempting to correlate these data with the maturation of PS. This would mean that PS has an inhibitory function, preventing excitations of subcortical origin. Whatever the case, the fetus, like the mother, is flooded with hormones of which progesterone is the one whose action upon the central nervous system is best known.

Eye-movement Intervals

A total of 42,319 eye-movement intervals were measured. Only those below 1 second and those between 1 and 2 seconds were taken into consideration. Short intervals ($I \leq 1''$) occurred three to four times as frequently in the pregnant woman of 33 weeks' gestational age as in control subjects (Fig. 4). This difference is significant at a level of $p < 0{\cdot}001$. Intervals between 1 and 2 seconds are twice as numerous

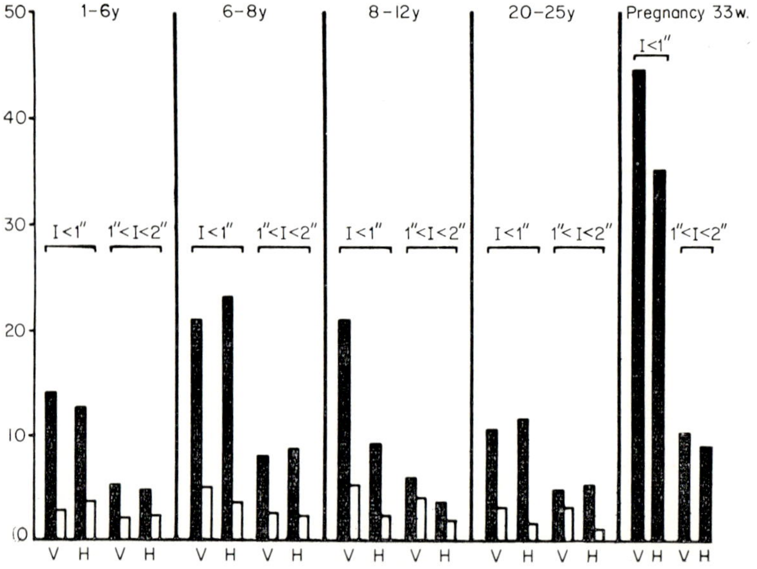

FIG. 4. Frequency distribution of intervals between eye movements. Columns 1, 2, and 3: (in black) normal control children; (in white) mentally retarded children. Column 4: (in black) normal adult control subjects; (in white) mentally retarded adult subjects; Column 5: pregnant women of 33 weeks' pregnancy. Frequency of the eye-movement intervals $\leqslant 1''$ and $1'' < I \leqslant 2''$ per period of $100''$ of PS during total night-sleep recordings. I = intervals. V = vertical eye movements. H = horizontal eye movements.

in the pregnant woman. Intervals above 2 seconds are almost equally distributed in the two groups of subjects. One wonders whether the bursts of rapid eye movements are not evidence of an excitatory state induced by hormones.

We compared the eye-movement intervals in normal subjects with those in oligophrenics of the same age. In normal subjects the frequency of intervals of less than 1 second was four times higher, and those between 1 and 2 seconds two to three times higher, than in the mentally retarded (Fig. 4). In each age group the differences are highly significant

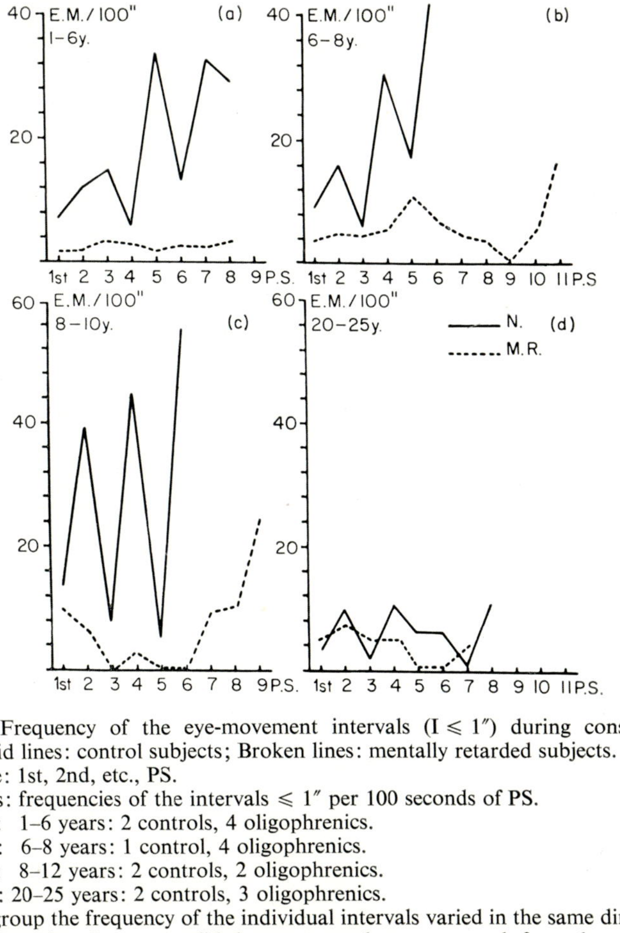

FIG. 5. Frequency of the eye-movement intervals (I ⩽ 1″) during consecutive PS epochs. Solid lines: control subjects; Broken lines: mentally retarded subjects.
Abscissae: 1st, 2nd, etc., PS.
Ordinates: frequencies of the intervals ⩽ 1″ per 100 seconds of PS.
Group a: 1–6 years: 2 controls, 4 oligophrenics.
Group b: 6–8 years: 1 control, 4 oligophrenics.
Group c: 8–12 years: 2 controls, 2 oligophrenics.
Group d: 20–25 years: 2 controls, 3 oligophrenics.
In each group the frequency of the individual intervals varied in the same direction from one PS to the other. In no case did the represented averages result from the accumulation of values varying in the opposite direction.

($p < 0{\cdot}001$). In addition, the frequency of occurrence of short intervals oscillates from one epoch of PS to the next. It is as if the mechanism responsible for the periodicity of PS, or, more exactly, for the periodicity of the rapid eye movements of the PS epochs during the night, passes successively through phases of excitation and inhibition (Fig. 5). The mentally retarded seemed to miss the phases of excitation even when they were approaching puberty, although the eye movements then spread over a frequency distribution similar to that of the mentally normal. Indeed, below the age of 15, the percentages of PS per night do not differ much in the two groups of subjects (Fig. 6). The normalization of PS towards puberty is thus only an appearance and accounts for the large eye-movement intervals only. Nevertheless, this normalization is also observed in the other sleep-stages (Fig. 7). In the adults the levels

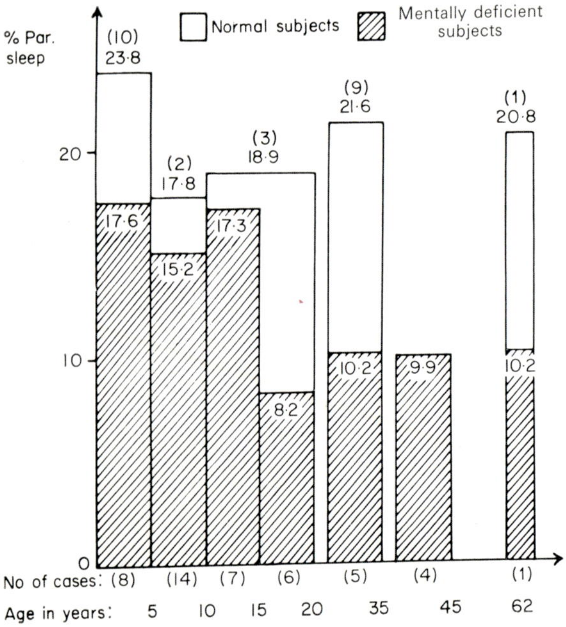

FIG. 6. Percentage of paradoxical sleep in night sleep as a function of age. Ordinates: percentage of PS in total night-sleep recordings. Upper levels: mean percentage of PS in normal subjects; number of cases in parenthesis. Lower levels: mean percentage of PS in retarded subjects (hatched columns). The white columns give the differences between the levels of PS in the normal subjects compared to the oligophrenic subjects. Abscissae: age groups (1 to 5 years, 5 to 10 years, etc.).

Age in years	0–5	5–10	10–15	15–20	20–35	35–45	62
St. 1, 2, 3 Norm. subj.	54·9	59	62·2		69·8	—	76·5
Ment. def. subj.	45	49·7	62·6	68	71·8	75·1	64
St. 4 Norm. subj.	19·2	18·5	16·5		7·5	—	0
Ment. def. subj.	14·1	14·7	18·5	17·8	11·9	11·8	24

FIG. 7. Evolution with age of the mean percentage of stages 1, 2, and 3 (taken together) and of stage 4, in normal and oligophrenic subjects.

of the eye-movement discharges did not differ much between the normal and the mentally retarded but the durations of night-PS were then clearly reduced in the retarded (Fig. 5d).

In the normal subjects the periods of abolition of muscle tone during sleep diminished with age (Fig. 8). In the mentally retarded these periods were much longer, particularly in the infants. Percentage estimates of abolition of EMG activity in the retarded approach normal

Age	*Normal subjects*	*Mental def. subjects*
3m.–5y.	14·7 (10)	55 (8)
5–10y.	9 (4)	55·7 (14)
10–15y.		12·8 (7)
15–20y.	2·4 (8)	30 (6)
20–25y.		30·4 (5)
25–30y.		
35–40y.		37·5 (4)
62y.	0·9 (1)	56·1 (1)

FIG. 8. Mean value (in %) of EMG abolition during the 4 sleep stages in total night-sleep recordings. Number of cases in parenthesis.

values for subjects between the ages of 10 and 15 years; before and after this, there is a much wider deviation.

As mentioned by Reiss (1961), endocrine disorders in childhood may lead to mental retardation. It is probable that secondary endocrine disorders develop from a single disorder—through a lack of stimulation of the brain-endocrine feedback mechanisms. Some endocrine disorders may possibly act in this way even during intra-uterine life.

CONCLUSION

It is reasonable to look at humoral and hormonal changes for the origin of the sleep variations of the pregnant woman. First we see an increase in spindles. Heuser and associates (1967) observed that progesterone produces an increase of spindles in the cat.

Sawyer and Kawakami (1959) have shown that in the female rabbit injected progesterone produces an EEG after-reaction characterized by a frequential association of spindles and PS. Moreover, progesterone has a biphasic effect: first an induction of PS by lowering of its threshhold, then a rise of this threshold. Such a biphasic effect of progesterone or another hormone may explain the paradoxical sleep variations at the end of pregnancy.

After delivery the increase in the amount of PS at 1—2 days and the subsequent marked decrease at 5—15 days is probably due to the contribution of a second hormone, prolactin, which also seems to have a biphasic effect.

It has been demonstrated that in hyperthyroidism the percentage of PS increases up to 45 per cent (Passouant *et al.*, 1966) and that spindles are markedly reduced in number, increasing after thyroxine has been given (Schultz *et al.*, 1968).

The increase of both PS and spindling activity in the pregnant woman seems thus to be evidence of a non-specific reaction of the central nervous system to some hormonal activity. The correlations between fetal movements and the mother's sleep suggest a common humoral factor. The similarities between the sleep of the newborn and that of the woman after delivery suggest a similar cerebral mechanism.

Autoradiographic studies (Michael, 1965) have shown that steroids localize preferentially in the hypothalamic, preoptic, limbic, and septal areas—that is, in the area extending from the limbic system down to the midbrain where sleep mechanisms have been identified.

According to Hamburg (1966) hormones should provide some kind of general disposition upon which learning factors would operate. Does the presence of PS indicate such a disposition? Our observations would fit this hypothesis, but the sleep data in oligophrenia have posed more problems than they have solved.

REFERENCES

Aserinsky, E. and Kleitman, N. 1955. A motility cycle in sleeping infants as manifested by ocular and gross bodily activity. *J. appl. Physiol.* **8,** 11–18.

Dement, W. C. and Kleitman, N. 1957. Cyclic variations in EEG during sleep and their relation to eye-movements, body motility and dreaming. *Electroenceph. clin. Neurophysiol.* **9,** 673–690.

DITTRICHOVÁ, J. 1962. Nature of sleep in young infants. *J. appl. Physiol.* **17,** 543–546.

HAMBURG, D. A. 1966. Effects of progesterone on behavior. In R. Levine (Ed.), "Endocrines and the central nervous system". *Res. Publs Ass. Res. nerv. ment. dis.* **43,** 251–265.

HARTMANN, E. 1966. Dreaming-sleep (the D-state) and the menstrual cycle. *J. nerv. ment. Dis.* **143,** 406–416.

HEUSER, G., LING, G. M. and KLUVER, M. 1967. Sleep induction by progesterone in the preoptic area in cats. *Electronceph. clin. Neurophysiol.* **22,** 122–127.

JOUVET, M., BOBILLIER, P., PUJOL, J. F. and RENAULT, J. 1967. Suppression du sommeil et diminution de la sérotine cérébrale par lésion du système du raphé chez le chat. *C.r. hebd. Séanc. Acad. Sci., Paris* **264,** 360–362.

MICHAEL, R. P. 1965. Oestrogens in the central nervous system. *Br. med. Bull.* **21,** 87.

NAUTA, W. J. H. 1958. Hippocampal projections and related neural pathways to the midbrain in the cat. *Brain* **81,** 319–340.

PARMELEE, A. H., BRÜCK, K. and BRÜCK, M. 1962. Activity and inactivity cycles during the sleep of premature infants exposed to neutral temperature. *Biologia. Neonat.* **4,** 317–339.

PARMELEE, A. H., WENNER, W. H., AKIJAMA, Y., SCHULTZ, M. and STERN, E. 1967. Sleep states in premature infants. *Devl Med. Child Neur.* **9,** 70–77.

PASSOUANT, P., PASSOUANT-FONTAINE, T. and CADILLAC, J. 1966. L'influence de l'hyperthyroide sur le sommeil. Étude clinique et expérimentale. *Rev. Neurol.* **15,** 353–366.

PETRE-QUADENS, O. 1965. Étude du sommeil chez le nouveau-né normal. In *Le sommeil de nuit normal et pathologique*. Nouvelle série. (Vol. 2). Électroencéphalographie et Neurophysiologie Clinique. Masson, Paris. Pp. 149–155.

PETRE-QUADENS, O. 1966. On the different phases of sleep of the newborn with special reference to the activated phase or phase *d. J. Neurol. Sci.* **3,** 151–161.

PETRE-QUADENS, O. and JAUDOUL-LAMBRECHTS. 1965. L'ontogénèse de la phase de sommeil correspondant au rêve. *Acta neurol. psychiat. belg.* **65,** 971–977.

PETRE-QUADENS, O., DEBARSY, A. M., DEVOS, J. and SFAELLO, Z. 1967. Sleep in pregnancy: evidence of foetal sleep characteristics. *J. Neurol. Sci.* **4,** 600–605.

PRECHTL, H. F. R. 1965. Problems of behavioral studies in the newborn infant. In D. S. Lehrman, R. A. Hinde, and E. Shaw (Eds.), *Advances in the study of behavior*. Vol. I. Academic Press, New York and London. Pp. 75–98.

REISS, M. 1961. Endocrine research in psychiatry. In *Proceedings*, Vol. I, Third World Congress of Psychiatry, 1961, Univ. of Toronto Press and McGill Univ. Press. Pp. 121–127.

SAWYER, C., KAWAKAMI, M. and KANEMATSU, S. 1966. Neuroendocrine aspects of reproduction. In R. Levine (Ed.), "Endocrines and the central nervous system". *Res. Publs Ass. Res. nerv. ment. Dis.* **43,** 59–85.

SAWYER, C. and KAWAKAMI, M. 1959. Characteristics of behavioral and electronencephalographic after-reactions to copulation and vaginal stimulation in the female rabbit. *Endocrinology* **65,** 622–630.

SCHULTZ, M. A., SCHULTE, F. J., AKIYAMA, Y. and PARMELEE, A. H. 1968. Development of electroencephalographic sleep phenomena in hypothyroid infants. *Electroenceph. clin. Neurophysiol.* **25,** 351–358.

STERMAN, M. B. and JEANNEROD, M. 1967. Relationship of fetal activity to maternal EEG sleep stage. *Electroenceph. clin. Neurophysiol.* **23,** 81.

Discussion

ROBINSON: Can Petre-Quadens explain her classification of different states of sleep?

PETRE-QUADENS: In 1962 Delange and Passouant in Montpellier first described a sleep-stage in the newborn resembling paradoxical sleep (PS), or rapid eye-movement (REM) sleep, in adults. (1962. Revue Neurol. **107,** 271.) However, closer analysis showed that active sleep in the newborn, or sleep associated with eye movements, is not a homogeneous state, but two states which differ in respect of EEG, EMG, and the grouping of eye movements. We have designated these two stages of active sleep stage *a* and stage *d*. Stages *b* and *c* then refer to quiet sleep, or sleep without eye movements.

Stage *d* resembles paradoxical sleep in the adult. The EEG amplitude is at its lowest, and eye movements appear in bursts as in the adult. Muscle tone in the jaw muscles is often, but not always, abolished in the mature newborn.

Stage *a* is an ill-defined stage which Parmelee described at the same time as us. He called it "undifferentiated sleep". During this stage there are strong sucking movements, and positive muscle tone at the level of the notch of the jaw. Isolated eye movements occur. The amount of stage *a* is greater at low gestational ages in premature infants whereas the amount of stage *d* or paradoxical sleep is less at low gestational ages.

Stages *b* and *c* comprise quiet sleep. They are characterized on the EEG by slow waves, and fast waves, respectively. In both stages there are spindles: in stage *b* they occur at 6—7 c/s, in stage *c* at 13—14 c/s. During stages *b* and *c* the babies have only a few jerks and no eye movements. The muscle tone at the level of the notch of the jaw is generally positive. It is impossible to distinguish between these two stages of quiet sleep by observations other than the EEG. Some newborns during quiet sleep have an EEG essentially of type *b*, others essentially of type *c*. Whatever the EEG aspect of quiet sleep might be, its amplitude is always higher than during the other sleep stages.

In adults, paradoxical sleep has the same polygraphic characteristics as in the newborn (where I have called it stage *d*). Quiet sleep in the adult is subdivided into stages 1, 2, 3, and 4 on the basis of differing EEG characteristics:

Stage 1 is characterized by a low-voltage EEG in which the alpha waves are absent.

Stage 2 is still characterized by the absence of alpha waves but spindles of 14 cycles per second appear.

Stage 3 is characterized by spindles but they are mixed with delta waves of high amplitude.

Stage 4 is characterized by continuous delta activity of high amplitude.

During all these 4 stages of quiet sleep in normal young adults, EMG activity is present at the level of the chin muscles.

KAUFMAN: You found less REM sleep, less paradoxical sleep, in the premature than in the fullterm infants. This is in contrast to the findings of Roffwarg and other people?

PETRE-QUADENS: Yes, but Roffwarg assimilates the rapid eye movements and the isolated eye movements into the same stage. That is to say, he includes both stages *a* and *d* in one stage called "active sleep". This explains why he obtains a curve showing 100 per cent active sleep in the young prematures.

We pay more attention to the grouping of the eye movements and we describe as paradoxical sleep only those periods where bursts of rapid eye movements occur. This explains why, instead of having a curve showing 100 per cent paradoxical or stage *d* sleep in the young premature, we obtain a curve showing that sleep characterized by rapid eye movements is rare in the very young premature and that it increases progressively to reach its highest proportion at 36 weeks of gestational age. Incidentally, Roffwarg did not study any very immature babies.

BERGSTRÖM: How do you define isolated eye movements?

PETRE-QUADENS: The paper runs at a speed of 15 millimetres, and one page represents 20 seconds. When we have two or more eye movements per page we call it REM sleep (that is, stage *d*), and when we have less than two we regard it as stage *a*. There were more sucking movements and gross startles in stage *a*—where there were less than 2 eye movements per 20 seconds—than in true paradoxical sleep. The pattern of eye movements as recorded by the electro-oculogram is also different. The isolated eye movements are mainly vertical.

ROBINSON: And stage *a* with the isolated eye movements usually occurs when the baby first goes to sleep?

PETRE-QUADENS: Yes. Stage *a* precedes—and follows—paradoxical sleep.

SCHULTE: Don't you think that you should divide the mentally retarded children into several groups according to the aetiology of their mental retardation? For example, we found that in quiet sleep hypothyroid infants had fewer spindles, whereas infants with phenylketonuria have a great amount of spindles. If one takes all these mental retardation cases together the result might be misleading because in the individual groups the findings are different. For this reason, in the last few years our approach has been to take a group of children with the same condition for example phenylketonuria, at the same age, and to compare the results with those from another group, for example children with hypothyroidism, at a similar age.

PETRE-QUADENS: We did not have enough cases of individual conditions in each age group. However, in any particular age group the data on all the mentally retarded children taken together fell in a Gaussian distribution, and that is our justification for considering them together.

SCHULTE: The connection between steroids and sleep states is interesting. There is evidence now that some steroids have a considerable effect on the membrane excitability of neurones and on certain brain structures. If one feeds pregnant rats with steroids the newborn infants are hyperexcitable and have a low threshold for convulsions.

Development of Sleep in Infancy

JAROSLAVA DITTRICHOVÁ[1]

Institute for the Care of Mother and Child, Prague

DEVELOPMENT OF QUIET SLEEP

THE TASK OF our laboratory is to study the development of, and the individual differences in, the higher nervous functions in early life—approximately in the first half year. We study development from different points of view in order to assess the factors which might influence it either positively or negatively.

I would like first to show some examples of our analysis of the development of quiet sleep, or state 1 according to Heinz Prechtl's terminology. The polygrams were recorded about 8 p.m. after the evening feed and we tried to catch three sleep cycles in each child. Besides that, we observed a group of children for the whole period from 4.30 p.m. until 5.30 a.m., but in these observations we recorded only body movements, respiration, and observed eye movements; we did not record EEG, EMG, or EOG. Figure 1 shows a portion of a polygraphic recording of state 1 in a newborn child: you can see *tracé alternant* in the EEG, the presence of EMG activity at the chin, the regularity of respiration, and the absence of eye movement. In children about 4 weeks old *tracé alternant* disappears, and irregular, slow waves prevail. One can then see runs of waves at 12 to 15 cycles per second which later—in approximately 2 weeks—develop into typical sleep spindles.

Figure 2 shows a portion of a polygraphic recording of state 1 in a 20-week-old child. Slow, high amplitude waves prevail. In the fronto-parietal leads one can see some spindles. EMG activity is present at the chin, respiration is regular, and there are no eye movements.

[1] Dr. Karel Paul also took part in these studies.

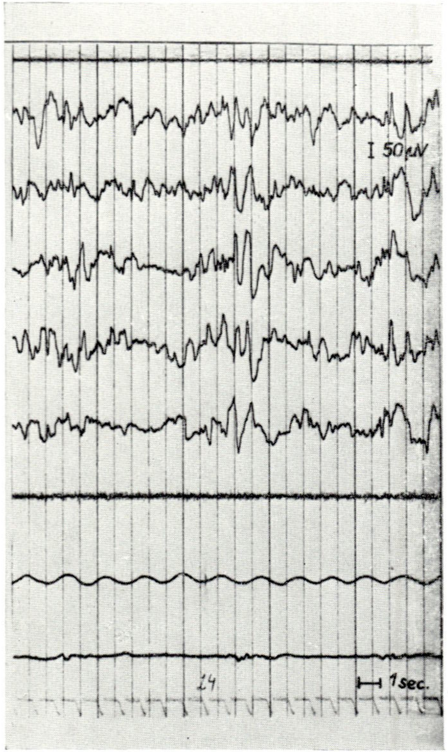

FIG. 1.

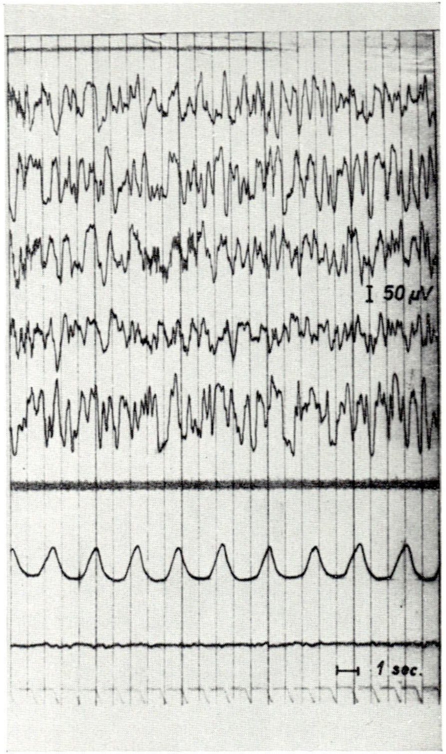

FIG. 2.

FIG. 1. Polygraphic recording made during quiet sleep in a newborn child. The first five lines are EEG. The sixth line is the EMG of the chin muscles, the seventh line respiration and the eighth line the electro-oculogram.

FIG. 2. Polygraphic recording made during quiet sleep in a 20 week old child. Key as for Fig. 1.

The respiratory rate in quiet sleep diminishes with age. Figure 3 shows the average respiratory rate during quiet sleep in children aged from 2 to 24 weeks. The average respiratory rate in the 2-week-old children is approximately 40, and it diminishes significantly by the tenth or twelfth week of life to approximately 30 per minute.

I would now like to show you the developmental changes in the total amount of state 1 and in the duration of individual periods of state 1 in the first half year. Figure 4 represents the average duration in

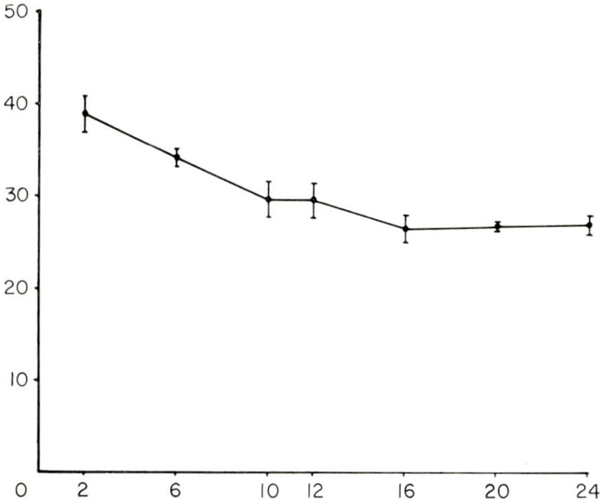

FIG. 3. Changes of respiratory rate during quiet sleep with age. Ordinates: respiratory rate per minute. Abscissae: age in weeks.

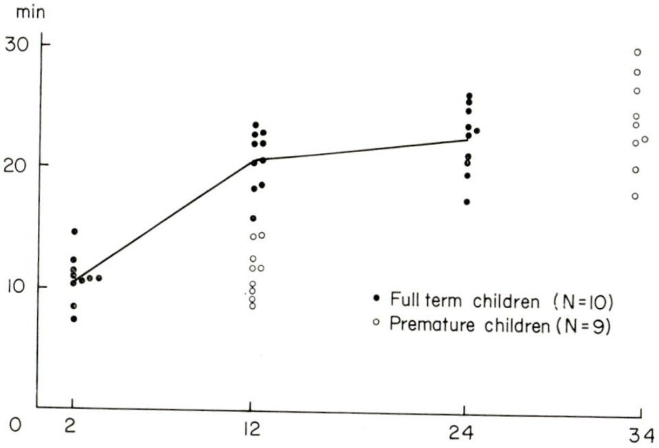

FIG. 4. Duration of individual periods of quiet sleep in premature and fullterm infants. Ordinates: duration in minutes. Abscissae: age in weeks.

minutes of individual periods of quiet sleep in ten children born at term, and in nine born prematurely. In the infants born at term the average duration of individual periods of quiet sleep is about 11 minutes in the second week of life and about 22 minutes in the twelfth week. This difference is significant, but the difference between the twelfth and the twenty-fourth week of life is not significant. We can compare the data from nine premature children with those from the children born at term. Seven of the premature children were born 10 weeks before term and we started observation in the twelfth week of life, that is, in the second week of their corrected age. We included data also from two premature children born 8 weeks before the expected date; their corrected age was also 2 weeks. Comparison of the premature children with fullterm children shows that the duration of individual periods of quiet sleep is different; but if we use the corrected age of the premature children, and therefore compare these results with the results of the fullterm children in the second week of life, there is no significant difference between the two groups. The same is true if we compare the 34-week-old premature children with 24-week-old fullterm children.

Observations were made on babies continuously from 4.30 p.m. till 5.30 a.m. at ages from 2 to 34 weeks. Figure 5 shows the percentage of this observation time which the baby spent in quiet sleep (state 1) at different ages. Both in the fullterm children and in those born prematurely, the percentage of time spent in quiet sleep increased significantly with increasing age. If we compare these two groups according

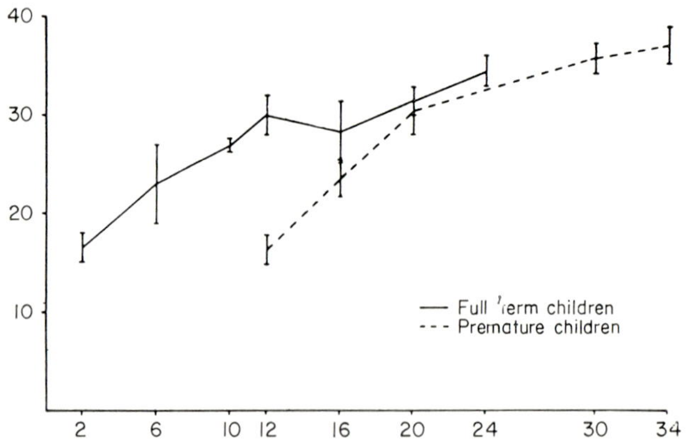

FIG 5. Percentage of total sleep time spent in quiet sleep during the period 4.30 p.m. to 5.30 a.m. in premature and fullterm infants. Ordinates: quiet sleep as percentage of total sleep. Abscissae: age in weeks.

to their chronological age we can see the difference between them. However, if we compare the premature children according to their corrected age (making allowance for their prematurity) with fullterm children, the difference between these two groups disappears.

These results show that the total duration of quiet sleep and also the duration of individual periods of quiet sleep is related to the gestational age or to the maturity of the central nervous system rather than to chronological age from birth.

DEVELOPMENT OF PARADOXICAL SLEEP

I would now like to discuss the development of state 2 in our children. Figure 6 shows a polygraphic recording made during state 2 (using Prechtl's terminology) in the first week of life. The left side of the figure shows the characteristic features of state 2. The EEG is low and irregular with a voltage of 15 to 30 microvolts and there is no difference between the recording from the dorsal and from the frontal areas of the head. In

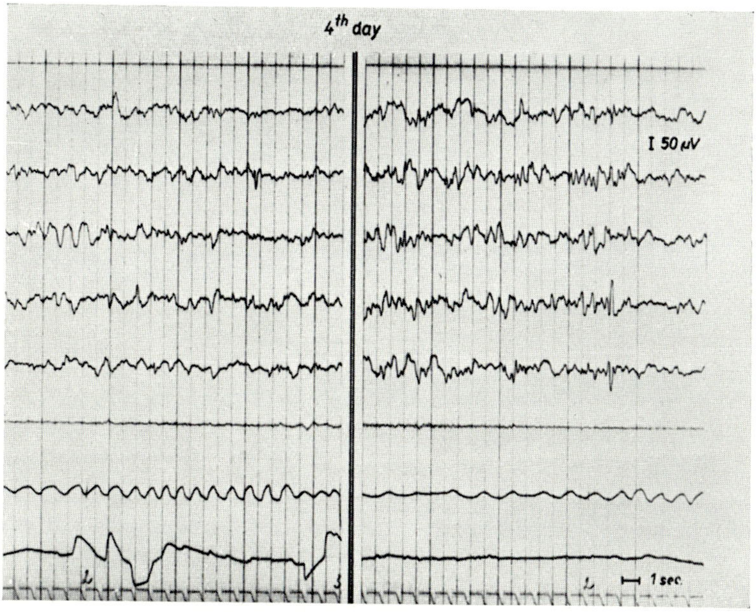

FIG. 6. Polygraphic recordings made during paradoxical sleep (left) and transitional sleep (right) in a 4-day-old child. Key as for Fig. 1.

the frontoparietal lead one can see waves of higher amplitude at 1 to 2 cycles per second. EMG activity of the chin muscles is reduced and respiration is irregular. One can see eye movements. The right side of Fig. 6 shows, according to our criteria, a transitional state from paradoxical sleep into quiet sleep. Figure 7 shows a child in the same states at 6 weeks.

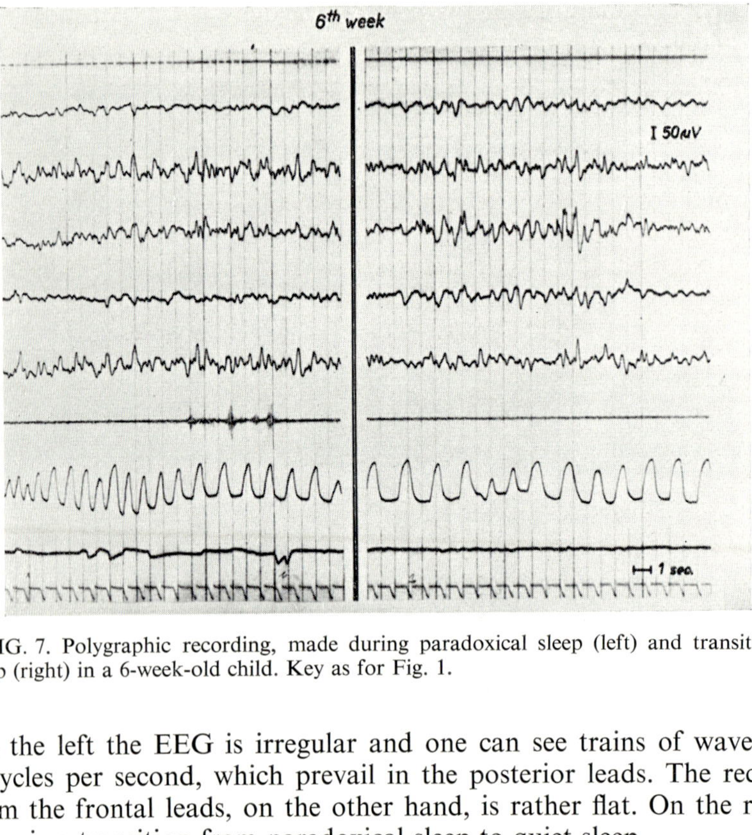

FIG. 7. Polygraphic recording, made during paradoxical sleep (left) and transitional sleep (right) in a 6-week-old child. Key as for Fig. 1.

On the left the EEG is irregular and one can see trains of waves at 2 cycles per second, which prevail in the posterior leads. The record from the frontal leads, on the other hand, is rather flat. On the right there is a transition from paradoxical sleep to quiet sleep.

Figure 8 shows a similar recording from an infant of 16 weeks, which would be typical for ages 12-20 weeks. On the left, during paradoxical sleep, rhythmic activity prevails. Its frequency varies from 2 to 4 cycles per second, and its amplitude is about 80 microvolts. Respiration is irregular and there are eye movements. The right side portrays the transition from paradoxical sleep into quiet sleep.

Figure 9 shows the mean duration of reduced EMG activity, of the presence of rapid eye movements (REMs), and of EEG activity characteristic of paradoxical sleep. The bottom row shows the total duration of rapid eye movements occurring simultaneously with EEG changes. The data are derived from two or three sleep cycles in six children. One can see that the changes in EMG activity last longest. We could observe the reduced EMG activity in nearly all cases before the changes in other parameters were present, and again after the end

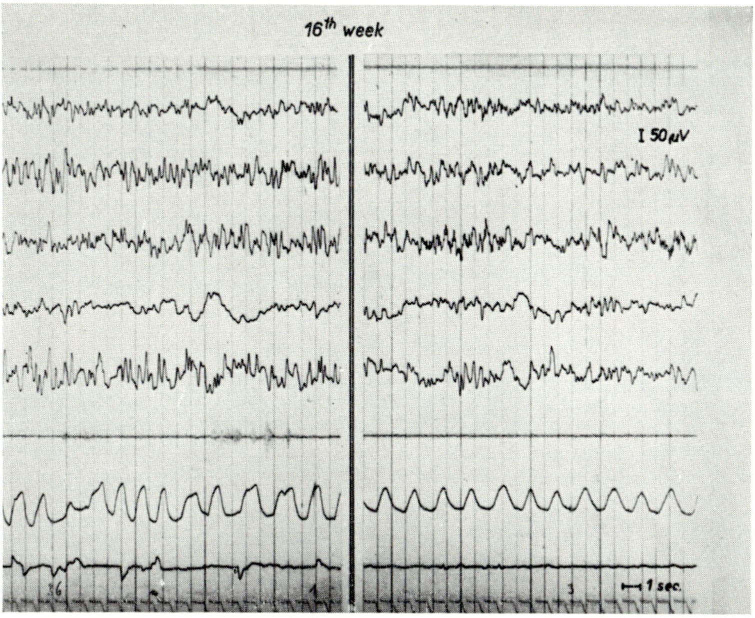

FIG. 8. Polygraphic recordings made during paradoxical sleep (left) and transitional sleep (right) in a 16-week-old child. Key as for Fig. 1.

of REMs and EEG changes. It sometimes persisted even when the EEG or respiration were already characteristic of quiet sleep. For this reason it seems to us that the changes in EMG activity are less suitable than the other two criteria for the differentiation of paradoxical sleep from transitional states. The length of the periods of REMs diminishes with age. The same is true of the EEG: in the second week the changes of paradoxical sleep last 30 minutes, diminishing to approximately 11 minutes in the twentieth week. If we examine periods in which REMs and EEG changes occur simultaneously, we can see again that their duration is related to age.

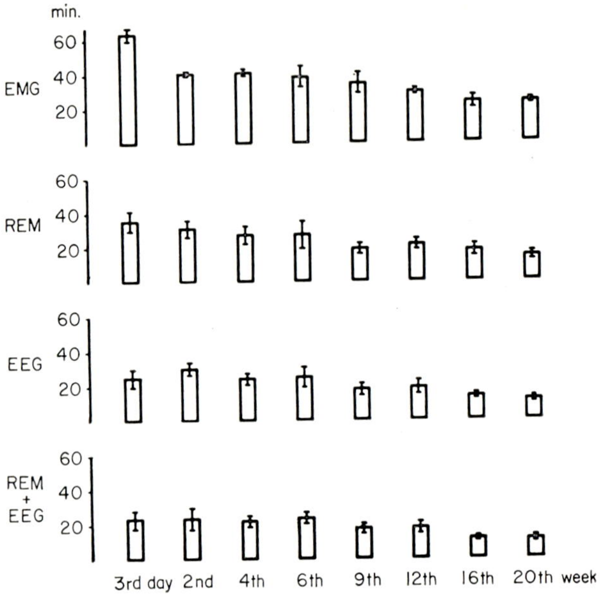

FIG. 9. Mean length of individual periods during which particular criteria of paradoxical sleep are present at different ages. Ordinates: time in minutes. Abscissae: age in weeks. EMG: absence of EMG activity in chin muscles. REM: rapid eye movements. EEG: changes characteristic of paradoxical sleep. REM + EEG: simultaneous presence of characteristic EEG changes and of rapid eye movements.

CONCLUSION

Our results showing the differences in the duration of changes in different parameters might lead to the question: Which state is to be considered as paradoxical sleep or state 2? Is it the state during which changes are expressed in only one parameter or the state during which changes are present in more than one parameter? A second question which seems to us more important is: How frequent is the state during which there are changes in only one parameter and under what conditions is the paradoxical state expressed in more than one parameter simultaneously? This method of analysis seems likely to be fruitful for assessment of the development of sleep and of its disturbances.

Though we are able to assess the development of sleep in our children and to complement the data obtained by other methods, it is difficult to explain the changes or even to know what level of explanation should be used in interpreting these results. There are similarities between state 1 or quiet sleep in infants and synchronized sleep in animals, and we know something about the mechanisms and areas which control synchronized sleep in animals. Our results show that with increasing age the proportion of sleep occupied by quiet sleep becomes longer, as do the individual periods of quiet sleep. It may be that the areas of the brain responsible for quiet sleep become more mature with age, but this is only a very rough impression and only very hypothetical. The prolongation with age of the individual periods of quiet sleep is very important for sustaining sleep. We know from the work of Moruzzi (Magnes *et al.*, 1961) that parts of the brain stem reticular formation, interacting with certain regions of the cortex, are necessary for maintaining synchronized sleep. It is possible that these areas have become more mature in the older child who has a greater ability to sustain the period of quiet sleep. But this is very hypothetical and I wonder how much we really know about the brain mechanisms which underlie the development of sleep in children.

REFERENCE

MAGNES, J., MORUZZI, G. and POMPEIANO, O. 1961. Electroencephalogram-synchronizing structures in the lower brain stem. In G. E. W. Wolstenholme and M. O'Connor (Eds.), *The nature of sleep.* Ciba Foundation Symposium. Churchill, London. Pp. 57–78.

Discussion

SCHULTE: In the infants of 24 weeks' chronological age, you had a decrease of respiration rate in state 1, that is, in quiet sleep. But at 24 weeks of age there are at least three stages of quiet sleep according to the EEG. Is there a difference in the rate of regularity or respiration between these different EEG stages?

DITTRICHOVÁ: I think so. We compared the respiratory rate and the rhythm of respiration during the spindle stage and during the high amplitude stage, and there was a difference. It therefore seems that, in the analysis of development of quiet sleep in young children, it is useful to separate EEG stage 4 from stage 3 or 2.

PRECHTL: One danger in discussion of state is forgetting that our state concept is a matter of agreement on criteria, so that it is a very artificial thing. First we must stick to very strict criteria and, secondly, when we analyse the duration of the various states, we must be quite sure what the environmental conditions are. I can think of at least two which have a considerable effect on the duration of the various states: environmental temperature and clothing. There are probably many more, but I always need to know these two, at least, before I understand data on duration. What were Petre-Quadens' and Dittrichová's conditions?

PETRE-QUADENS: In our studies the children slept in a bed, in a quiet but not sound-proof room where the EEG of course was functioning, and it makes a noise. All our data were collected on the second night, to avoid "first night" effects.

DITTRICHOVÁ: The important question is what can influence the duration of particular states. We tried to keep the conditions constant. The room temperature was 22° C and the children were clothed. The humidity was about 50 to 60 per cent.

WOLFF: By what mechanism does the mean length of periods of quiet sleep increase with age? After a feed the first period of restful sleep is the longest, and subsequent ones become successively shorter. Even the newborn baby has the initial long period of quiet sleep. What happens with increasing age is that the subsequent periods become relatively longer. One would miss this effect by looking only at the mean duration of quiet sleep.

DITTRICHOVÁ: We compared the duration of individual periods of quiet sleep during the whole night, too. We saw that all periods of quiet sleep became longer with increasing age. There was also a significant difference between the first period after evening feeding in newborns and in 12- to 24-week-old children: the first period lasted approximately 17 minutes in newborns and 30 minutes in older infants.

MACKEITH: Does the frequency of feeding make a major difference to the long periods of quiet sleep?

WOLFF: I haven't persuaded mothers to feed their babies more often to see if it will increase the periods of long sleep, but what we have tried is to apply "white" noise to prolong these periods. If you put on a white noise during irregular sleep you can put the baby into regular sleep again. However, if you use the noise in the middle of a period of restful sleep, the most you can do is to extend that period by about 3 or 4 minutes beyond the usual duration of quiet sleep. I have the impression that there is a natural cycling which is not easily manipulated.

PRECHTL: We have tried to feed babies in regular sleep or in irregular sleep states, and the cycles are not shifted by more than 3 to 5 minutes.

BERGSTRÖM: Can one explain the development of quiet sleep from the point of view of inhibitory influences from the cortex? We know there are suppressive areas in, for instance, the premotor cortex, the extrapyramidal cortex. If this quiet state could be the result of active inhibition, then perhaps one could think that the cortical inhibitory systems are maturing and then inhibiting the whole system.

DITTRICHOVÁ: That is possible but very hypothetical. Probably the maturation of the whole system and the developing interplay between various parts of it play a role in the development of quiet sleep.

PLOOG: Is it still thought to be true that Jouvet's paradoxical sleep has its localized focus in the rhombencephalon? If Jouvet's findings in cats can be applied to humans, this might be a take-off point for discussing the maturation process.

PETRE-QUADENS: Jouvet's work is especially concerned with the abolition of the electromyogram, because he agrees that even if we destroy the rhombencephalic area, rapid eye movements remain. Jeannerod and Sterman have found evidence of prefrontal inhibition during REM sleep. (M. Jeannerod *et al.*, 1965. *Electroenceph. clin. Neurophysiol.* **18,** 554; M. B. Sterman and C. D. Clemente. 1962. *Expl Neurol.* **6,** 103.)

PLOOG: Both the prefrontal areas and the rhombencephalic area have to be functioning to produce the phenomenon of rhombencephalic sleep?

PETRE-QUADENS: Yes.

PRECHTL: I doubt these ideas concerning the neurophysiological organization of regular sleep. It is not simply that the reticular formation does something and the cortex inhibits it. The organism has difficulty in building up regular respiration, regular heart rate, and the high-amplitude EEG. It takes a much longer time to build this up than to disrupt it. The EEG amplitude certainly depends, among other things, on the P_{CO_2} in the brain: increase the P_{CO_2} and you get a high amplitude, reduce it and you get a low amplitude. We need to know, for instance, what the P_{CO_2} is. It might be that the regular, relatively shallow respiration brings the baby into hypercapnia and hence this sudden switching to the other state. There is obviously less of the stable, regular state—quiet sleep—in the early stages of development than in the later stages. This must be a maturational effect. If there is something wrong in the system—in whatever area—you get a disappearance or a significant decrease of regular sleep. We see this in both apathetic babies and hyperexcitable babies. The apathetic babies have significantly fewer rapid eye movements and a markedly prolonged irregular sleep. We must be careful in transferring data from the adult cat to the human newborn. The stages look very similar, but the organization must be different because the response patterns you get to various stimuli are completely different.

ROBINSON: The mean arterial P_{CO_2} tends to be lower in preterm infants with very irregular breathing in the form of periodic breathing than in those with more regular breathing (Chernick *et al.* 1964. *J. Pediat.* **64,** 330.).

The Infant:
development of vision

Vision in Infancy: Structure-function Relationships

G. BRONSON

Mills College, Oakland

DR. BOWER'S PAPER (p. 211) will present hard data, but first it might be well to note some kinds of early visual behaviour, and suggest how these phenomena might be interpreted. I want to try to relate the development of the central nervous system to the development of visual behaviour, with the general hypothesis that more complex visual functioning will emerge as higher levels of the CNS become functional.

Unfortunately, we have a difficulty in that there is no direct evidence on the functional development of various parts of the nervous system, and therefore I find that one must rely almost exclusively on Conel's anatomical analyses (Conel, 1939, 1941, 1947). There is, however, a certain advantage to Conel's work. Since this massive piece of research was done by one man we are not confronted by the problem of trying to equate different techniques or different criteria used in studying development, coming from different laboratories which explored different parts of the nervous system at different ages. It's all of a piece. Conel analysed the histological development of neural cells within the neocortex of infants at various ages after birth. He selected his subjects as being normal from a neurological point of view. He had just a handful of cases available at each age, so one must take his normative statements as being approximations: they could well be a week or two off from the modal level of development of the population from which he was sampling. He studied infants shortly after birth, at 1 month, 3 months, 6 months, and 15 months, and then at 2 and 4 years. Throughout the first year the general ordering of development within various areas of the cortex seemed to follow the same pattern: the primary motor areas were most developed; the primary sensory areas came second; sensory association areas were third; and the prefrontal lobes were markedly retarded for the first 2 years. Now the main point that seems significant is that Conel found little change in the neocortex during the first month of life; however, when he examined the 3-month infants he found that marked development had occurred during the second and third months. One can't really say from his data when the neocortex begins to play a significant functional role, but one can use the course of anatomical development as a perspective from which to view behavioural development.

Let me turn briefly to the behavioural evidence on visual development, which seems to match rather well the thesis that throughout the first month there is little change, and then between 1 and 3 months a marked developmental advance.

At birth, visual behaviour includes pupil dilatation, which is probably subcortical in meditation, and visual following which, I suggest, is also subcortical. I suggest this partly on evidence from studies of other mammals—adult dogs, for example, seem to follow a target better if you remove the visual cortex. Also there are reports that human infants born without a neocortex still show this visual pursuit phenomenon (Jung and Hassler, 1960).

During the second month you find evidence of visual pattern recognition. Visual pattern recognition implies two things: firstly, the ability to perceive complex patterns, and secondly, the capacity to encode patterns, since recognition implies that previous experience is affecting reactions to the contemporary input. The development of visual recognition in the second month seems to fit very well with Conel's finding that marked neocortical development begins in this period. The smiling response is a useful index of pattern recognition; beginning at around 6 weeks an infant will smile on presentation of a face. And I think it is most relevant that premature infants who have had an additional 10 weeks of visual experience do not smile earlier than fullterm infants (*see* p. 165)—evidence that the age at which visual pattern recognition is achieved is not determined only by the accumulation of a prerequisite amount of visual experience. Something else must be delaying the development of smiling, and I suggest that this is neocortical maturation.

Finally, I want to make a brief reference to the work of Fantz (1964), who has a technique for simultaneously presenting two visual targets to infants and observing the length of fixation on one target or the other. He finds, in the first 2 weeks of life, what he calls "pattern discrimination": the infants stare longer at one target than at another. He may present, for example, a blank circle as opposed to a bull's eye, or a bull's eye compared with stripes, and the amount of time spent looking at one or the other target is not random: there is a preferential fixation on one target. I would like to suggest, however, that this does not necessarily indicate pattern perception in the sense that adults perceive patterns. It seems likely to me that this ability to discriminate between visual patterns, which you find in the first weeks of life, is not the anlage of pattern perception, but is mediated by a more primitive process; true pattern perception—the ability to encode, to remember complex visual patterns—requires neocortical mediation and is probably not present at this early age. How then does one account for Fantz's material? Some time ago Sackett (1963) pointed out that the organizational capacity of the bipolar cells at the retinal level is probably sufficient to distinguish the contour qualities of Fantz's stimuli. If that is the case, then you could have pattern discrimination without really having pattern perception. Feedback from visual input to eye muscles, which determines fixation, could be entirely at a subcortical level without involving neocortical mediation. There is one piece of evidence from Fantz himself which seems to support this interpretation, although as far as I know, Fantz has not discussed this possibility. He found that during the third month infants began to prefer looking at novel visual patterns. He was using the same kinds of patterns as before, but he would present one pattern to infants for a considerable period, and then present simultaneously the "familiar" and a novel pattern; the infant would shift his gaze to the novel one. This implies that the previously exposed pattern had been encoded. Fantz did not find this phenomenon until age 2 months. Before that, visual preference seemed to be stimulus-bound: it was not a function of how much past experience the infant had had with the visual targets. This indicates that there was no encoding of these patterns; you could predict the pattern on which the infant was going to fixate from knowledge of the stimulus object without having to know the infant's previous visual experience.

This is as much as I want to present, at this time. I have made a very crude dichotomy here between neocortical processes and subcortical processes, and I am sure we can refine this somewhat further.

REFERENCES

CONEL, J. L. 1939. *The postnatal development of the human cerebral cortex.* I. *Cortex of the newborn.* Harvard Univ. Press, Cambridge, Mass.

CONEL, J. L. 1941. *The postnatal development of the human cerebral cortex.* II. *Cortex of the one-month infant.* Harvard Univ. Press, Cambridge, Mass.

CONEL, J. L. 1947. *The postnatal development of the human cerebral cortex. III. Cortex of the three-month infant.* Harvard Univ. Press, Cambridge, Mass.

FANTZ, R. L. 1964. Visual experience in infants: decreased attention to familiar patterns relative to novel ones. *Science* **146,** 668–670.

JUNG, R. and HASSLER, R. 1960. The extrapyramidal motor system. In J. Field (Ed.), *Handbook of physiology.* Sect. I: *neurophysiology.* Vol. II. American Physiological Society, Washingto D.C. Pp. 863–927.

SACKETT, G. P. 1936. A neural mechanism underlying unlearned, critical period, and developmental aspects of visually controlled behavior. *Psychol. Rev.* **70,** 40–50.

Perceptual Functioning in Early Infancy

T. G. R. BOWER

Harvard University

MOST OF MY work has been on supposedly more complex visual functions than perception of brightness, colours, lights, and so on. It has been concerned with concepts like shape constancy and size constancy. Not only are such visual functions considered much more complicated but, among American psychologists at least, they are also thought to involve learnt skills. I shall not spend much time on techniques: that aspect will be discussed later (p. 225). Because of the rather crude techniques that I am currently using, the age of the infants in most of my studies is about 6 weeks. It is possible to work with much younger ones, and I plan to do so in the future.

The standard procedure, as in any conditioning study of perception, is that you train the infant to respond in the presence of one stimulus, reinforcing only when that stimulus is present. The stimulus is an object which the infant can see; the conditioned response is a head turn in one direction or the other. I try to bring the infants up to a high rate of response, and I am attempting to get all the infants in the experiments to meet the criterion of one response every 2 seconds, for that rate wipes out any need to look at state variables. In terms of response strength and response rate, all the infants we finally included in the perception tests were the same, and they responded very similarly in the tests. We have had very little trouble with individual differences. A practical difficulty which limits the number of studies one can carry out is lack of subjects. We find these experimental sessions cannot be much more than a day apart to get good conditioning, and not too many people can bring their babies in for 10 consecutive days at the same time every day without a break—minimum requirements for good conditioning.

The first series of experiments was on size constancy. The problem is illustrated in Fig. 1. According to the viewer's distance from them,

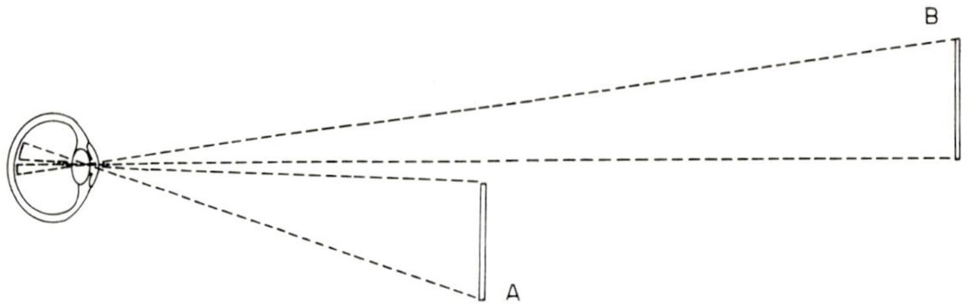

FIG. 1. Size constancy. Two objects of the same physical size may produce very different retinal image sizes and yet be seen as the same size. Reprinted with permission. Copyright © 1966, by Scientific American, Inc. All rights reserved.

two objects of the same physical size project images of very different size on the retina. An object of a particular size projects an image three times as large when it is 3ft away from the viewer as when it is 9ft away. The question is: Can infants recognize the identity of size despite variations in the size of the retinal image? In other words, can they perceive distance and can they use distance in combination with the retinal image size to pick up the true size of objects?

The structure of the experiment is shown in Fig. 2. We trained an infant with a cube which was 1ft on each side, side-presented, 3ft away. The infant was trained to respond in the presence of this stimulus;

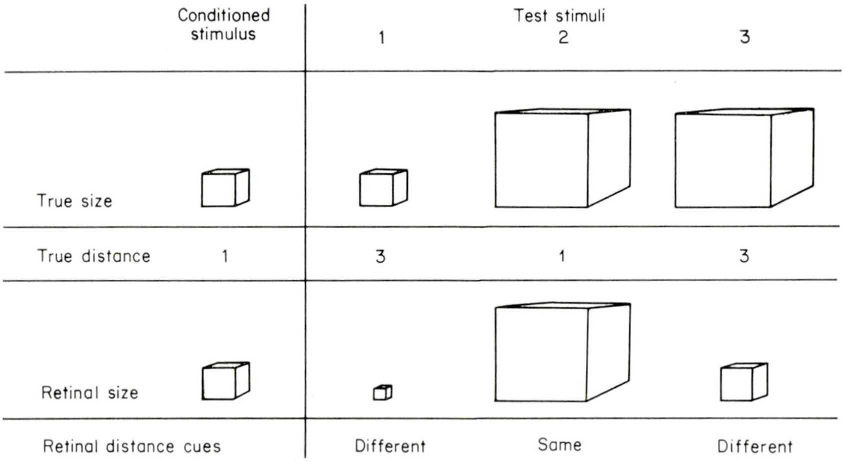

FIG. 2. Similarities and differences between the CS and the three test stimuli used in the experiment on size constancy. Reprinted with permission. Copyright © 1966 by Scientific American, Inc. All rights reserved.

he learnt never to respond when the cube was not there. After the discrimination had been well established and the infant was responding at a high rate, we shifted it into a generalization test. During generalization testing no reinforcement is ever given. We used four stimuli in the generalization testing: the conditioned stimulus which was shown in its original position, at its original distance and, presumably, with the same retinal size; a cube of the same size at three times the original distance, so that the retinal image was very small (test stimulus (1)); a new stimulus which was larger (three times the size of the conditioned stimulus) shown at the same distance as that at which the conditioned stimulus had been shown, and projecting a much wider retinal image (test stimulus (2)), and the same cube as in test stimulus (2) shown at three times the distance of the training distance so that it projected the same size of retinal image as the conditioned stimulus.

In terms of physical size, we can see that the conditioned stimulus and test stimulus (1) are the same physical size, and that test stimulus (2) and test stimulus (3) are completely different sizes. Now, if we look at the retinal sizes, we can see that the conditioning stimulus and test stimulus (3) have the same retinal size. Their retinal images are virtually identical. All four stimuli were presented, one after another, in a counter-balance order—four times each, counter-balanced with every one of the subjects. The problem was whether the infant would distribute the responses according to real physical size or according to retinal size; in other words, would the generalized responses be to the conditioned stimulus, that is, to the same physical size, or would the response split so that the infant responded to the retinal size only? The results were that the infant responded with a total of something like 90 responses to the conditioned stimulus; about 55 responses to test stimulus (1) which is the same physical size as the conditioned stimulus but a different retinal size; about 50 responses to test stimulus (2) which is a different physical size but at the same distance; and approximately 20 responses to test stimulus (3) which was the same retinal size but a different physical size at a different distance. This discrimination pattern shows very clearly, I think, that whatever the infants were responding to, they were not responding to the simple retinal variable. In fact, they seemed to be responding almost perfectly to physical size and physical distance, with the retinal variable playing almost no role at all.

The next series of studies was on shape constancy—a very similar problem in that a rectangle is projected on the retina as a rectangle only when it is in the frontal parallel plane. As soon as it is rotated away from the subject in the third dimension to any extent, it becomes a trapezoid. The question is: Are these infants of 6 weeks of age able to distinguish a rectangle from a trapezoid? Fig. 3 shows a true rectangle with a rectangular retinal image, a rectangle which has been rotated and gives a trapezoidal retinal image, and a trapezoid in the frontal parallel plane projecting a trapezoidal image on the retina like that projected by the rotated rectangle.

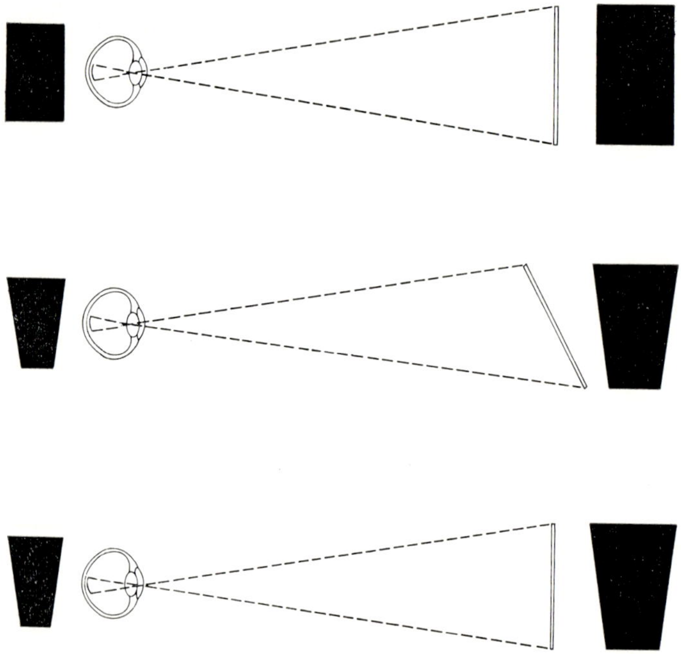

FIG. 3. Shape constancy. The retinal image of a rotated rectangle is more like that of trapezoid than that of a rectangle in the frontal parallel plane, yet adults and, to some extent, infants seem able to recognize a rotated rectangle as a rectangle. Reprinted with permission. Copyright © by Scientific American, Inc. All rights reserved.

We trained the infants in this task just as we did for the size task and came up with some very strange findings. The first was that infants had no difficulty perceiving the difference between a retinal trapezoid projected by a physical rectangle and a retinal trapezoid projected by a physical trapezoid. However, they were completely unable to discriminate between a retinal trapezoid projected by a physical rectangle and a retinal rectangle projected by a physical rectangle. We found it impossible to train infants of 6 or 7 weeks of age to discriminate between these two presentations. The response was entirely determined by the physical stimulus. The retinal differences did not enable the infants to make this discrimination. However, we were able to prove that infants can recognize orientation very well. If we showed them a surface in the frontal parallel plane they could discriminate this from a surface which had been turned to 45 degrees. By surface I mean something which has no edges. As soon as we let the edges of the surface become visible, the orientation discrimination went down. For instance, if we showed the infants only the centre portion of a rectangle rotated to 45° they could discriminate between those surfaces very well, but as soon as we let them see the edges—the shape—then the discrimination disappeared. Again, the gigantic retinal difference was just no use to them; their response was entirely controlled by the physical stimuli.

Currently I am working on a rather bizarre constancy which is usually called existence constancy, though Piaget calls it object permanency. This is the kind of constancy which we demonstrate whenever an object disappears from our view. For example, I have a box of matches here which you can all see. I move the box behind my hand and of course you know perfectly well that the box of matches is still there. Piaget claimed that existence constancy is not present in young infants. He claimed that for the young infant when an object disappears it is functionally no longer present. It really is gone for good. Piaget's original monograph on object permanence is fascinating and I have no wish to denigrate it, but he was not concerned with stimulus control. He would make an object disappear in any way he could—by dropping a hat on it, throwing it away, and so on. However, existence constancy depends on precise stimulus sequences which I will illustrate. For example, imagine a movie in which an object appears in two frames, and in the third frame there simply no longer is an object (Fig. 4). It just disappears

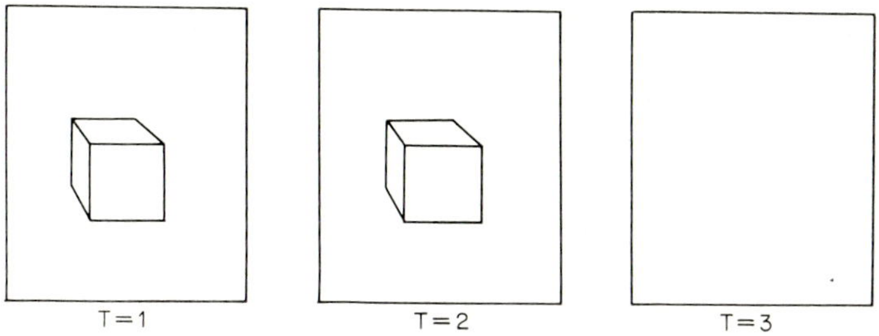

FIG. 4. An instantaneous disappearance sequence which leads to a failure of permanence for infants and adults.

instantaneously. This is the kind of disappearance which even in human adults would lead to loss of perceptual constancy. The object is perceptually gone; there is no existence constancy. Let us compare this with another sequence in which you start off with an object in the first frame, in the second frame you see half an object, in the third frame you see a small piece of that object, and in the fourth frame nothing (Fig. 5). Permanence occurs in this case. If we show this sequence to an adult he believes that the object is still there, behind a screen or something of the sort.

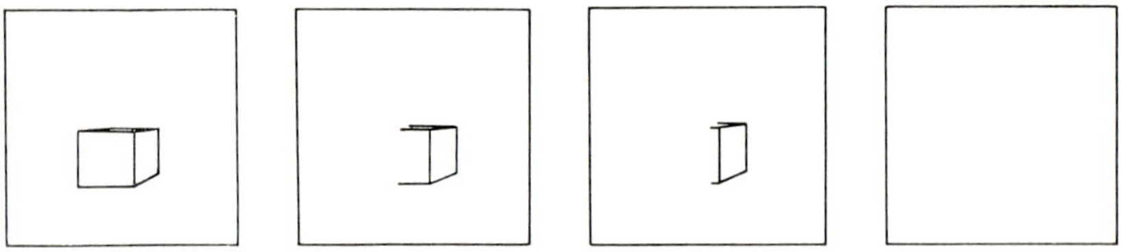

FIG. 5. A local perspective disappearance, simulating gradual passage of an occluding screen, leads to permanence in infants and adults.

We trained infants to respond to an object, reinforced them for responding to the object, and then made the object disappear in a number of ways. It disappeared suddenly, or it disappeared in the gradual way seen in Fig. 5, or it stayed there and was not reinforced. Infants whose conditioned stimulus disappeared gradually responded for quite some time, although not nearly as much as an infant whose conditioned stimulus did not disappear at all. That the infants who were shown this kind of slow disappearance sequence continued to respond, indicates, I think, that the conditioned stimulus, although no longer present in stimulation at all, was still functionally present for them. This is existence constancy, or object permanence as Piaget has described it. This is one of the few things that we have studied in proper developmental perspective, starting with young infants and following them up for a year. Although with the very youngest infants we have studied, at about age 2 weeks, there is always this kind of existence constancy, it has very grave limitations. The first is that if we make this disappearance sequence very rapid, then the object is gone for good. As infants grow older there is always a continuous monotonic increase in the disappearance speed at which they will continue to behave as if the object were present. We have also studied memory parameters with this design and found that, as the rate of disappearance speed which they can tolerate increases, so does the duration of the memory—the length of time at which they can remember that the object is there. With these two parameters and a third one, response latency, we can account for 99 per cent of Piaget's data on object permanence. The residual 1 per cent is the most important, of course. It seems to consist of learning to disregard perceptual information completely.

We also have carried out some studies on the development of Gestalt perception and what the developmental effect of the Gestalt was. Gestaltists have used a number of laws with which to explain perception. An important ability of our perception is to see an object such as a wire triangle with a bar over part of it. (Fig. 6) and to perceive that the triangle is continuous behind the bar, that there is not a gap. We trained

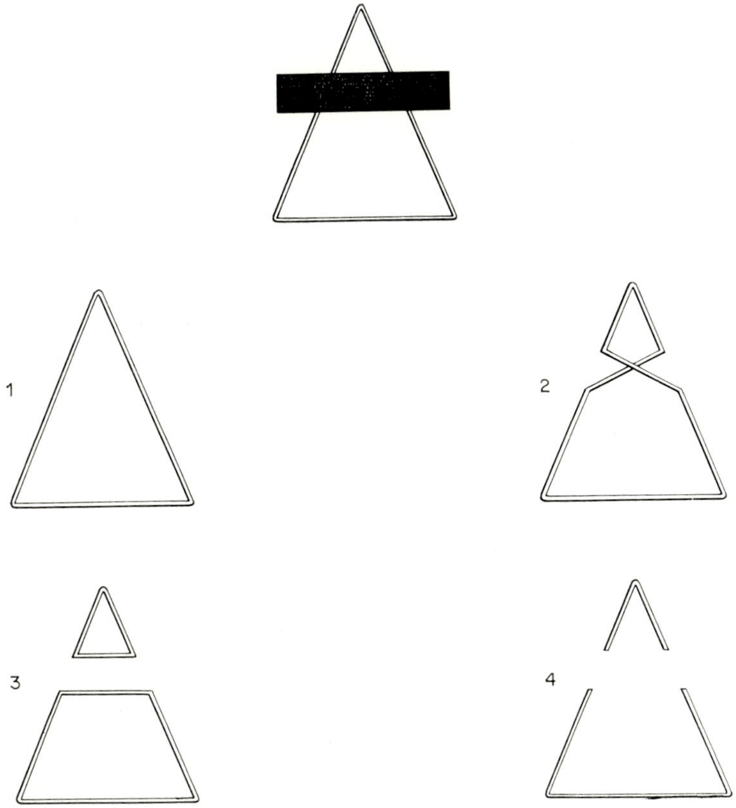

FIG. 6. Good continuation. The top figure could be any of the four below. However, infants and adults see it as a complete triangle. Reprinted with permission. Copyright © 1966 by Scientific American, Inc. All rights reserved.

an infant to respond to the complete stimulus, triangle with the bar, and then gave him a generalization test with the four other stimuli shown in Fig. 6.

We discovered that a number of Gestalt laws were operative. The 6-week-old infants who were trained with the triangle with the bar over it, when given the other stimuli, transferred most of their responses to the complete triangle. They did not transfer to any of the other physically possible stimuli. Again, I found that the law which is called "continuation" is operative, and also that the law which is called "common motion" is operative. The latter states that if two or more elements in an array move together, they will be seen as a unit; that was also found to be operative very early. The one thing for which I can find no evidence by operant method or any other method until infants are really rather old is proximity. By proximity I mean that those elements that are closer to one another than to any other will be seen as a unit. We tested this ability in a conditioning situation to find out what effect it had on the response if we broke up a unit so that two units became three. For example, in Fig. 7a, A and B appear as a unit, and C is seen as a unit by itself. In Fig. 7b, by contrast, A, B and C are equally units, with no

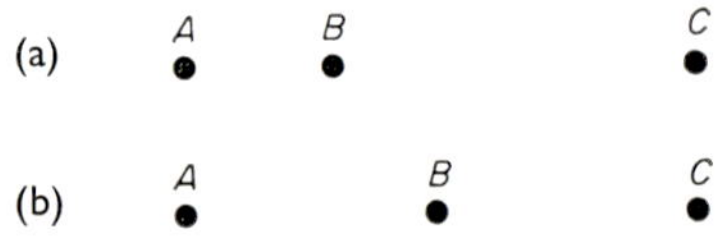

FIG. 7. (a) Proximity: adults see this display as two units, (AB) and (C) Infants apparently do not. Infants confuse the array shown in (a) with the display shown in (b).

coalescence at all. I can obtain no evidence that infants discriminate between these two presentations, although different stimuli might give better results.

Figure 8 is taken from an experiment on heterogeneous summation. The law of heterogeneous summation states essentially that a whole is equal to the sum of its parts. It has always been used by ethologists as a

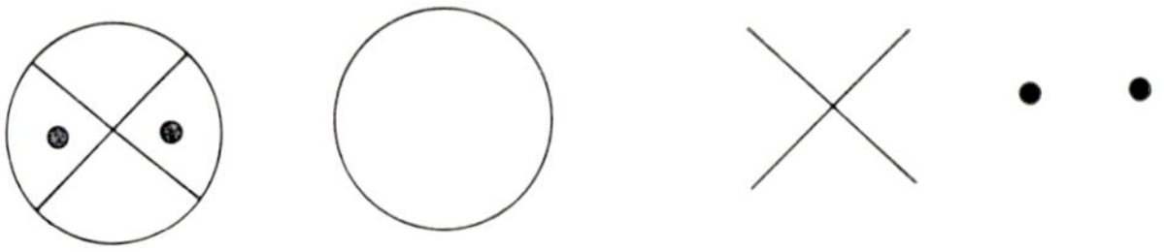

FIG. 8. The whole and its parts used in the experiment on heterogeneous summation.

law governing the elicitation of both innate and learnt responses. Ethologists have pointed out that young organisms operate according to the law of heterogeneous summation but older organisms operate according to Gestalt principles. Gestalt principles, of course, argue that the whole is a great deal more than the sum of its parts—that it is somewhat different from the sum of its parts. Heterogeneous summation has always fascinated me because it is so simple, unlike the Gestalt laws which are mathematically complicated to apply. So I trained babies to respond to the left-hand pattern in Fig. 8 and then gave them generalization tests in which all four stimuli were presented. I simply counted the responses to all the stimuli and then added up the number of responses that each part elicited. I compared the sum with the number of responses that the whole pattern elicited to discover if there was any significant difference. In infants up to 10 weeks, there was none. The whole was essentially equal to the sum of its parts. By 14 weeks, this was no longer true and it appeared that a whole may be equal to something like one and one-third of its parts. Somewhere between 10 and 14 weeks of age the infant's visual system began to follow a completely new law of operation, a new law of pattern discrimination. The pattern is no longer just a collection of elements, but is, in fact, a whole in a mysterious sense, in the Gestalt sense. This is an important experiment because the results show that there are qualitative differences in perceptual functioning at different ages in infancy. When you look at such things as shape and size constancy, there is no qualitative difference, only a quantitative difference: the capacity increases as the infant gets older. Pattern perception is different: somewhere about 10 to 14 weeks of age there is a qualitative shift along with the quantitative shift.

As far as brain mechanisms are concerned, my initial encounters with neurologists were rather unhappy. In terms of structural maturation, most of these functions were supposed to be impossible. I think the important thing for us now is to try to see what the responses really represent. Observers of older infants will find that they are all very sensitive to motion, and that they can use motion gradients very effectively. I find no evidence that they can make use of static arrangements. There is no evidence of pattern perception. "Heterogeneous summation" is the opposite of pattern perception. In these older infants there is a kind of space perception which is dependent on motion dynamics. I do not know about other species, but if you look at Torsten Wiesel's work on the neonate or premature cat cortex, one thing that is very evident is that the motion analysers are very mature already. I think if we just gave the human infant a set of motion analysers, he would be able to produce behaviour which would look like space perception and size constancy and all the rest of it without pattern perception, which is something that comes much later. Looking at the inability of the infant to handle patterns, one is almost, regardless of one's feelings, forced to think about the amount of information that the infant can carry. In most of these studies we use very refined stimulus situations. Think of the shape experiment—an infant can discriminate shape and he can discriminate orientation, but he cannot discriminate shape and orientation simultaneously. There seems to be a limit to the way in which he can handle multiple sources of information at one time. If we think back to the disappearance sequences, infants show good existence constancy with a stimulus which disappears slowly, but if the stimulus disappears quickly they just do not pick this information up. So, once more, we have some evidence that infants cannot use multiple pieces of information simultaneously. The response of very young infants to approaching objects, which is speed-dependent, again suggests that there is an upper limit to the information that can be handled.

Dr. Bergström has already discussed informational processes in development. What is the neural substrate of increasing ability to handle information? Is myelination perhaps involved? I should be grateful for any clues.

Discussion

BRONSON: Visual adaptive mechanisms must have operated in primitive organisms; with evolution, more complex visual capacities emerged that served analogous adaptive purposes but at a higher degree of sophistication. We might view the human nervous system from this perspective. The visual system consists of a hierarchy of increasingly complex mechanisms; from the developmental perspective, the first weeks of life represent a transitional period during which more complex systems become sufficiently mature to override the more simple visual mechanisms. Now to link this with Dr. Bower's material: I made a distinction between primitive mechanisms, which are largely precoded, and more complex mechanisms which are able to encode complex visual patterns. As a working hypothesis I think of neocortical tissue as being basic to the visual experience. More primitive visual reactions—those of the neonate—would involve pathways from the retina through the superior colliculi and back to the eye muscles. I don't know how much reticular structure would be involved in this subcortical system, probably relatively little. It should, therefore, have little capacity for the encoding of visual patterns. Thus it is difficult to explain Bower's "fading reaction", where the infants seem to distinguish between a sudden and a gradual disappearance, which seems to require visual memory but which was present during the first weeks of life. In the light of this evidence, and my belief that neocortical visual systems are essentially non-functional during the first weeks, I suggest that two levels of complexity might be distinguished among subcortical visual mechanisms: the very primitive one involving the pathways through the superior colliculi, and perhaps a somewhat more complex one, involving what Pribram has called intrinsic areas, within the thalamus. This latter system might provide the basis for some of the very early visual behaviour which seems to require the encoding of visual patterns.

BERGSTRÖM: Why do you need reticular structures in the visual system in this connection?

BRONSON: I assume that learning of any complexity requires a diffusely interconnected network in which the initial connections are largely random.

PLOOG: The same functions can be achieved in very different organisms. The octopus is able to discriminate so as to perform rather complex learning tasks. I am just referring to this because of the general questions of neuronal structure and perception. To a turkey (which again has a very different brain) the Lorenz-Tinbergen T-shaped dummy bird "flying" in one direction represents a bird of prey and in the other direction represents a goose or something like that. Schleidt solved this by showing that the cue is not Gestalt perception but the angular velocity and the distance. So there are two physical functions which create that response. I don't think there is a direct correlation between the organization of the nervous system and Gestalt perception or any developmental aspect of this perception. Nevertheless, I think that if one sticks to human perception, one can correlate certain functions with certain stages of performance or ability to perform.

BOWER: Consider space, which is as much a condition of our life as the composition of the air we breathe. If there were any perceptual capacity which ought to be the same throughout phylogeny and the same throughout ontogeny, it would have to be the spatial behaviours and spatial responses. Adaptively we know that it is almost impossible to go far enough down in the phylogenetic scale to define an organism which does not display properly co-ordinated spatial behaviour, with size constancy, shape constancy, etc. My colleague, Trevarthen, an anatomist, who has been working on the mapping of the external, visual world in the nervous system, claims that it is essentially identical in all mammals. It is functionally identical even in fish. The argument is that as far as physical stimulation is concerned there is a great deal of identity, as far as function is concerned there is identity for space, and as far as anatomy is concerned there also seems to be some identity. Now this is, I think, the sort of thing Lorenz had in mind when he said that space had to be built into us before any other behaviour could take place. I think we must separate this aspect of perceptual function from, for example, the human response to the face—which is probably species-specific; or the fowl's response to the hawk, which is again probably species-specific—because why should I be afraid of a hawk? I think we can make a clear distinction between things which should be functionally and structurally identical across phylogeny, and things which probably are species-specific. We must look at development only within a species, unless it is for perception of something like space.

ROBINSON: Bronson said that visual pursuit did not depend on neocortical function. Others have said quite categorically that it does (B. Brazelton *et al.* 1966. *Pediatrics, Springfield* **37,** 284).

BRONSON: My statement is a working hypothesis derived from evidence that infants without a neocortex demonstrate visual pursuit. This does not imply that visual pursuit is not mediated by the neocortex later on, only that the pursuit reaction of the neonate need not imply a functional neocortex. I refer to Jung and Hassler's observations.

MACKEITH: "Later on" might be at 36 weeks' gestation or at 6 weeks after birth.

BRONSON: There is clear evidence of marked postnatal growth in the visual areas of the neocortex, but the question remains: when do they become functionally significant? The evidence of a shift in the visual behaviour of infants during the second month makes me suggest that this is the point when these areas become functionally important. It is a tenuous hypothesis but it is useful as an initial position.

BOWER: Can we distinguish "gaze-capture" vision? If you move an object across the visual field and the child can't draw his eyes away from it, this is different from active looking around, in which the child actually searches a visual field for objects. Certainly by one month the head and eye movements of the neonate are not reflex—it will look around for an object.

ROBINSON: Is this obligatory nature characteristic of a number of neonatal responses? The grasp is obligatory at birth but by 3 or 4 months it is under voluntary control. Perhaps what you say suggests that this happens much earlier with vision than it does with other items of motor behaviour.

WOLFF: Somewhere between 3 and 6 weeks. If you build a tower of cans for a baby, there is first a tendency to look at the top, that is, wherever the border is. About a week after this starts, there is up-and-down scanning. This kind of looking around is still in a sense stimulus-fixed but it can leave a certain border and scan up and down.

PRECHTL: When does the hand-eye co-ordination develop?

BOWER: Various different studies give essentially the same answer: the main developmental change in simple reaching is that the latency of the response becomes less. Gesell restricted his infants to a 30-second period within which the baby could reach. In Bruner's laboratory they have completely different results from Gesell, and they have shifted the whole range just by giving the infants a minute to reach and strike. We have found that a baby of 4 weeks will strike very rapidly and accurately at an object at certain distances. These are not just tonic neck reflexes.

The Infant:
learning and conditioning

Learning Capacities of the Human Infant[1]

LEWIS P. LIPSITT[2]

Brown University

INTRODUCTION

Historical Orientation

THE FIELD OF child development has traditionally relied on psychometric or "maturity-measuring" techniques. Though these are founded on the use of morphological models borrowed from structural biology (Gesell, 1954; Harris, 1957), they have been used even for assessing the behavioural properties of the young organism and for seeking principles explaining the origins of later behaviour in the history of the organism (Lipsitt, 1963). It has been implicitly assumed that intellectual endowment is genetically determined and essentially constant; proper attention has not been paid to the behavioural consequences of experimental precursors. These attitudes and assumptions have almost preempted the search for, and discovery of, the special capacities of infants to receive sensory stimulation in all modalities and to learn. The studies of Pratt (1954), Irwin (1943), and Marquis (1931, 1941) were notable exceptions.

No thoughtful observer or researcher of infant behaviour would deny the obvious fact that some behavioural differences are related to age. Nevertheless the human newborn can no longer be regarded as a spinal creature who can have no capacity for learning or cognitive activity because of absence or reduction of myelination or cerebral convolutions (Elkonin, 1957).

The normal human infant shows an exceptional talent for differential responding, conditioning, and discrimination learning. These are often

[1] The research reported here and the writing of the present paper were supported largely by a grant to the author from the U.S. Public Health Service, National Institutes of Health (Grant No. HD 03911).

[2] The author expresses his gratitude to the staff of Providence Lying-In Hospital, where so much of the newborn research reported here has been carried out.

achieved in a matter of minutes, particularly when the responses are relevant to the maintenance of life, or to evolutionary selection, or when they provide opportunity to explore the environment. I hold no brief for any particular mode of learning or for any special theoretical model for the understanding of specific learning effects that may be induced in the immature organism. A constricted view of the possible mechanisms whereby experimental circumstances may work their wonders would limit the accumulation of knowledge in this area, as did the premature conclusion that the structural properties of the immature organism could not possibly permit learning to occur. It would be equally senseless to allow a monolithic learning-theory orientation to shut off possible lines of inquiry as it was to permit the tyranny of an exclusive developmental-structural dogma. Indeed, it may well be that we are only beginning to understand some of the very special learning skills of the young human (Hinde, 1966).

It should no longer surprise us that organisms do not inevitably get better and better at whatever they do with increasing age. Of course there has always been acceptance of a statute of limitations for the aged in this connection; but apologists have generally considered the frailties of age to be the result of a superimposition of disease and deformity rather than a "true" developmental effect. The effectiveness of some types of stimulation, and the organism's capacity for response, become diminished in many different ways with increasing age; with respect to some human attributes the developmental decline or social destruction of a response may begin at birth. The human newborn is as good at the palmar grasp, at the Babkin response, at rooting, and even at sucking soon after birth as he will ever be again. Some of the body's glands decrease proportionately in size from birth on, while others increase and then decrease in both size and function. So, too, may certain behavioural capacities of the "growing" organism either "atrophy" or wax then wane with increasing age. It is perhaps time for someone to present the thesis that the newborn human creature is about as competent a learning organism as he can become.

Research Programme

For the past decade, I have been fortunate to have a laboratory for sensory assessment and conditioning in one of the larger U.S. maternity hospitals. Many of the infants first studied during the newborn period, along with small populations of infants from private paediatric practices, have been available subsequently for behaviour studies at various intervals throughout the first year. The eventual aim of this research programme is to document longitudinal changes (or constancies) in the learning and sensory properties of the child at least through the first year of life. The success of such studies depends heavily upon the prior development of appropriately reliable experimental stimulation techniques and upon the initial documentation of behaviour-phenomena worth pursuing across an extensive age-span. For these reasons, and because longitudinal data-cells require more time to fill, the results available thus far are concerned predominantly with the behaviours that occur at specific young ages and with the stimulating conditions necessary to elicit them. Although our concern is with processes or changes in behaviour occurring over periods of time or with repetitive stimulation, the time courses to which I shall refer here will, with two exceptions, be of relatively short duration.

The newborn laboratory in which much of this research is carried out is equipped with a stabilimeter crib (Lipsitt and DeLucia, 1960), a six-channel polygraph for the permanent recording of behavioural and autonomic responses, timing units and stimulating devices for the automatic presentation of stimuli and polygraphic monitoring of such presentations, sterilization equipment, and so on. Sensing devices include electrodes for recording heart rate, a pneumobelt and associated pressure transducer for recording respiration, and an automatic nipple device (DeLucia, 1967) with associated transducer enabling analogue recording of the infant's sucking activity and providing for controlled feeding. A cardiotachometer records heart rate, and an integrator associated with the stabilimeter enables the cumulative recording of amount of body-activity in the presence or absence of stimulation.

Brief Review of Previous Findings

As a background for the present paper, some of the previous studies carried out in these laboratories and reported in detail elsewhere will first be reviewed. Several studies (Lipsitt, 1967; Engen and Lipsitt, 1965; Engen, Lipsitt, and Kaye, 1963) have clearly demonstrated that habituation occurs in the human newborn; repetitive presentation of stimulation of moderate intensity, in this case odorants, produces response decrement over successive trials, and subsequent recovery of response whether to totally new odorants or to olfactory stimuli which were components of previously habituated compounds. Such behaviour suggests that the human newborn processes information in a rather sophisticated way, suppressing response to non-threatening stimulus signals but alerting once again if a novel stimulus, even in the same sensory modality, should be introduced suddenly. Moreover, the phenomenon of response recovery to components of previously habituated compounds indicates that some central nervous system mechanism is probably involved in the discrimination, since peripheral factors and fatigue are ruled out by the technique.

With respect to sucking behaviour, it has been established that the human newborn is keenly sensitive to momentary differences in intra-oral stimulation and that reinforcing circumstances associated with the sucking act may increase (or diminish) sucking-response frequency. In a study (Lipsitt and Kaye, 1965) which compared the sucking behaviour of infants who were administered either nipple, tube, or nipple-tube-alternation sequences of trials, it was shown that the sucking rate is greater with an ordinary nipple than with a less flexible and less rounded tube, that nipple-sucking is adversely affected by the previous administration of the tube, and that tube-sucking is made easier by previous nipple-sucking. The evidence of these lasting effects of previous experience brings us closer to an understanding of the role of prior experience in the determination of infants' behaviour.

Using the tube as a conditioning stimulus, Lipsitt, Kaye and Bosack (1966a) gave one group of infants a dextrose solution through the tube on specified trials so that these subjects received dextrose in association with tube-sucking. A control group was fed the same amount of dextrose and was provided the same experience with the tube, but tube-sucking and dextrose intake were not permitted to occur simultaneously. The first group showed a reliable increase in tube-sucking, and response decrement in extinction; the control group showed only a gradual waning of sucking in response to tube insertion in the mouth.

Also relating to mouth-opening and other feeding-like activity in the newborn, Kaye (1965) has demonstrated that it is possible to condition infants in the first days of life to make Babkin-type responses in the absence of the unconditioned stimulus (palm-pressing) initially necessary to elicit the Babkin response. Kaye produced this effect by moving the baby's hands from the hips to a position near his ears, then pressing the palms. After a series of conditioning trials of this sort, the arm movement alone was sufficient to precipitate mouth-opening reliably more often than in control subjects receiving just the arm-transport or the palm-press conditions.

The work of our laboratory has recently been increasingly concerned with the exploration of conditioning techniques using responses of the infant that may be presumed to have functional significance for the survival of the organism and for the maximization of exploratory arousal. The human infant seems capable of making many responses which have the consequence of increasing stimulus input. The assimilation of such stimulus input often results in arousing still further "searching" activity. When this relationship between the organism and the environment has progressed to a maximum (to be determined for each subject, for each type of stimulus, and for various reinforcing conditions) the stimulation loop is often "turned off" by the subject who now manifests satiation, fatigue, or habituation. This cycle of events can perhaps be best understood in operant behavioural terms, but it must be acknowledged, if not insisted, that respondent behaviour has an important role in the cycle.

RECENT STUDIES

The Newborn Infant

Conditioned head-turning. Elaborating upon techniques earlier reported by Papoušek (1959, 1960, 1961), Siqueland and Lipsitt (1966) used both tactile stimulation and nutritive reinforcement to condition head-turning in neonates. The general procedure requires tactile stimulation of the infant at the corner of the mouth, a procedure that characteristically elicits ipsilateral head-turning in 25—35 per cent of the trials prior to conditioning. Such "rooting" is usually considered to be respondent behaviour, since it requires a specific eliciting stimulus. The procedure used in these studies involved the systematic reinforcement of the respondent as if it were an operant or instrumental behaviour. Thus, on conditioning trials in which the infant turned his head appropriately in response to the tactile stimulus, a nipple was quickly placed in the baby's mouth, allowing it to suck and to be nutritively reinforced. In all these studies, auditory stimuli preceded and occurred simultaneously with the tactile stimulus, in order (1) to determine whether classically-conditioned anticipatory head-turning might increase in frequency over conditioning trials, and (2) to afford an opportunity to study discriminative behaviour as well as non-differential conditioning behaviour.

In our first study the procedure was to sound a buzzer for 5 seconds, during the latter half of which the left cheek of the subject was stroked. If the infant responded ipsilaterally, dextrose was administered for 2 seconds. Eighteen subjects in the second and third days of life received thirty trials of conditioning, with 30-second inter-trial intervals, while another 18 matched control subjects received the same programme of stimulation, subject for subject, but were given the dextrose, on appropriate trials, 8—10 seconds after termination of the tactile stimulus.

Response to the tactile stimulus increased strikingly in the experimental group—from approximately 30 per cent to 80 per cent—while the matched control group merely declined in the frequency of ipsilateral head-turning.

In an elaboration of the technique, two groups of infants 2—4 days old were studied to see whether differential reinforcement for two responses, left versus right head-turning, would lead to discriminative responding. Now two auditory stimuli were used, a tone and the buzzer, and trials were alternated between the left and the right cheeks, the buzzer being associated with touch to one side and tone with touch to the other. The tone and buzzer were each the positive stimulus for a random half of the subjects, and a basal assessment period enabled application of the positive stimulus to the less favoured head-turning side. For the 20 experimental subjects, reinforcement was presented after ipsilateral turns to the positive stimulus (R^{S+}), but not after turns to the negative stimulus (R^{S-}). Twenty control subjects received the same total number of reinforcements, subject for subject, but dextrose reinforcement was presented 8—10 seconds after tactile stimulation and was not contingent upon head-turning. Learning was reflected in relative shifts in percentages of R^{S+} and R^{S-} over trials. The shift occurred in the experimental group, which rose in R^{S+} responding from approximately 20 per cent to 75 per cent, while the control group declined from 20 per cent. Learned differentiation of head-turning behaviour in the newborn was thus substantiated.

Next, in an attempt to induce a still more difficult differentiation, the two auditory stimuli served as positive and negative cues for reinforcement at one side only. Sixteen infants, aged 48 to 116 hours, were divided into two groups: for one the tone was positive and the buzzer negative, while for the other the designations were reversed. Turns to right-sided stimulation in the presence of one auditory stimulus were reinforced, while right turns in the presence of the other auditory stimulus were not. After original training $S+$ became $S-$, and $S-$ became $S+$ in each group. As previously, stimulus presentations occurred on a 30-second inter-trial interval basis, and tactile stimulation overlapped the last half of the tone or buzzer. Under such conditions, responding to the positive stimulus increased sharply, from approximately 25 per cent to 70 per cent, while response to the negative stimulus changed negligibly. Upon reversal of the stimulating conditions, the expected shift in behaviour was such that the previously negative and now positive stimulus eventually generated reliably more ipsilateral responses than the previously positive and now negative stimulus.

In none of these three studies did conditioned subjects demonstrate a reliable increase in classical anticipatory responding during the sound-stimulus presentations, but it is apparent from the differential behaviour established in the third study that the auditory stimuli had discriminative signal functions.

Free-operant head-turning. In a further study of reinforcement patterns and extinction in human newborns Siqueland (1968) demonstrated large differences in free-operant head-turning behaviour, during extinction, as a function of differences in reinforcement schedules during acquisition. An apparatus for the continuous polygraphic monitoring of head-turning activity was used, and a 10° head-turn arc in either direction was adopted as the required operant. Three groups of eight newborns each in the third and fourth days of life were given 5-second presentations of a non-nutritive nipple as reinforcement. Conditioning procedures involved a 3-minute baseline period, 25 reinforcements, a 5-minute extinction period, 15 additional reinforcements, and a second extinction period of 3 minutes. Training in one group was on a continuous (100 per cent) schedule, and a Ratio group received one reinforcement for every two responses early in learning and one for every three responses later. A third group received reinforcement for each 20-second period in which a head movement was *not* made (that is, a 10° movement delayed reinforcement for 20 seconds). The groups were thus equated on total number of reinforcements, prior to each extinction period, while their patterns of reinforcement varied.

The analysis of data was concerned with extinction behaviour. It is very clear that the three groups varied greatly in frequency of head-turns during both of the extinction conditions. The Ratio group gave reliably more responses than the Continuous Reinforcement group, and the third group produced the fewest responses. In fact, reliable increases in responding over the course of extinction were evidenced by the third group, as would be expected by the fact that for this group conditioning involved the suppression of head-turns.

While the Siqueland-Lipsitt studies demonstrated strong learning effects in a situation involving nutritive reinforcement, the Siqueland study shows very clearly that opportunity to suck non-nutritively may also serve as a powerful reinforcing event. This study is also the first clear demonstration of free operant conditioning in a situation that does not rely on eliciting stimulation as in the Papoušek and the Siqueland-Lipsitt studies.

Temporal conditioning. Marquis (1941) has shown that human infants within the first 10 days of life are capable of adjusting their activity patterns and sleep-waking cycles (Irwin, 1930) to temporally controlled feeding schedules. To explore the capacity of the neonate for short-term temporal conditioning Ambrose and Lipsitt (unpublished) studied temporal responsivity under three different modes of stimulation: auditory, vestibular, and olfactory. Two methods were used to assess whether temporal conditioning occurred: (1) presentation of mock or test trials after a series of stimulations to determine whether responses would occur at the accustomed time of stimulus presentation, and (2) examination of increased responding, over training trials, to determine whether there is an increased tendency for anticipatory responses to be made in the interval immediately preceding the customary stimulus presentation time. To provide vestibular stimulation Ambrose designed a motor-driven baby rocker which automatically moves the baby up and down through an excursion of 3 inches at controlled rates of speed. Besides the vestibular stimulation of rocking, the infants in the present study received olfactory stimulation from anise oil on a cotton-swab, and sound stimulation produced by dropping a pegged wooden ball through a constant distance to a wooden surface. The auditory stimulus was an 87-dB clack of noise, of essentially momentary duration, while the odorant presentation and rocking stimulation lasted 5 seconds on each trial. Three groups, each of five infants, received the stimulus types in different orders: (1) sound, odorant, rocking, (2) odorant, sound, rocking, and (3) rocking, sound, odorant. Each of the three stimuli was presented to each infant on eight successive occasions, then was followed by three "mock" trials during which the polygraph record was marked at the regular 30-second interval (the interval between all stimulations). No stimulation whatever was administered on mock trials.

The analysis of responding was concerned with respiration, heart rate, and motility, the latter represented in either the electromyographic or stabilimetric records (these being almost perfectly correlated). The response of greatest concern was that occurring during the nine mock trials. The period for response-assessment was a 5-second unit of time. The first such period began 30 seconds after the previous stimulus presentation and the subsequent ones were at 30-second intervals. A response was defined simply as any change in pattern form or frequency relative to a baseline period. Baseline was the 5-second interval immediately preceding this time unit, unless an anticipatory response occurred, in which case the 5-second unit immediately preceding that interval was used. When two judges were unable to make identical judgements concerning the occurrence of response on mock trials, the trial was scored "uncertain". In the case of heart-rate change a stringent criterion was adopted:

a change of two beats or more per 5-second interval (24 beats per minute) was required. Responding during the mock trials was compared with control intervals which were of comparable duration but which followed each mock trial by 15 seconds. Each subject then had nine opportunities to respond during mock trials and nine opportunities during control intervals. The mean number of responses made during mock trials was 4·53, as compared with mean control-interval responding of 2·46, a difference resulting in a t of 4·55, significant at the ·01 level (df = 14).

Although the magnitude of the temporal-conditioning effect as found here is not great, further corroboration of infant capacity for such learning has been found by Fitzgerald and associates (1967) for pupillary responding (although not for eyelid blinking), and further study of such phenomena seems warranted.

The "Bronshtein effect". Ever since the reports of Bronshtein and his colleagues (1958) American researchers in neonatal behaviour have been fascinated by the possibility of suppressing ongoing behaviour by external stimulation. This phenomenon is now commonly referred to as the Bronshtein effect; for example, if an infant has a nipple in his mouth and is sucking ordinarily (that is, is engaging in sucking behaviour dictated by his idiosyncratic congenital patterns under no special conditions of external stimulation), the sudden introduction of an extraneous stimulus such as a sound, visual stimulus, or odour will tend to disrupt the sucking pattern. The phenomenon has been interpreted as one of external inhibition or the arousal of orienting behaviour which competes with other ongoing behaviour (Sokolov, 1963; Lynn, 1966).

In connection with the disruption of ongoing behaviour through the introduction of external competing stimulation, Bronshtein reported that habituation of such disruption occurs over successive stimulus presentations. Thus although the introduction of a tone at first had a marked effect upon the sucking pattern this effect diminished progressively with increasing experience. In our laboratory two studies have failed to replicate the Bronshtein suppression effect (Kaye and Levin, 1963), but other investigators (Keen, 1965; Haith, 1966) have been able to document it clearly.

Semb and Lipsitt (1968) completed an investigation in which the Bronshtein suppression effect without habituation has been clearly demonstrated in newborns. The study was designed to provide optimal conditions for its occurrence in that the tonal stimulation was introduced on specific occasions when the child was sucking, not on a random-presentation or a temporally locked basis. At the same time, and in the same subjects, the obverse response to that of sucking-suppression was studied. On occasions when the infant was not sucking, the same tone was systematically introduced. Under these conditions activation of sucking is readily induced; in fact activation of sucking in the presence of a non-sucking state of the infant occurs about twice as frequently as the sucking-suppression phenomenon.

In this study, 30 normal newborns were subjected to a series of 91-dB acoustic stimuli, each lasting 1 second. Continuous polygraphic records were taken of the infant's respiration and bodily activity, and a manually operated marker simultaneously recorded presentations of acoustic stimulations. The baby's sucking activity was also continuously monitored by the automatic nipple in the mouth and this provided the pertinent response measure for the experiment. Control trials were interspersed throughout the test session in order to provide a basal level of change in sucking behaviour in the absence of acoustic stimulation, and these "mock" trials were also recorded on the polygraph record. A suck was defined as a minimum of 5-mm pen deflection. On any given trial the infant could be sucking and either stop or not upon presentation of the tone, or could be not sucking and either start or not. Any infant who did not suck at a minimum rate of 20 responses per minute during a pre-test period was eliminated from the study. A trial period was initiated 13 seconds after the previous tone stimulation, and the tone was administered if, and only if, the infant had been either actively sucking or not sucking for at least 2 seconds. Following such a 2-second observation period, the tone was administered (or a mock trial occurred). Thus whether the trial was to be a suppression or an activation trial depended solely upon the sucking behaviour of the baby at the moment of stimulation. The data were treated in terms of probability of change of sucking state as a result of stimulus presentation. Overall, response of either type was reliably greater on stimulus-presentation occasions than on mock trials, and two major methods for analysis of the suppression and activation effects demonstrated both effects reliably, with the probability of activation being reliably greater than the probability of suppression (with numbers of trials in which each could occur ruled out). An interesting additional finding of the study was that there was no habituation either to sucking suppression or to sucking-activation.

The Semb-Lipsitt study provided the impetus for a study now in progress, on which I can report preliminary results. It appeared from the polygraph records of the previous study that when the tone happened to occur in the early portion of a sucking-burst the probabilities that sucking-suppression would occur were higher than if the tone fortuitously occurred later in a burst. Haith's (1966) study used this procedure. A study was therefore designed to make use of this observation and is now in progress. Tones of the same intensity as in the study reported above (Semb-Lipsitt) are administered with a minimum 15-second inter-stimulus interval but only when the infant is at the beginning of a burst of sucking (that is, after approximately three full-amplitude sucks of a burst). Thus after each tone a 15-second interval occurs; then the record is monitored for the next occurrence of a burst, after three sucks of which tone is delivered. This occurs over a series of ten trials, following two basal periods in which (1) the infant's resting respiration, heart-rate, and body activity are recorded for 3 minutes and (2) the nipple is placed in the infant's mouth for a 3-minute no-stimulation period. Preliminary data indicate that sucking suppression does clearly occur under the aforementioned conditions, and it also appears that habituation of such sucking suppression occurs over a series of trials, at least in some subjects. Further analyses of these data will be directed towards the question of whether infants with different basal levels of sucking, or different sucking patterns, behave differently in the presence of external acoustic stimulation. An ancillary finding which is already apparent from this study is that the heart rate is clearly dependent upon sucking activity; during each burst of sucking, the heart rate is elevated until an inter-burst interval ensues, at which time the heart rate diminishes until the next burst.

Older Infants in the First Year

Conjugate reinforcement. At this point I should like to leave consideration of the newborn to discuss recent advances in techniques for studying behaviour in the older infant. It is our eventual aim to have techniques for longitudinal study of learning proficiency and for the study of specific stimulating circumstances and their short-term effects on behaviour. In studies of learning in infants, various environmental events must be sought which promote and sustain some measured behaviour. Although it is apparent to most investigators of child behaviour that infants and children engage in much behaviour that seems "self-reinforcing" only recently have there been systematic attempts to incorporate such behaviour into basic psychological theory or to study its origins parametrically. White (1959) introduced the term "competency striving", Butler (1953) the term "curiosity motivation", and Harlow, Harlow and Meyer (1950) spoke of the "manipulation drive" to refer to behaviour occurring in the absence of apparent or traditional primary drives. Hunt (1965) has spoken of infants as having a need for sensory input and opportunity to experience "recognitive familiarity", and in a physiological context Pfaffmann (1960) spoke of "the pleasures of sensation". However, in studies involving sensory input as reinforcement rather than more vital consequences of response, reinforcers often lose their effectiveness, due to adaptation or boredom, before the associative process has been demonstrated or explored extensively (Lipsitt, 1963). Recently Lindsley and co-workers (1961) and Lindsley (1962, 1963) implemented and investigated a type of reinforcement that shows promise in infant conditioning.

Conjugate reinforcement involves the presentation of a continuously available event contingent upon response, such that the event's intensity varies directly and immediately with response strength (for example, rate or intensity). The prototype is the hand-generator flashlight in which illumination intensity is controlled directly by the response rate and pressure on a trigger or dynamometer handle. Compared with episodic schedules in which reinforcement is provided either by delivery of pellets or candies, or by punitive circumstances with discrete onsets and offsets, the conjugate type of response-consequent permits (1) closer analysis of periodic changes in the value of reinforcing stimuli, and (2) maintenance of the subject in the observation situation for fairly long periods of time.

In our first use of the conjugate reinforcement technique (Lipsitt *et al.*, 1966b) 12-month-old subjects were seated in an infant chair attached to a box containing a manipulandum, a clear plastic panel. Response to the manipulandum activated a power supply which was designed to vary the light intensity inside the box according to changes in the response rate. Opportunity to see inside the box, which was otherwise dark, was proportionate to the response rate, and transition from low to high brightness and *vice versa* was gradual rather than sudden. In the box a colourful clown picture was rotated continuously. An electrical counter enabled cumulative recording of response every 15 seconds. The procedure involved the use of a basal period of no reinforcement for responding, followed by a conditioning session in which visual reinforcement was available, followed by extinction, then reconditioning, then re-extinction. The behaviour of infants in this situation even for as short a period as 15 minutes supported the efficacy of conjugate reinforcement in the study of infant learning; response rates increased from basal levels through conditioning and decreased when reinforcement was withheld.

Mobiles for conjugate reinforcement. Recently a former student of our laboratory conducted a study using her own 2-month-old infant and five other children of the same age. Following suggestions of Uzgiris and Hunt (1965), Rovee and Rovee (1969) hung a mobile over the infants' cribs. The infants were familiarized with the mobile for several weeks before the experimental procedure began. For four of the infants, the experimental session lasted 27 minutes, and for two others the session lasted 46 minutes. For the experimental session, the infants were loosely clothed with legs exposed and feet bare. Observations were made from the foot of the crib, with the observer out of view of the child. The 27-minute procedure involved a 3-minute baseline period during which the operant level of right-foot kicks was established, a 15-minute acquisition period involving conjugate reinforcement wherein the mobile was linked to the child's leg via a light string, and a 5-minute extinction period in which the string connecting the child's limb with the mobile was detached. The two subjects serving in the 46-minute session received a 10-minute re-acquisition period followed by 5 minutes of re-extinction. The operant response conditioned was that of leg flexions, and the reinforcement was that of visual feedback from the moving mobile. It should be emphasized that the mobile always remained in position during the basal and extinction phases, but limb movements during these phases were not instrumental in activating movement of the object.

Reliability tests indicated that limb movement increased, relative to the basal level, when the mobile could be moved by the leg and that detachment of the string connection resulted in diminution of leg activity.

The Rovees observed that the behaviour of the infants changed qualitatively as well as quantitatively over the course of the sessions. Gross, diffuse body activity occurred early in the sessions, but after experience in operating the mobile the infant used smooth direct thrusts of the limb to which the cord was attached. During the reinforcement phases intense kicking was often followed by rather long pauses, during which the infant remained still but kept his gaze fixed on the swaying figures.

Following the Rovees' work, another study was conducted by Leslie Smith on her own child between the ages of 2 and 5 months. She tested the infant with a multitude of mobile objects varying in colour and form; some were offered with associated sound stimulation. In this study, movements were registered by an automatic counter. As in Rovee's study, it was shown that a 2-month-old infant quickly learns to move his limb appropriately to activate the visual reinforcer, and that limb movement increases during reinforcement periods and diminishes during extinction periods. Interesting findings from this pilot investigation include the strong suggestion that with increased experience in the situation the infant begins to "test" the effect of the response, so that after some training the infant comes to recognize quickly when his responses are effective and when not and adjusts his behaviour accordingly and rapidly. The mobile-reinforcement situation provides a potentially sensitive procedure by which to assess infants' preferences for various types of stimulation. For example, when the child in the Smith study was presented with a red mobile its response rate was consistently higher than when it was presented with an otherwise identical but white mobile.

The Smith data show clearly that infants will behave in a mobile-movement situation for very long periods of time without apparent fatigue or satiation except as indicated by occasional pauses. To be sure, the technique is hampered by the occasional occurrence of fussy or crying behaviour—such activity increases limb-movement responses considerably—and for purposes of assessing cognitive processes it would appear that the procedure ought to be "shut off" during fussy periods of this sort. On the other hand these studies suggest that crying itself might become an important subject for study. It seems that crying occurs rather frequently some minutes after the onset of an extinction condition, as if the crying may be generated by the frustration of expectation. It was noted that the crying could sometimes be abated by re-institution of a conditioning period.

Sucking and visual stimulation. Over the past 2 years Siqueland has developed a line of research in which infants as young as 3 months of age can control the visual input which they receive by sucking on an automatic nipple linked to a slide projector. The presentation of visual stimuli or the experimental withdrawal of these stimuli is contingent upon the infants' making high-amplitude sucking responses. When high-amplitude sucking is required to activate the projector light, infants rapidly adjust the intensity of sucks to produce higher illumination, much as previously described in the conjugate reinforcement situation.

In one experiment Siqueland sought to determine whether non-nutritive sucking could be studied in 4-month-old children by the use of visual reinforcers. Subjects were 30 infants assigned to one of three groups: *Gp C* (control baseline), *Gp R* (reinforcement group), and *Gp W* (stimulus withdrawal group). The first group provided a baseline reference for 10 minutes of non-reinforced sucking, and the other groups received a 13-minute session consisting of conditioning, extinction, reconditioning, and re-extinction. For *Gp R* reinforcement was contingent on sucking during the conditioning periods, and for *Gp W* sucking resulted in withdrawal of the visual stimulus, each criterion suck resulting in a 5-seconds delayed onset of the visual stimulus. For both groups, eight chromatic 35 mm slides showing geometric forms, cartoon figures, and human faces were presented for 30 seconds each in 4-minute conditioning blocks.

The reinforcement group showed rapid acquisition of criterion sucks, while the baseline group showed negligible change in such behaviour. *Gp W* showed a slight decrease in the ratio of high-amplitude sucking. The evidence clearly shows that heterogeneous visual stimulation may function in a reinforcing capacity to maintain sucking behaviour in infants of 4 months.

Another of Siqueland's studies compared the sucking behaviour of three age groups (4-, 8- and 12-months) in the visual reinforcement situation again using the sucking response as the operant. Highly reliable differences in sucking rates were obtained among the three age groups during a baseline-assessment session lasting 5 minutes.

Siqueland next attempted re-establishment of sucking behaviour in 12-month-old infants when such behaviour is operative in enhancing visual stimulation. Two groups of ten infants received different sets of visual stimuli. One group was shown four coloured slides four times each over two 4-minute sessions, and the other group was shown a set of eight slides twice each. The results showed dramatic increases in sucking rate for both groups as compared with baseline controls of the same age. Reliable response decrements were also obtained after reinforcement ended. Moreover, although predicted differences between the two groups were not obtained during initial conditioning and extinction phases, apparent stimulus familiarization (satiation) effects were reflected in a decreasing response rate for the 4-stimulus group during reconditioning as compared with high stable rates for the 8-stimulus group. Siqueland's work continues to explore which stimulus parameters, including comparisons across modalities, are influential in controlling an infant's sucking behaviour. The apparent case with which infants learn to control their visual environment by appropriate sucking behaviour is interesting because many observers of infants have noted that visual exploratory behaviour is often most intense in a child that is engaged in sucking. Many a mother has reported that she can most easily attract the child's gaze to hers when the infant is feeding. In the earliest days of life, sucking and visual exploratory behaviour seem to have an intimate relationship.

PROSPECTS FOR THE FUTURE

It only remains to be said that as we progress in our studies of human behaviour in the first year of life some of the seeming complexities become better understood through experimental analyses and careful measurement of the relationships between the response and the environmental feedback. Experimental techniques based on some traditional notions about the reinforcing functions of environmental stimulation have been immensely useful in leading to knowledge about the control of behaviour by stimuli. However, it must also be admitted that experimentalists must pay more attention to the ordinary non-laboratory circumstances under which the human organism generally lives and to which he seems, all things considered, remarkably well adapted. The ecologists in America (for example, Wright, 1960; Barker, 1951) and the ethologists in Europe (for example, Hinde, 1966; Eibl-Eibesfeldt, 1967) have done the field of experimental child psychology a great service in calling for increased attention to the naturalistic habitat and the built-in response repertoire of the human child. A healthy consequence is that conjugate reinforcement phenomena, for instance, are now being seriously explored by child experimentalists.

It does appear at present that modifications and embellishments of traditional classical and operant conditioning techniques seem quite in order for the further advance of understanding of infant learning behaviour. The enormous amount of effective learning which takes place during the first year of life in infants reared "naturally" is seldom accomplished under conditions exactly like those used in the laboratory to study basic acquisition and extinction processes. In real life learning trials are almost never deliberately spaced, the stimulating conditions are seldom well-controlled, and much of the infant's learning gives the appearance of occurring fortuitously.

The proper scientific study of a natural phenomenon is not usually the exploration of the fortuitous. Nevertheless it is quite possible that by taking advantage of the changing state of the baby from moment to moment, including the momentary changes in its condition of curiosity, and by using variant rather than constant stimulation conditions experimenters might understand better some of the learning processes that have often proved refractory in the well-controlled laboratory situation. It is apparent to me, for instance, that most early learning is neither of a purely classical conditioning nor of a purely operant variety, but is some sort of amalgamation of these. The Siqueland-Lipsitt finding with respect to conditioned head-turning is a case in point, inasmuch as the procedure fulfilled both respondent and operant requirements, providing both eliciting and emitting stimulus conditions. It is sometimes necessary or desirable to use an eliciting stimulus to potentiate a response which can then be reinforced operantly, thus increasing the probability of the occurrence of that response in the absence of the eliciting stimulation on future occasions. For example, the process of conditioning the sucking behaviour of a newborn with an initially low-probability level of sucking might be facilitated by pressing the infant's palms when the nipple is in the mouth, thus eliciting a higher sucking rate. This higher sucking rate may then be reinforced through feeding, eventually allowing the eliciting stimulation of the palm-press to be faded out. In a sense, we might most readily engender learned behaviour in the immature organism by violating the basic requirements of the classical and operant conditioning paradigms. The head-retraction response in the presence of a smothering stimulus may well be of this type, whereby it first occurs as an elicited or respondent behaviour but becomes a learned operant in the course of development; thus the older child positions his head so as to preclude smothering even before an actual threat of respiratory occlusion occurs. Similarly, it is not unlikely that smiling behaviour in children first occurs primarily as respondent behaviour which is supplanted or overshadowed later in ontogeny by a predominantly operant mode of occurrence (Bijou and Baer, 1965).

REFERENCES

BARKER, R. G. 1951. *One boy's day*. Harper, New York.

BIJOU, S. W. and BAER, D. M. 1965. *Child development II: Universal stage of infancy*. Appleton-Century-Crofts, New York. Pp. 3–7.

BRONSHTEIN, A. I., ANTONOVA, T. G., KAMENSTKAYA, A. G., LUPPOVA, N. N. and SYTOVA, V. A. 1958. On the development of the functions of analysers in infants and some animals at the early stage of ontogenesis. In *Problemy evolyutaii fisiolgicheskikh funkisii*. Academiya Nauk, Moscow and Leningrad. Transl. (Off. of Tech. Servs. Report No. 60–61066, 1960. Pp. 106–116) obtainable from U.S. Dept. of Commerce, Office of Technical Services, Washington, D.C.

BUTLER, R. A. 1953. Discrimination learning by rhesus monkeys to visual exploration motivation. *J. comp. physiol Psychol.* **46,** 95–98.

DELUCIA, C. A. 1967. A system for response measurement and reinforcement delivery for infant sucking-behaviour research. *J. exp. Child Psychol.* **5,** 518–521.

EIBL-EIBESFELDT, I. 1967. Concepts of ethology and their significance in the study of human behaviour. In H. W. Stevenson, E. Hess, and H. L. Rheingold. (Eds.), *Early behavior: comparative and developmental approaches*. Wiley, New York. Pp. 127–146.

ELKONIN, D. B. 1957. The physiology of higher nervous activity and child psychology. In B. Simon (Ed.), *Psychology in the Soviet Union.* Routledge & Kegan Paul, London. Pp. 47–68.

ENGEN, T. and LIPSITT, L. P. 1965. Decrement and recovery of responses to olfactory stimuli in the human neonate. *J. comp. physiol. Psychol.* **59,** 312–316.

ENGEN, T., LIPSITT, L. P. and KAYE, H. 1963. Olfactory responses and adaptation in the human neonate. *J. comp. physiol Psychol.* **56,** 73–77.

FITZGERALD, H. E., LINTZ, L. M., BRACKBILL, Y. and ADAMS, G. 1967. Time perception and conditioning of an autonomic response in human infants. *Percept. Mot. Skills* **24,** 479–486.

GESELL, A. 1954. The ontogenesis of infant behavior. In L. Carmichael (Ed.), *Manual of child psychology.* Wiley, New York. Pp. 335–373.

HAITH, M. M. 1966. The response of the human neonate to visual movement. *J. exp. Child Psychol.* **3,** 235–243.

HARLOW, H. F., HARLOW, M. K. and MEYER, D. R. 1950. Learning motivated by a manipulation drive. *J. exp. Psychol.* **40,** 228–234.

HARRIS, D. B. 1957. (Ed.), *The concept of development.* Univ. of Minnesota Press, Minneapolis.

HINDE, R. A. 1966. *Animal behaviour: a synthesis of ethology and comparative psychology.* McGraw-Hill, New York.

HUNT, J. McV. 1965. Traditional personality theory in the light of recent evidence. *Am. Scient.* **53,** 80–96.

IRWIN, O. C. 1930. Amount and nature of activities of newborn infants under constant external stimulating conditions during the first ten days of life. *Genet. Psychol. Monogr.* **8,** 1–92.

IRWIN, O. C. 1943. The activities of newborn infants. In R. G. Barker, J. S. Kounin, and H. F. Wright (Eds.), *Child behavior and development.* McGraw-Hill, New York. Pp. 29–47.

KAYE, H. 1965. The conditioned Babkin reflex in human newborns. *Psychon. Sci.* **2,** 287–288.

KAYE, H. and LEVIN, G. R. 1963. Two attempts to demonstrate tonal suppression of non-nutritive sucking in neonates. *Percept. Mot. Skills.* **17,** 521–522.

KEEN, R. 1965. Effects of auditory stimuli on sucking behavior in the human neonate, *J. exp. child Psychol.* **1,** 348–354.

LINDSLEY, O. R. 1962. A behavioral measure of television viewing. *J. advert. Res.* **2,** 2–12.

LINDSLEY, O. R. 1963. Experimental analysis of social reinforcement: terms and methods. *Am. J. Orthopsychiat.* **33,** 624–633.

LINDSLEY, O. R., HOBIKA, J. H. and ETSTEN, B. E. 1961. Operant behavior during anesthesia recovery: a continuous and objective method. *Anesthesiology.* **22,** 937–946.

LIPSITT, L. P. 1963. Learning in the first year of life. In L. P. Lipsitt and C. C. Spiker (Eds.), *Advances in child development and behavior.* Vol. 1. Academic Press, New York. Pp. 147–195.

LIPSITT, L. P. 1967. Learning in the human infant. In H. W. Stevenson, E. H. Hess, and H. L. Rheingold (Eds.), *Early behavior: comparative and developmental approaches.* Wiley, New York. Pp. 225–247.

LIPSITT, L. P. and DELUCIA, C. A. 1960. An apparatus for the measurement of specific response and general activity of the human neonate. *Am. J. Psychol.* **73,** 630–632.

LIPSITT, L. P. and KAYE, H. 1965. Changes in neonatal response to optimizing and non-optimizing sucking stimulation. *Psychon. Sci.* **2,** 221–222.

LIPSITT, L. P., KAYE, H. and BOSACK, T. N. 1966a. Enhancement of neonatal sucking through reinforcement. *J. exp. Child Psychol.* **4,** 163–168.

LIPSITT, L. P., PEDERSON, L. J. and DELUCIA, C. A. 1966b. Conjugate reinforcement of operant responding in infants. *Psychon. Sci.* **4,** 67–68.

LYNN, R. 1966. *Attention, arousal and the orienting reaction.* Pergamon, Oxford.

MARQUIS, D. P. 1931. Can conditioned responses be established in the newborn infant? *J. genet. Psychol.* **39,** 479–492.

MARQUIS, D. P. 1941. Learning in the neonate: the modification of behavior under three feeding schedules, *J. exp. Psychol.* **29,** 263–282.

PAPOUŠEK, H. 1959. A method of studying conditioned food reflexes in young children up to the age of six months. *Pavlov J. Higher Nerv. Activ.* **9,** 136–140.

PAPOUŠEK, H. 1960. Conditioned motor alimentary reflexes in infants. *Cesk. Pediat.* **15,** 861–872, 981–988.

PAPOUŠEK, H. 1961. Conditioned head rotation reflexes in the first months of life. *Acta paediat., Stockh.* **50,** 565–576.

PFAFFMANN, C. 1960. The pleasures of sensation. *Psychol. Rev.* **67,** 253–268.

PRATT, K. C. 1954. The neonate. In L. Carmichael (Ed.), *Manual of child psychology.* Wiley, New York. Pp. 215–291.

ROVEE, C. K. and ROVEE, D. 1969. Conjugate reinforcement of infant exploratory behaviour. *J. exp. Child Psychol.* **8,** 33–39.

SEMB, G. & LIPSITT, L. P. 1968. The effects of acoustic stimulation on cessation and initiation of non-nutritive sucking in neonates. *J. exp. Child Psychol.* **6,** 585–597.

SIQUELAND, E. R. 1968. Reinforcement patterns and extinction in human newborns. *J. exp. Child Psychol.* **6,** 431–442.

SIQUELAND, E. R. and LIPSITT, L. P. 1966. Conditioned head-turning in human newborns. *J. exp. Child Psychol.* **3,** 356–376.

SOKOLOV, E. N. 1963. Higher nervous functions: the orienting reflex. *A. Rev. Physiol.* 545–580.

UZGIRIS, I. and HUNT, J. MCV. 1965. A longitudinal study of recognition learning. Paper read at the biennial meeting of the Society for Research in Child Development, Minneapolis, Minnesota.

WHITE, R. W. 1959. Motivation reconsidered: the concept of competence. *Psychol. Rev.* **66,** 297–333.

WRIGHT, H. F. 1960. Observational Child Study. In P. H. Mussien (Ed.) *Handbook of research methods in child development.* Wiley, New York. Pp. 71–139.

Discussion

PAPOUŠEK: This paper is an excellent example of how one can show a rather high level of learned behaviour in the neonate. Using operant conditioning this is a bit easier to show than with classical conditioning —in particular, milder criteria are needed and that is the difference between Lipsitt's studies and ours. For example, the degree of rotation of the head which is used as the criterion at which you start reinforcing is less in Lipsitt's studies. We use 30°, whereas he uses 10°. We too have studied discrimination in the newborn. If you test discrimination before conditioning, it takes much longer for the baby to acquire than if you first condition the babies and then start discrimination. So conditioning actually facilitates discrimination; the total time spent for establishing the conditioned responses first, and discrimination second is less than if you start with discrimination. Have you any similar data?

LIPSITT: We were impressed by the remarkable speed with which the newborns developed discrimination. I can't really imagine facilitating it via a straight conditioning technique; it happens so quickly in the course of the 30-minute session.

BRONSON: Is there a two-stage learning process, one stage being more permanently coded than the other? To what degree can learning on one day still be demonstrated on the day following?

LIPSITT: We are now working on a longitudinal study of learning over the first 4 days of life, but we first had to acquire the appropriate techniques whereby we could get learning in one day. I can only quote at present the habituation data in which there was a carry-over effect from the first day of learning to the second (R. E. Keen, *et al.* 1965. *Psychon. Sci.* **2,** 265).

PRECHTL: In your first study head-turning was elicited by tactile stimulation, which means it was a rooting response. And you got responses in about 25 per cent of subjects. This puzzles me because provided babies are awake, and that it isn't just 10 minutes since they were fed, rooting is an obligatory response. What is the state of your babies?

LIPSITT: They are in state 1, 2, or 3. They are midway between two feedings at the time of the experiment.

PRECHTL: They are asleep?

LIPSITT: Yes, sometimes, although they are awake at the outset.

WOLFF: Do you stimulate them while they are still asleep?

LIPSITT: We are not controlling terribly well for state, but we ought to have a more thorough discussion of what state is all about. A large part of conditioning may actually involve changing the infant's state; obviously, you change his state of learning.

PRECHTL: We are mixing up terminology. Every change in the nervous system could be called a change in the state, but that is not what we mean. There are five different behavioural states of the newborn baby: State 1. Eyes closed, regular respiration, no movements. State 2. Eyes closed, irregular respiration, more or less rapid eye movements, small twitches. (This is what Wolff calls irregular sleep.) State 3. Eyes open, no gross movements. State 4. Eyes open, gross movements, no crying. State 5. Crying.

There are various other possible ways of classifying states in the newborn. This one is convenient and avoids confusion.

ROBINSON: These are descriptions of particular states; can you give a general definition of state?

PRECHTL: State was defined very helpfully by Ashby: "By a state of a system is meant any well defined condition or property that can be recognized if it occurs again." (W. R. Ashby. 1956. *An Introduction to Cybernetics*, p. 25. Chapman & Hall, London.) We have defined the parameters as respiration, and eyes open or closed, and movement.

LIPSITT: None of my comments about state disparages the obvious usefulness of this concept. But let us not put the concept of state in a separate category of behaviour from all other behaviours. When one conditions an organism, one is not necessarily doing something different from changing its state. That is, one effect of conditioning could very well be to disrupt an infants' respiratory activity in response to a given stimulus like the tactile stimulus. However, remarkable changes in state of our infants—in the sense in which Prechtl uses the term—did not occur over the course of conditioning. True, sometimes their eyes opened, true that sometimes their respiration became increasingly disrupted over the course of time. But we deliberately used experimental conditions that would minimize changes in what you would call state: that is, we had these children closely bundled in order to keep them in a condition of relative quietude for the duration of the study.

WOLFF: If you get rooting in 80 per cent of babies who are awake and in only 25 per cent of those who are asleep, that makes a considerable difference, regardless of how we conceptualize it. Whether the conditioning stimulus wakes the baby up is an important question.

LIPSITT: It is quite possible that one of the consequences of conditioning is a change in state. However, regardless of any such changes the nature of our experimental designs, particularly in the third of the Siqueland-Lipsitt studies, was such as to preclude state changes as an explanation for the conditioning obtained.

SCHULTE: You said the babies were swaddled in order to prevent them from changing from one state to another. The main changes of state occur whether the baby is swaddled or not. We have looked for differences in the duration of each state—while the baby was swaddled, while the baby was not swaddled, while the baby was under neutral temperature conditions, while not, and whether the baby was hooked up with all the polygraphic apparatus or not. There are some differences but they are very, very minor. The main cycle of states is well preserved provided the conditions are reasonably normal whether the baby is swaddled or not.

LIPSITT: This differs from older studies comparing clothed with unclothed babies, swaddled with unswaddled (O. C. Irwin and L. A. Weiss. 1934. *University of Iowa Studies in Child Welfare* **9,** 149).

PRECHTL: Barbiturates have a very marked effect on rooting in the first 10 days. Did the mothers receive drugs at delivery?

LIPSITT: Yes.

PETRE-QUADENS: Is the medication of the women just before and during labour always constant?

LIPSITT: No, it varies according to the obstetrician.

PETRE-QUADENS: In our clinic many women have no drugs during labour. We have found considerable difference in sleep patterns between the children born by Caesarian section—whose mothers had therefore had anaesthesia—and children born normally. I don't know how long this effect lasts on the baby.

LIPSITT: We are getting remarkable conditioning even under adverse conditions of neonatal physiology; in a population such as yours one might get even more marked conditioning. We have less conditionable subjects.

ROBINSON: How old were your oldest babies for the neonatal studies?

LIPSITT: Four days.

BRONSON: Have you ever tried to reverse Siqueland's conjugate reinforcement studies (in which the presentation of visual stimuli was contingent on the infant's performing high amplitude sucking) so that the operant behaviour is essentially a quietening one in order to get a certain reinforcement?

LIPSITT: Siqueland has done this with the sucking response. He has taught infants to stop sucking in order to get the lights on. It does occur both ways, but it takes longer to get the child to stop responding, rather than to respond more in order to get the reinforcement. It is very difficult to get an animal to stop moving around the cage in order to get a pellet of food. We got a child to reduce the intensity of his sucking in order to see better, though not to stop sucking entirely. Similarly, when I say that we got him sucking in order to turn on visual stimulation I mean we got him sucking at a higher amplitude. We can pick up any sucking intensity level and make that the criterion of responses required for sucking to activate the visual stimulation.

KAUFMAN: Does conjugate reinforcement change the sucking rate at all?

LIPSITT: The rate of sucking stays the same—just the amplitude is influenced.

PRECHTL: Have you ever recorded the course of sucking without stimulation over a long period of time? Do these sucking bursts occur throughout an hour or so under normal conditions?

LIPSITT: Yes, we have extensive basal data on sucking activity without stimulation (G. R. Levin and H. Kaye. 1964. *Child Development* **35,** 749; G. R. Levin and H. Kaye. 1966. *J. Exp. Child Psychol.* **3,** 146). Non-nutritive sucking we have found, goes down very, very little in the course of a 20-minute sucking period, and within an individual the burst characteristics with which a child sucks on the second day of life look very much like the burst characteristics on the fourth day of life—though there are differences between infants because they have individual differences in the rhythm of sucking bursts.

Individual Variability in Learned Responses in Human Infants

HANUŠ PAPOUŠEK

Institute for the Care of Mother and Child

WE HAVE ALREADY heard from two contributors who have studied head movements because these provide an easily conditionable response in newborn and young infants. We have used the method of conditioned head turning for different purposes, and also in a different modification representing a combination of Pavlovian and instrumental conditioning.

In the first studies we used milk presentation as a reinforcement of correct responses to acoustic stimuli: the sound of an electric bell (CS_1) or a buzzer (CS_2). The response we taught our subject first was to turn his head to the left with CS_1. After establishing a conditioned response to CS_1, we also studied conditioned discrimination, that is we taught the subject to turn to the left with CS_1 and to the right with CS_2. In each daily experimental session the two stimuli were each applied five times in random order. It is unnecessary to go into the details now, because I explained our methods in November 1967 (Papoušek and Bernstein, 1969).

We were mainly interested in the problems of individual differences in the higher nervous functions. First we analysed the role of age differences that appeared very significant, particularly in the first 6 months of human life. For this purpose we compared the rates and the courses of the establishment, extinction, and re-establishment of the conditioned response as well as of the establishment of conditioned discrimination in several groups of infants with different initial ages.

Then, analysing the variability of the data relating to homogeneous age groups, we tried to evaluate the role and the determination of the inborn, genetically fixed individual differences which seemed to be characteristic for each child and which appeared quite early after birth (Papoušek, 1967a, 1967b).

We found two aspects of the determination of the conditioned responses interesting when we analysed their variability in a particular individual. The first concerns the role of the general state. We studied learning only in waking subjects, but soon we noticed differences in the level of waking and its relation to the level of the conditioned responses. This relationship is reciprocal: the level of the behavioural state can influence the course of the conditioned response, but it can itself be influenced by the conditioned responses or by the course of conditioning in general (Papoušek, 1961). Our state criteria were different from those recommended by other authors in more recent studies and at this meeting.

With the help of polygraphic recording of respiration and general motility, as well as observational coding of the quality of movements, vocalization, and the state of the eyes, we differentiated the following four states of wakefulness:

State I: Regular breathing, no other movements or vocalization, eyes open.

State II: Irregular breathing, quiet movements of eyes, head or distal parts of extremities, no vocalization.

State III: Vivid movements of whole extremities or trunk and/or vocalization other than fussing or crying.

State IV: Upsetness, uncoordinated gross movements and/or fussing or crying.

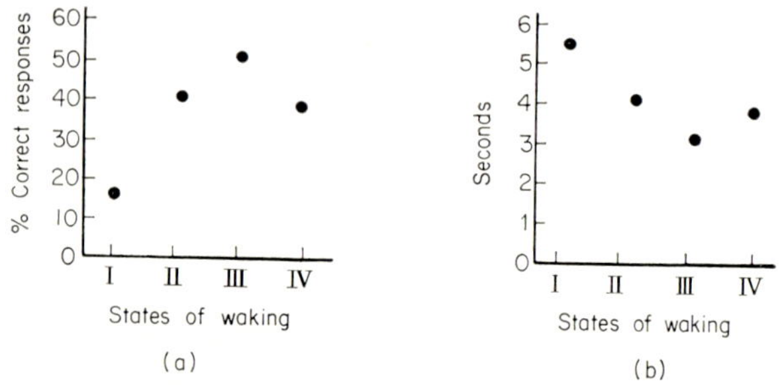

FIG. 1. Effect of different states of waking on conditioned responses. (a) Frequency of correct responses and (b) latency in the four waking states described in the text.

Figure 1 shows the influence of different waking states preceding the CS upon the course of the conditioned response.

Significant differences related to the states of waking were found both in the frequency of 4,287 correct responses and the latencies of 1,521 responses. I think that States II and particularly III can be considered the optimal waking states, whcreas States I and IV represent two different types of deviation from the optimal waking state. The maximum proportion of correct responses and the shortest latencies appear in State III.

Emphasis must be put on the reciprocity of the relationship between the conditioned responses and the behavioural states: the conditioned responses themselves can cause changes in the behavioural state. Figure 2 is an example of our polygrams. It shows a typical micro-

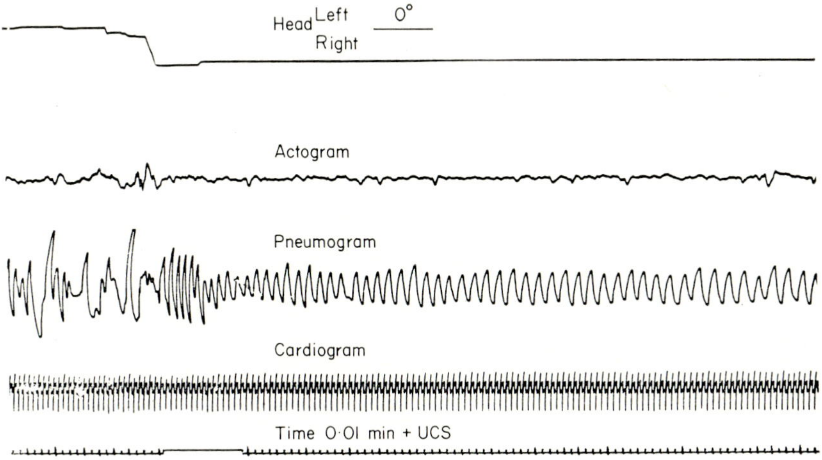

FIG. 2. Effect of conditioning on state. The polygram represents from above downwards: head movement, general body movement, respiration, heartbeat, and time. The time at which the conditioned stimulus was applied is shown on the time marker.

cycle of a sudden change in the general state connected with the application of CS. The abrupt drop in movements, the rhythmical breathing and the slow heart rate resemble the changes seen in sleep, but the eyes are open, and the cycle lasts only a fraction of a minute.

Conditioning techniques can be used for showing an inhibitory effect on the conditioned stimulation (Fig. 3). In this case conditioned head responses were established to two different auditory stimuli *A* (bell) and *B* (buzzer). Then stimulus *A* was applied without reinforcement, so that the conditioned response to it was extinguished. Under these conditions stimulus *A* is not irrelevant as it was before the beginning

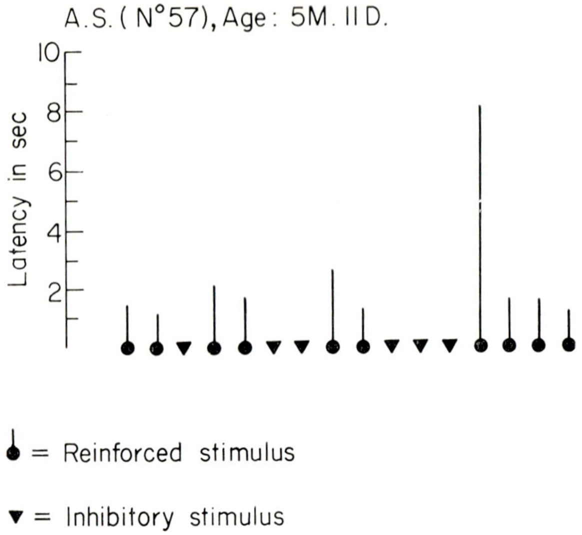

FIG. 3. Inhibitory effect of a stimulus to which the conditioned response has been extinguished. The vertical bars indicate the latency of response. The latency of response to the reinforced stimulus is greater following the inhibitory stimulus.

of conditioning, but instead shows inhibitory qualities. It changes the behavioural state so that general movements and vocalization decrease or stop, and breathing and heart rate become slower and more regular. If stimulus *A* is applied alternately with stimulus *B* the inhibitory effect of *A* can also be shown in the prolongation of latencies in the response to *B* (Fig. 3). The greater the number of consecutive stimuli of type *A* which precede stimulus *B*, the more marked the prolongation of latency. In fact by cumulating consecutive inhibitory stimuli it is possible to induce sleep in infants—as occasionally happens during extinction of the conditioned responses.

Another topic I wish to comment on concerns the problem of specific human patterning or organizing of responses.

If one pays attention not only to the analysis of whole samples, but also to the course of individual responses and their emotional and facial accompaniments, one starts thinking of some higher mental processes behind the responses. This happened when we studied conditioned discrimination. Here and there, we saw something suggesting a strategy in the infant's responses.

The conditioned discrimination was designed so that we used a bell for signalling milk presented from the left side, and a buzzer for signalling milk presented from the right. Both signals were applied from the midline and in a random order to avoid any "time conditioning" or any regularity in the sequence of responses. Yet the infants seemed to pick up an occasional accidental sequence of the conditioning signals suggesting a regular schema, and carried out the next responses in accord with this schema and regardless of the real meaning of the signals. For instance, some infants turned regularly once to the left and once to the right. An accidental congruence of the reinforcement with their "strategy" elicited signs of pleasure in their behaviour, whereas an incongruence elicited signs of displeasure. In another case, they always turned to the side from which the milk had been presented the previous time.

Another surprising observation was made when we tested the effects of hunger and satiation upon the level of conditioned responses. In an infant with well-established conditioned responses we applied 39, 40, or more signals during one session. He accepted milk as a reinforcement until he had taken twice as much milk as usual. Then he started refusing it, but he continued performing excellent conditioned responses with very short latencies and with obvious signs of pleasure. With every conditioning stimulus he turned to the correct side, smiled, and bubbled, but as soon as we tried to give him milk he turned away and would not take a drop more. So it looked as if some motivation other than hunger was involved—some demand to respond correctly or to solve a problem. And the congruence between the infant's plan or expectation and the real events seemed to please him. There may be other psychological terms for it, but this was the basic observation.

Thus we became interested in the question whether infants were able to detect some rules, systems or strategies in the environmental stimulation and adapt their behaviour to them. Bernstein and I therefore modified our method in an operant conditioning way, to some extent similar to that described by Bower. Conditioning stimuli were not used, but during 2-minute periods of time every head turn corresponding to certain criteria was reinforced with a visual reinforcement represented by 10 colour bulbs blinking in a random order for 5 seconds. The bulbs were placed in the midline above the infant lying in the supine position. In order to be able to watch the reinforcement the infant had to turn his head back to the midline.

Under these conditions 4-month-old infants soon learn a new peculiar type of head movement which we call "switching-on movements". They turn to the appropriate side, let us say to the left, and then quickly back to the midline in order to see the visual reward. Switching-on movements can easily be distinguished from normal spontaneous head

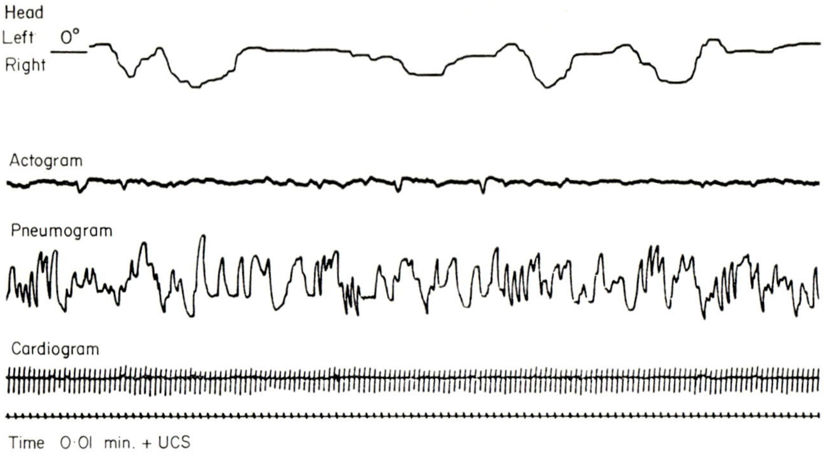

FIG. 4. Polygram showing spontaneous head movements. Channels as in Figure 2.

movements in our records. Figure 4 gives an idea of the normal type of spontaneous head movement. With a left turn of the head the uppermost record is deflected upwards; with a right one it turns downwards.

Figure 5 illustrates distinct shaping of the irregular head movements to the typical switching-on movements in an experiment where left turns of at least 30 degrees of rotation were reinforced. The conditions for reaching the visual reward can be modified according to different

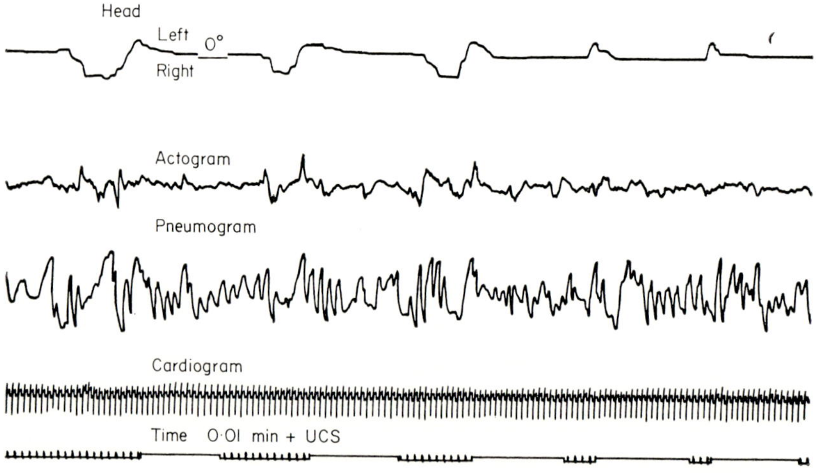

FIG. 5. Polygram showing head movements of "switching-on" type. Channels as in Figure 2.

schemes or rules. No instruction is given to the infants. In 4-month-old infants we tried to apply the following conditions for reinforcement:

(i) two turns to the given side carried out consecutively and through at least 30 degrees;
(ii) three such consecutive head turns;
(iii) regularly alternating turns to the left and to the right;
(iv) regularly alternating double turns to the left and to the right;
(v) two turns to one side and three turns to the opposite side.

Figures 6 to 9 illustrate adaptation of the head movement to some of these rules. Figure 6 shows an experiment in which we reinforced every second turn to the left provided there was no right

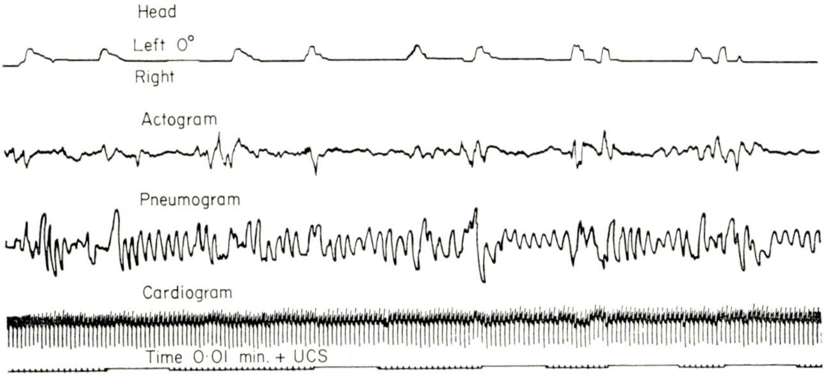

FIG. 6. Grouped pairs of head movements to the left when every second consecutive head turn to the left is reinforced. Channels of polygram as in Figure 2.

turn between the first and second left turns. You can see how the switching-on movements became grouped into regular pairs of quick movements. Similarly, Fig. 7 shows grouping of head movements into triads, when every third head turn to the same side was reinforced. This is a more difficult task, but in this study our babies were mostly children of university students, and knew how to count up to three. In another case, we reinforced regularly one turn to the left side and one to the right side. In Fig. 8 the head movements are well adapted to this sequence.

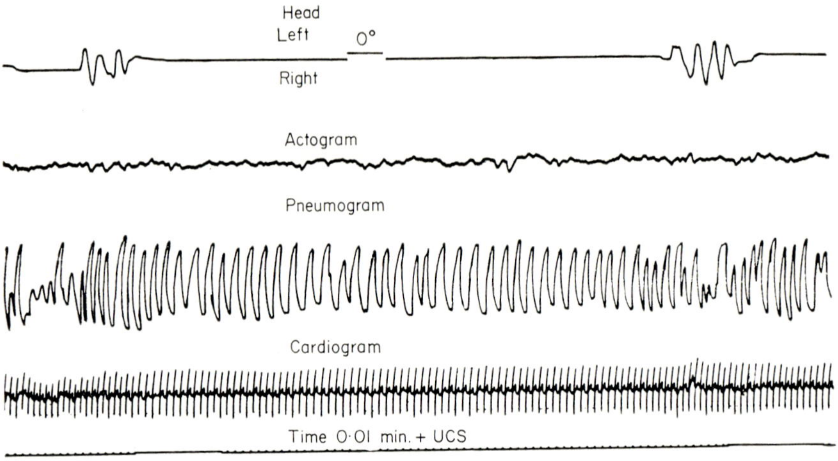

FIG. 7. Grouped triads of head turns to the right when every third consecutive turn to that side is reinforced. Channels of polygram as in Figure 2.

We have not yet been able to teach the infants to turn twice to the left and three times to the right. That is obviously too difficult. Indeed it is no easy task for an adult to find out why some movements are reinforced but others are not: our adult assistants or visitors could confirm how difficult it is. The stricter you are in respect to standardization of experimental conditions the harder it is. For instance, it is very puzzling

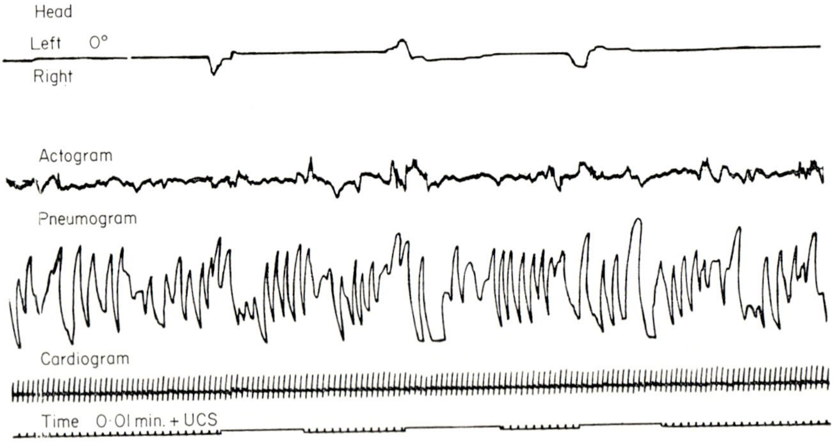

FIG. 8. Alternating head turns to left and right, when reinforcement is provided for this sequence. Channels of polygram as in Figure 2.

for the infant if he carries out three head turns but he is not rewarded—because one of the movements does not reach 30 degrees of rotation.

Figure 9 raises the question of what is the actual reward in these experiments: whether it is the blinking lights themselves or the congruence between expectation and its confirmation. Here you see an infant

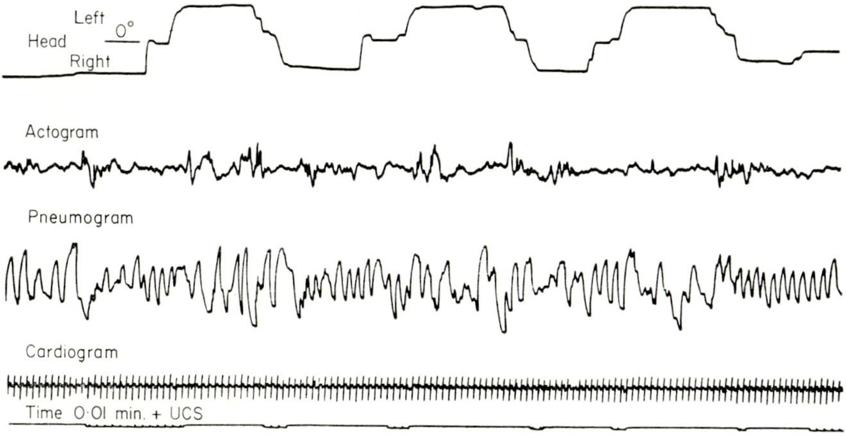

FIG. 9. The infant keeps its head turned sharply towards the side which had produced a reward, despite the fact that the visual reward is offered in the midline. Channels of polygram as in Figure 2.

who was taught, so to say, to turn regularly once to the left and once to the right. He does so, but as you see, he turns up to 90 degrees to the left and leaves his head in this position even during the visual reinforcement coming from the midline. He cannot watch it, although he may have partial information about it since the blinking lights change the whole illumination around him. As soon as the reinforcement is finished, the infant turns back to the midline and carries out the next correct response to the right, again up to about 90 degrees. And again he does not watch the visual reward but he seems to be pleased by carrying out the correct responses. His smiles and bubbling at least indicate pleasure.

This explains how we came to the question of the mental processes involved in structuring the responses. What we know about the linkage between brain functions and these higher forms of behavioural adaptation may still be vague. Nevertheless, the mere fact that we can now make a behavioural study of the earliest development of these functions seems to me to be an important step forwards which can stimulate people studying other aspects, in morphology and physiology. This way, we can also approach the brain functions specific for the human species.

The older theories did not pay attention to cognitive mediation in the preverbal stage of mental development. However, the relation between speech and cognitive functions may be such that cognition has to develop to a certain level in order to make the development of speech possible. The modern theory of information, and advances in brain engineering, can explain in terms of mechanisms used in cybernetic devices and computers some basic processes important for cognition. There is evidence from neuroanatomy and neurophysiology that some mechanisms of processing the informational input in the nervous system may be organized in this way. For instance, the functions maintaining constant body temperature, oxygenation, homeostasis, etc., can be considered analogues to the servomechanisms constructed to the principle of TOTE (test-operation-test-exit) systems.

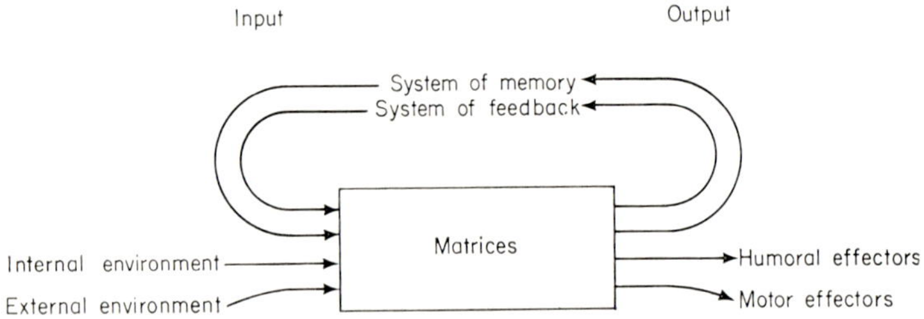

FIG. 10. The TOTE system. For explanation *see* text.

Figure 10 shows a scheme of the CNS as an organ which processes information. The input comes from four main sources: from sensory organs giving information about the external environment, from organs controlling the internal environment of the organism itself, from the system of memory, and from the system of feedback giving information about the course and outcome of responses. On the other side, the output goes to the system of motor effectors, to the humoral effectors, to the memory, and to the feedback system.

We should keep in mind (and Prechtl underlines this aspect) that on both the input and output sides, we always deal with very complex phenomena. The simpler our research methods, the greater the risk of our missing the specifically human features of behaviour. Unfortunately we cannot observe many phenomena at the same time. Even as complex an analysis of behavioural states as Prechtl presents covers only the motor responses. It does not touch the humoral responses, although the interaction of motor and humoral responses is very important. The same is also true on the input side.

We usually try to isolate one particular stimulus and observe one adequate response. However, both the input and the output represent enormous constellations of informational particles—molecules, if you like. It is no random constellation; the parts exist in spatial, causal, temporal, and other relations which are detectable. The probability of individual combinations is also an important factor.

The black box in the centre of Fig. 10 which receives the input represents those parts of the nervous system where the information is analysed and whence sets of commands are sent down to different effectors. We know that on different levels of the nervous system there are simple loops, or more complicated connections of the feedback system, controlling realization of these commands.

In the TOTE system of self-control of a device, the first step is to test the congruence of a critical aspect of the controlled phenomenon to some given standard, for example, to measure the temperature of the air and to signal any deviation beyond the limits within which the oscillations of temperature are considered negligible. Any incongruence between the test and the standard starts operations preventing damage caused by an abnormal temperature. That is the second step. The third one is to test whether the effect of the operations is sufficient according to other given standards. Any incongruence resulting from this testing keeps the operations in function. A congruence leads to the final step, that is, to ending the operations.

We assume that in a similar way in the brain, different aspects of the incoming information are tested and compared to standards coded in some way in the memory. Any incongruence starts operations enabling an adaptation to the signalled change, and keeps them functioning as long as necessary. Let us suppose that somewhere in the memory there are "matrices" containing standards for the most important life conditions, and instructions for different ways of adapatation to changes in life conditions. Thus we may have matrices for maintaining body temperature, for homeostasis, for satiating hunger or thirst, for reproduction, for social communication, etc. Each of them provides specific responses to specific stimuli. But I think there is another special matrix which provides a very general response to any incongruence resulting from matching a piece of information to standards, or to neuronal models if we use the Sokolovs' term. Apart from specific operations, such an incongruence starts non-specific operations for gaining more information and improving its analysis. These operations appear when a piece of information is unfamiliar or when a subject's response does not lead to the expected result. Such operations may consist of orientation reflexes, or of mechanisms for increasing one's attention, or for testing new hypotheses in problem situations. On the other hand a congruence between information and standard reduces or switches off such operations. According to our experience with infants I would say that these non-specific operations influence emotional behaviour, too, eliciting increased tension and eventually upsetness and signs of displeasure in the case of incongruence, and relief with signs of pleasure in the case of congruence. I believe that in man this type of matrix is closely related to cognitive functions. We ought, therefore, to pay more attention to its human peculiarities and to its early development.

Our idea about the structural development of the matrices is that they are systems open to constant and far-reaching adjustment. The basic forms of matrix, let us call them "the primary or innate matrices", are most probably coded in some way genetically. They are responsible for the inborn responses as represented by the Pavlovian unconditioned responses—or instincts—and also for the non-learned basic responses to specific releasing stimuli.

In accordance with new experience the primary matrices develop to secondary matrices and matrices of higher orders in the process of learning or cognition. The higher-order matrices organize learned responses to originally non-specific stimuli. They enable the organism to carry out conditioned responses, to respond to stimuli signalling future events, to become adapted in advance, to use verbal mediation, and to think.

I do not wish to suggest that we can interpret everything according to the TOTE system. I just want to say that some basic developmental forms of rather complicated functions may be analogous to this principle. This idea was used by Miller and associates (1960) to interpret some nervous functions and by Hunt (1966) in an attempt to explain intrinsic motivation.

To summarize, we believe that in the preverbal stage of human development information processing is developed to a relatively high level. The infant is able to analyse and categorize the informational input, to detect simple structural relations, schemes or rules in the input, and to adapt his behaviour to them. These basic forms of cognitive function can be studied experimentally in infants, and this may be a useful approach to the study of specifically human ways of organizing behaviour.

REFERENCES

Hunt, J. Mc.V. 1966. Intrinsic motivation and its role in psychological development. In D. Levine (Ed.), *Nebraska symposium on motivation 1965*. Univ. of Nebraska Press, Lincoln. Pp. 189–282.

Miller, G. A., Galanter, E. and Pribram, K. H. 1960. *Plans and the structure of behavior*. Holt, New York.

Papoušek, H. 1961. *Conditioned appetitional responses in infants*. SZdN (Thomayer's Collection No. 409), Prague. (Originally a dissertation, in Czech, Charles University, Prague, 1959.)

Papoušek, H. 1967a. Experimental studies of appetitional behavior in human newborns and infants. In H. W. Stevenson (Ed.). *Early behavior: comparative and developmental approaches*. Wiley, New York. Pp. 249–277.

Papoušek, H. 1967b. Genetics and child development. In J. N. Spuhler (Ed.). *Genetic diversity and human behavior*. Aldine, Chicago. Pp. 171–186.

Papoušek, H. and Bernstein, P. 1969. The functions of conditioning stimulation in human neonates and infants. In J. A. Ambrose (Ed.), Stimulation in early infancy. Academic Press, London.

Discussion

Bergström: Is your idea related to the simple reflex relationship between the input and output in the old Sherringtonian way? We can no longer explain the function of the whole nervous system by means of simple reflex mechanisms.

Papoušek: We can distinguish between different levels. I'm using the very general term "matrix" because it is not connected with the ideas of any particular school. The primary matrix would be something like the one which ensured the unconditioned reflex to unconditioned stimulation. With the example of thermoregulation, the direct change of temperature would be the unconditioned stimulus and all the responses which are organized at this level would be the unconditioned responses to it. Of course, the human organism has a remarkable ability to modify, and these matrixes are obviously open systems which many other signals and practically any kind of stimulation can enter—for example, in the form of a conditioning signal. This ensures behavioural responses adapted to the situation as it develops after birth. The organism can then respond not only to the immediate experience, but also to events before they happen. In the case of thermoregulation, it can respond not only to the immediate change in temperature, but also to the weather forecast. This is the notion of conditioned behaviour and can go in higher and higher orders.

Bergström: I'm not sure that we have the necessary concept of driving force in the concept which is based on a simple reflex.

PAPOUŠEK: There are testing organs which can detect changes in our environment. Why couldn't we have testing organs which would detect the incongruency between information on the one side and our response to it on the other? Whenever this feedback gave a warning that our way of response was not correct, that in itself would be a signal which would be tested by similar testing organs.

WOLFF: What Dr. Papoušek says is exactly the opposite of what would be implied by the reflex arc conception. Finding the congruency and incongruency implies an activity which is beyond the simple reflex arc conception. It is implied that there must be some kind of internal active organization or reorganizing activity.

KAUFMAN: The TOTE system comes from Miller, Galanter, and Pribram. The point of it is that this is not an organism at rest to which something has happened and which then sets homeostatic mechanisms working to bring about, or to restore, order. Rather it's an organism, equipped with a set of plans, that deals with matches and mismatches, congruencies and incongruencies in a very logical contingency-laden way, depending upon how experienced it is. So it's not in any way a simple homeostatic reflex mechanism. It starts out with a set of plans.

PAPOUŠEK: Yes, it's homeostatic at the level of primitive innate responses, but then there are plans of a higher and higher order and I think that this logically leads to a very general mechanism—the response to incongruency.

LIPSITT: I think we are now deeply into the question of what were called structuralized patterns and what has been previously referred to here as the organization of behaviour (*see* p. 307).

Structural Correlates of Conditioning

LIPSITT: With increasing development, there is obviously increasing cortical control over basically subcortical behaviour processes. Could it be that all conditioning in cognitive processes involves cortical elaboration of subcortical or reflexive response systems?

BRONSON: Firstly, there are conditioning phenomena which do not require the cortex, so not all conditioning would be a cortical elaboration.

LIPSITT: I take back the "all".

HUMPHREY: It depends on which animal you are conditioning. Conditioning probably does take place at a variety of levels in the nervous system. Conditioning a frog (and I presume you can) would not be a cortical phenomenon—it would probably occur at superior collicular levels.

PAPOUŠEK: There is now good evidence that cortical functions are not essential either for simple conditioning or for the simple forms of discrimination. The old studies were made on adult animals, and the recent studies on young animals. If you decorticate a very young animal these functions disappear for a time, but this period of stress is followed by the appearance of many functions which can occur as a result of co-ordination at lower levels. Nolokhov developed an interesting technique where fetuses are decapitated during intra-uterine development and then develop without the head to the end of the pregnancy. Here one can see the development of spinal functions without the interference of higher levels of co-ordination. The spinal functions are not inhibited by the higher orders but they are also not adaptive: the higher the levels of co-ordination, the better the adaptation. At the lowest level, there are economical or precise responses. At the lower level of co-ordination you can either facilitate or inhibit such responses, but you cannot see any finer adaptation of these responses. Certainly you wouldn't be able to see much learning at this level. The response is now more diffuse—and perhaps less organized. At the higher level you can again develop an economical carrying-out of the responses but in a sequence which can go through different pathways and become adapted to different situations in different ways, which could not occur at the lower level.

BRONSON: Following Papoušek's notion that perhaps learning can proceed at different levels and become more complex with maturation, what happens if you follow the development of a mechanism such as Dr. Lipsitt was demonstrating in the newborn? This presumably is learned or organized on a fairly simple level in the newborn, but would be mediated by more complex levels in an adult. If you followed the development of the ability to learn this reaction, from birth up to, say, 6 months, you might find that the neonate learned it fairly clearly. Then as higher levels began to mature but weren't yet really capable of efficient learning, you would have a developmental stage where this simple phenomenon was more difficult to learn, and then, at a somewhat older age, when the higher levels were more effectively functioning, you might go back to smoother learning, more like what you were able to achieve in the newborn. Has anyone ever followed longitudinally a very simple learning paradigm to see if there are periods when learning was disrupted as new centres began to take over but weren't really efficient?

LIPSITT: You have described essentially my view of conditioned head turning in the newborn. I believe that the newborn is probably more capable of that type of learning than he would be at 2, 4, or 6 months of age with respect to certain systems, but my idea about why it is more difficult later differs from yours. I think that the basic reflex on which that kind of conditioned head turning depends is not as intense at later ages as it is earlier, and that conditioned behaviour depends upon there being a very readily elicitable response. All conditioning depends on the basic reflex repertoire of the organism and capitalizes, as it were, upon the reflexes that are there at the outset. This is why so many of the responses that Humphrey is dealing with are very pertinent to the conditioner as well as to the neurophysiologist. The conditioner would wonder whether he might at 7 months' gestational age get from the fetus a conditioned response based upon that tickling type reaction or that head turning response which you get to the stimulation around the face.

PAPOUŠEK: Are neonates in some ways more perfect, and their capacities in some functions greater than later on? We probably have a similar situation with the development of speech—there comes a high level of organization, which for some time causes deterioration of the lower levels, and then as the higher level becomes more developed a new ability is gained at a much more advanced stage.

LIPSITT: Yes, the influence of higher levels or cognitive processes is well known even as it affects basic conditioning. Bring a person into a classical eyelid conditioning situation, tell him, "Now you are going to get a tone, and after the tone you are going to get an air puff delivered to your eye." Most people condition in such a way that after a while the tone will cause a blink. Then you say "But I don't want you to let it happen to you" and he can resist conditioning. This is the sort of high-level, cortical, cognitive, mediational control of behaviour that you are talking about.

MACKEITH: Another example of the change from a relatively well-organized stage to a badly organized stage and then to a stage even better organized than the first is the inhibition of primary walking. André-Thomas tried to train the child to continue primary walking, but he was unable to do it beyond about 4 months—it usually disappears around 2 months in ordinary children. (André-Thomas and S. Saint-Anne Dargassies. 1952. *Études neurologiques sur le nouveau-né et le jeune nourrisson*. Masson, Paris.) You still have this inhibition or damping down in order to allow the higher things to come in later.

WOLFF: With one unfortunate exception—didn't those children learn to walk faster than normal children do? (André-Thomas and S. Autguarden. 1953. *Presse méd.* **61,** 582.)

MACKEITH: I didn't think it was terribly well established. The children had a lot more attention.

Primate Studies

Early Communication Processes in Squirrel Monkeys

DETLEV PLOOG

Max Planck Institute for Psychiatry

INTRODUCTION

SINCE THIS IS the only paper dealing with non-human primate behavior during early development it was tempting to present as many comparative data as possible. However, in the space available it would be impossible to cover the whole field of behavioural development in subhuman primates without writing in such general terms as to stultify subsequent discussion. I shall therefore use some of the results obtained on my research animal, the squirrel monkey (*Saimiri sciureus*) in order to give examples of specific early communication processes. The specificity involved in the examples will shed light, I hope, on some key questions concerning the early developmental processes of primates in general.

Material and methods have been described elsewhere (Castell and Ploog, 1967; Maurus and Ploog, 1968; Ploog, 1966 and 1967; Ploog *et al.*, 1963 and 1967; Winter *et al.*, 1966.) Suffice it to say that the data are based on laboratory work over the last 6 years, conducted by four to seven co-workers and myself.

DEVELOPMENT OF SOCIAL BEHAVIOUR

Pregnancy and Delivery

The gestation period of squirrel monkeys is about 24—26 weeks (168—182 days), as in macaques and baboons: a 24-week squirrel monkey is probably premature. During the course of pregnancy locomotion becomes a little slower, aggressiveness towards the entire group increases, and certainly in the last months—sometimes for almost the whole period—sexual receptivity disappears. The amount of bodily contact decreases gradually, and while the mother is giving birth to the infant the members of the group, especially the males, leave her alone. During delivery she emits calls of "general aggression". In the early postpartum period calls of "directed aggression" increase and those of "general aggression" decrease (Fig. 1). This then is roughly the state of the mother when the first communication between mother and infant and between infant and group can be observed.

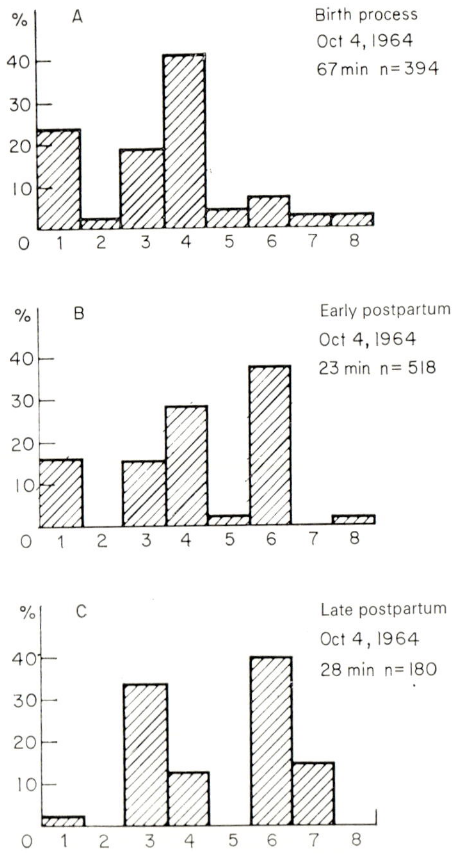

FIG. 1. Change of vocalization in a group of four animals during three stages of delivery (A, B, C). Most are vocal exchanges between the mother and a premature female (Winter *et al.*, 1966). For terminology of calls see Fig. 11.

1 = peeps and chirps; 2 = play peeping; 3 = twittering/trilling; 4 = cackling (general aggression); 5 = yapping; 6 = churr/purr (directed aggression); 7 = kecker; 8 = shrieking. n = total number of vocalizations. Reproduced by permission of Springer Verlag, Berlin.

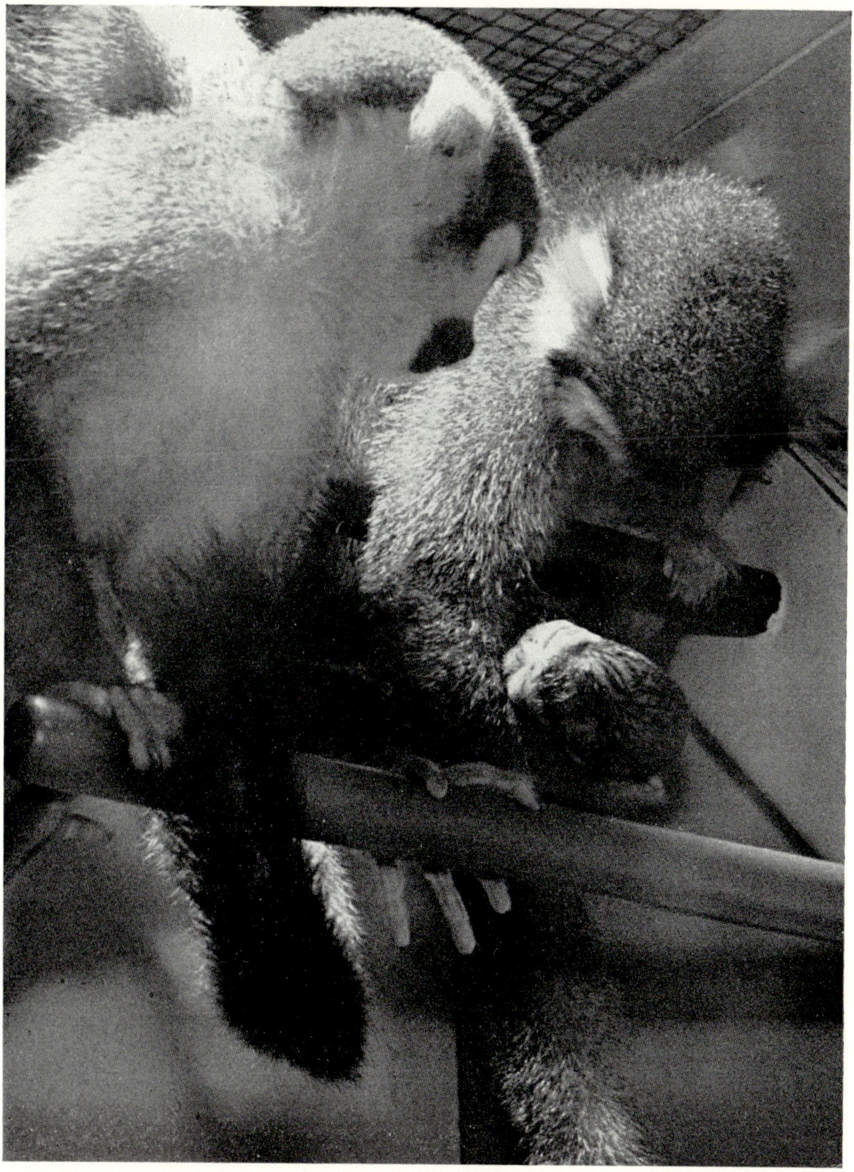

FIG. 2. Mother supports her motionless infant immediately after birth. (Bowden *et al.* 1967.) Reproduced by permission of S. Karger, Basel.

Just as there are considerable quantitative variations of maternal behaviour during pregnancy so there are variations of motility and vitality in the neonates; various aspects of the behaviour both of pregnant mothers and of neonates could be measured (Bowden *et al.*, 1967; Hopf, 1967). By means of telemetric methods it should be possible to investigate this problem more precisely. From comparative neuroanatomical studies on myelination one would, for instance, expect that the older fetus could respond to sounds.

First Mother-Child Interactions

During the period from the first appearance of the fetus to its complete emergence the mother assumes the squatting position characteristic of all primate species except modern man. She licks and nuzzles the

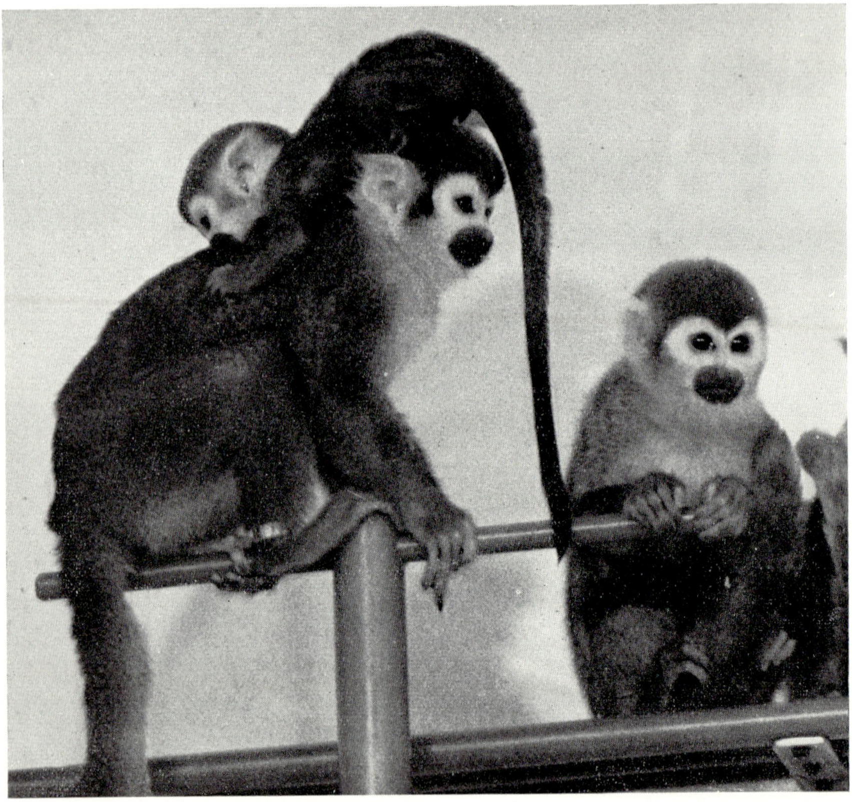

FIG. 3. 18-day-old infant using its mother as a "walking place".

half-exposed fetus but, unlike other primate mothers, she does not usually pull at it. The mature neonate may assist its own emergence by using its arms to climb up the mother's abdomen while the lower trunk and legs are still in the birth canal. Generally the mother's supportive role is minimal; however, there are cases which reveal maternal behaviour patterns capable of assuring support for many days, even to a totally unresponsive infant (Fig. 2).

Immediately after birth the neonate clings firmly, starts rooting, and displays not only the well-known head-turning component but also a vigorous head-up-down component, nodding against the mother's abdomen or chest. Since non-human primate mothers do not normally help the infant to find the breast, it is necessary for the neonate to be able to locate the nipple by its own efforts. Here an important feature of primate behaviour becomes apparent in squirrel monkeys. The baby obviously does not "know" where to climb and it frequently makes grave mistakes as it seeks the correct direction and position on the mother's body. However, certain regions—the groin, the axilla, and the neck—seem to provide directional cues. The groin cue usually sends the infant in precisely the wrong direction, so it ends up by clinging to the root of the mother's tail, which makes her increasingly restless. Only when its efforts are in vain does the mother assist the infant, by touching it softly. This immediately helps it orient itself on the maternal body. Such assistance may last up to the 12th day but has never been observed thereafter (Table I). The 18-day-old baby (Fig. 3) uses its mother as a "walking place". It no longer receives directional signals from the mother although she shows the characteristic posture and behaviour of passive attention. She rarely looks at the infant but guards her environment intently.

When infants are reared in partial isolation without a mother it can be demonstrated that angularity provides the directional cue which the infant uses to orient itself (Hopf, 1970). Figure 4 shows an infant of 4 weeks which has been exposed to a stuffed woollen sock as its substitute mother. At this age it still tried to reach the "ventral" surface of the sock, repeatedly rooting its nose into the angle between the floor and the curvature of the stuffed sock even immediately after bottle feeding. Its feeding posture precisely resembled that of a baby of 4 weeks raised normally (Fig. 5), and it was in this posture that the hand-reared baby preferred thumb-sucking, a behaviour never otherwise observed in squirrel monkeys. Note the angle between the mother's trunk and shoulder in the picture on the left. Within a few days of delivery a mother learns to lift her arm when the baby puts its nose in this angle.

TABLE I. CALENDAR OF DEVELOPMENTAL EVENTS

Behaviour patterns	*Period of first (last) appearance*	*Data of individual infants* ♀O	♀H	♀R	♂W	♂X	♂I
	Weeks						
Touching partner	1– 3	1	3	3			3
Grooming, active	3–12	3	12	4			
passive	1– 2	1	2	1			
self	5			5			
Object manipulation	1– 3	1	2	3			2
Oral activity	2– 3	3	2	3			3
Gnawing object	2– 5	3	2	3	5	4	4
Gnawing solid food	3– 9	3	9	6	6	4	4
Food stealing	3– 8	3	7	5	5	8	8
Eating solid food	7–10		10	9	8	7	
Urine washing, incomplete	2– 9	3	6	2	7	9	5
complete	5–13	5	13	9	12	12	7
Last orientation help from mother	1– 2	1		2			
Getting off mother	3– 5	3	4	4	5	4	
Mother pushes infant away	4– 7	7	5	6	6	4	
Genital display toward mother	4– 7	7	6	7	6	4	
Genital display toward other group mate	1–12	2	6	1	12	7	3
Playing with group mate's tail	5–12	6	12	5	5	8	
Leaping	6– 9	6	9	7	8		6
	Months						
Huddling	2– 5		3	5	4	2	2
Sleeping *beside* group mate	4– 6		4	6	4		
Approach-avoidance sequence before suckling, first time	4– 6		4	6		6	
last time	9					9	
Last suckling	13				13	13	
Last sleeping on mother's back	14					14	
Sexual activity (during play)	5– 9			9	9	5	
Rage	14				14	14	
Fighting	14				14	14	

The infant then learns to find its way more rapidly. A fully relaxed feeding posture is seen in the right-hand picture of Fig. 5: note the open hand of the baby which indicates satiation as it does in human babies.

The point I want to make here is that various features of neonate activity suggest the innate nature of certain fractions of the behaviour. These fractions are object-directed (for example, grasping the fur,

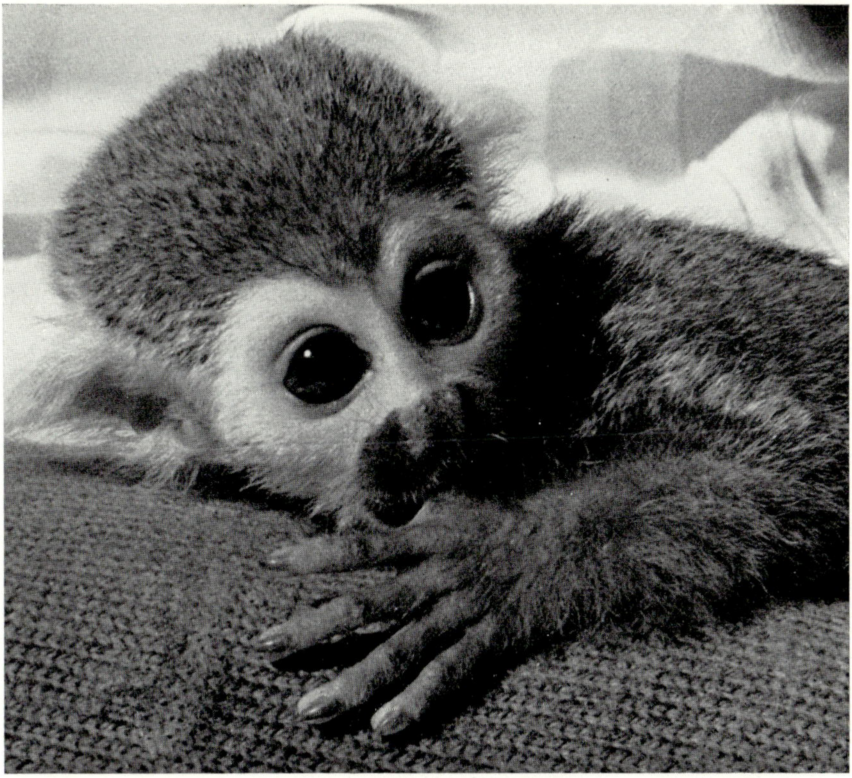

FIG. 4. Hand-raised infant of 30 days thumb-sucking on a stuffed woollen sock. (Ploog. *Nervenarzt* **37**, 1966.) Reproduced by permission of Springer Verlag, Berlin.

searching for and sucking the nipples), and they are guided by orienting cues of a very general nature such as angles, curvatures, and rather unspecific tactile stimuli from the mother. Similar observations have been made concerning lower mammals. These few corner stones form the base for the total behaviour. The rest is rapidly learned within a few days after birth. Only by careful observation is one able to distinguish between these fundamentally different mechanisms. Each built-in component of the infant's behaviour (such as response to an angle) serves as the natural reinforcer for the "in-between" parts (such as proper orientation on the mother's body), which must be learned. Exactly this sort of linkage of innate and learned or trained fractions of behaviour was described by Lorenz as early as 1932, mainly from observations on jackdaws (Lorenz, 1932; 1935). The difference in primates in this

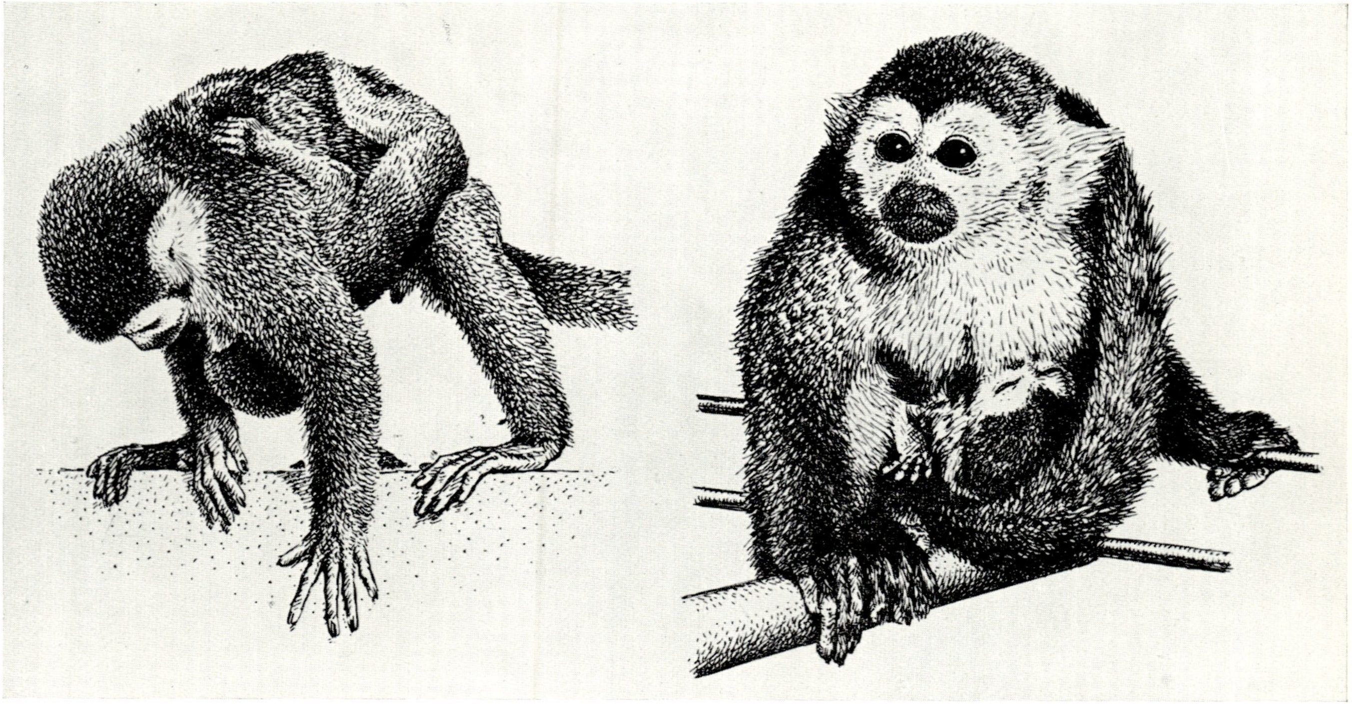

FIG. 5. Feeding postures. Left: Infant of 4 weeks. Right: Infant of 3 weeks. (Drawings by H. Kacher after photographs.) Reproduced by permission of Springer Verlag, Berlin.

respect is only of a quantitative nature in that the built-in fractions are fewer, less conspicuous, and less frequent, and that their release depends on more general sign stimuli than is the case for the rest of the vertebrates. But these sparse innate fractions are powerful reinforcers which rapidly promote the learning process. How powerful they are can best be seen where sucking and feeding occur separately in the case of the infant with a substitute mother.

The second point which I would like to emphasize is in contradiction to the common concept of early social communication. Especially in primate behaviour, the mother-infant dyad is considered to be the source and the beginning of social communication. My point of view is different. As mentioned earlier, the chained actions of the newborn are object-related and object-directed. The mother, therefore, is not really a social partner but rather a composite of objects consisting of fur, nipples, angles, curvatures, and warmth, which can be clasped and clung to. As we see in the substitute-mother experiment, although most of the stimulus properties have been greatly altered, the animal still performs almost perfectly. It even scratches the woollen sock—behaviour analagous to scratching the mother's fur, which is frequently observed in normally reared infants during the first few days. After that time they scratch only their own bodies. It is possible that the feed-back circuits are not fully functioning at birth. Even more striking is a specific defecation procedure which occurs only from the time when secure and skilled climbing on the mother's body is first evident until the infant leaves the "maternal home" for longer periods of the day. Within this time span the infant, when defecating, adjusts itself to the mother's body axis so that the faeces do not come in contact with her fur. Exactly the same behaviour during the same period in development has been observed in the motherless infant on the "back" of the sock.

Further evidence that the mother is a mere composite of certain stimulus properties is the fact that the infant tries out other animals for nursing. If the animal chosen is a lactating female she usually permits the infant to feed on her nipples. We have even seen a lactating female permit two infants to feed on her two breasts at the same time.

One also gains the impression, especially in primiparous cases, that the mother treats the neonate as a strange object, at least for the first week of life. She cares amazingly little about the newborn if its behaviour is "in order". After delivery she is completely engrossed in eating the placenta and in cleaning herself and her surroundings. Meanwhile the baby may suckle her nipples completely unguarded. She frequently rolls over on her back with the baby on it as if to get rid of this strange

TABLE II. SURVEY OF THE MAIN PHASES OF ONTOGENY IN THE SQUIRREL MONKEY

	Infant (I) and Mother (M)	*Infant (I) and Group*
First week	Progressing *M-I*-adaptation by means of tactile stimuli. Stabilization of *I*'s orientation on *M*'s body, depending on its state of maturation. *M* has nest function for *I*.	Social interactions with some females (mature or adolescent), which are attracted by the visual, vocal, and olfactory stimuli from *I*: Vocalizations, looking at, genital display toward, turning toward, and turning away from partners. Males defend *I* but have little or no interaction with *I*.
Second week	Training of motor coordination by climbing on *M*'s body.	Manual contacts with partner broaden *I*'s social behaviour.
Third to fourth week	*I* first leaves *M* for short intervals under her surveillance (enlargement of *I*'s territory as a result of motor training).	A female takes a special interest in *I* (so-called aunt-*I*-relationship) and subsequently forms a dyad with *M* that may outlast both *M-I*- and aunt-*I*-relationships.
Fifth to seventh week	Amount of daytime spent on own feet increases rapidly. *M-I*-behaviour is mainly composed of four characteristics: (1) *I* moving away from *M* (2) Strong *I-M*-ties (3) Onset of weaning (4) Strong protection by *M* Weaning: *I* runs toward *M*, *M* avoids *I*; this repeated many times until *M* allows sucking.	

	It seems that the four characteristics repeatedly occur without the influence of external stimuli. Visual interaction increases, *M-I*-relationship becoming more varied and "personal." First genital display toward *M*. This behaviour is seen frequently throughout weaning. Persistence of nest function. Fur on ventral side appears.	
Eighth week to fourth month	*M-I*-relationship remains stable. The four characteristics are balanced and are employed adequately. (1) Interest in environment (2) Loosening of *M-I*-ties (3) Continuation of weaning (4) Protection when necessary Feeding: both sucking and eating solid food.	Play with peers develops; aunt-*I*-relationship still present. *I* displays toward adult males without further interaction and toward unfamiliar group mates and humans.
Fifth to eighth month	*I* spends less time with *M*. *I* more independent. Characteristics (1) and (3) predominant: (1) *I* occupied with peers or objects (3) *M* avoids *I* for long periods	Intense play with peers including first copulatory behaviour, which starts during fifth to sixth or ninth to tenth months. In both periods of age *I* stops gaining weight. Male copulatory behaviour appears earlier than female. End of aunt-*I*-relationship. Frequent genital display toward the alpha animal.
Ninth to fourteenth month	Intense or sometimes aggressive weaning. End of *M*'s positive actions directed to *I*, except for her carrying *I* on back during nighttime; rare nursing and protection in violent danger.	

TABLE II—*continued*

	Infant (I) and Mother (M)	*Infant (I) and Group*
Second year	Juvenile-adult-interaction replaces former *M-I*-interaction. Long periods without any interaction.	Play with peers continues, but the now juvenile animal less frequently instigates play. More interaction with other group mates, especially the alpha animal: role of scapegoat, and play-fighting are exercised; alpha animal suppresses juvenile male. Frequency of genital display toward alpha animal decreases, threats toward juvenile increase in frequency and intensity. Juvenile male shows dominance toward females and exerts both sexual roles.
Third year		Stop in gaining weight. Sexual maturity in males at approximately 2 years, 9 months. Play decreases and is dependent on initiative of partner. Role of scapegoat continues. Intense suppression of juvenile male by alpha animal; fighting may result in injuries.

stimulus (Castell *et al.*, 1969). If a newly captured mother is frightened by her strange environment or if there are other reasons for emotional distress she may eat her baby and placenta or she may reject the baby, treating it aggressively like an enemy and even biting it. In this case the baby's cries enhance the aggression.

To summarize the essential characteristics of the first days of life: the neonate is not much bigger than Tom Thumb. It can grasp firmly and can hold its own body weight of about 100 grams with only one extremity. When it is not feeding it clings most of the time to the mother's back. For the first week the mother appears to be a composite of objects for the child, which soon learns to find the nipples and to adjust itself to the mother's body axis in a head-to-head and tail-to-tail position. It gradually gains skill in climbing. The mother is used as a "walking place". During the first 2 weeks of life there are very few interactions between the mother and child which resemble specific features of social behaviour, that is partner-directed interactions (Table II).

First Group Interactions

The situation between the neonate and the group is quite different. When the birth takes place in artificial light—in nature births always occur at night and therefore in darkness—the juveniles or adult females respond quickly to the visual appearance of the newborn. They attempt to nuzzle the infant (Fig. 6) and to pull its tail or sometimes its extremities. The infant tries to withdraw from these advances and the mother tries to drive the group members away. When the birth takes place in darkness (being observed in infra-red light) the group remains sleepy and merely responds with a few vocalizations to the first calls of the newborn. Already during the first day of life the infant exhibits curiosity for the group, follows individual members with its eyes, and exchanges glances and vocalizations with them. The females and the juveniles of the group are actively involved in these communications but the adult males remain aloof. They react only if the young is in danger, when they display rage and even attack humans—behaviour otherwise unknown, no matter how great the danger.

Specific Modes of Social Communication

Genital display. The phenomenon of genital display has been studied in detail and under various experimental conditions. It is a powerful social signal which contributes decisively to the formation of group structure. It is used in various ways in accordance with the standing

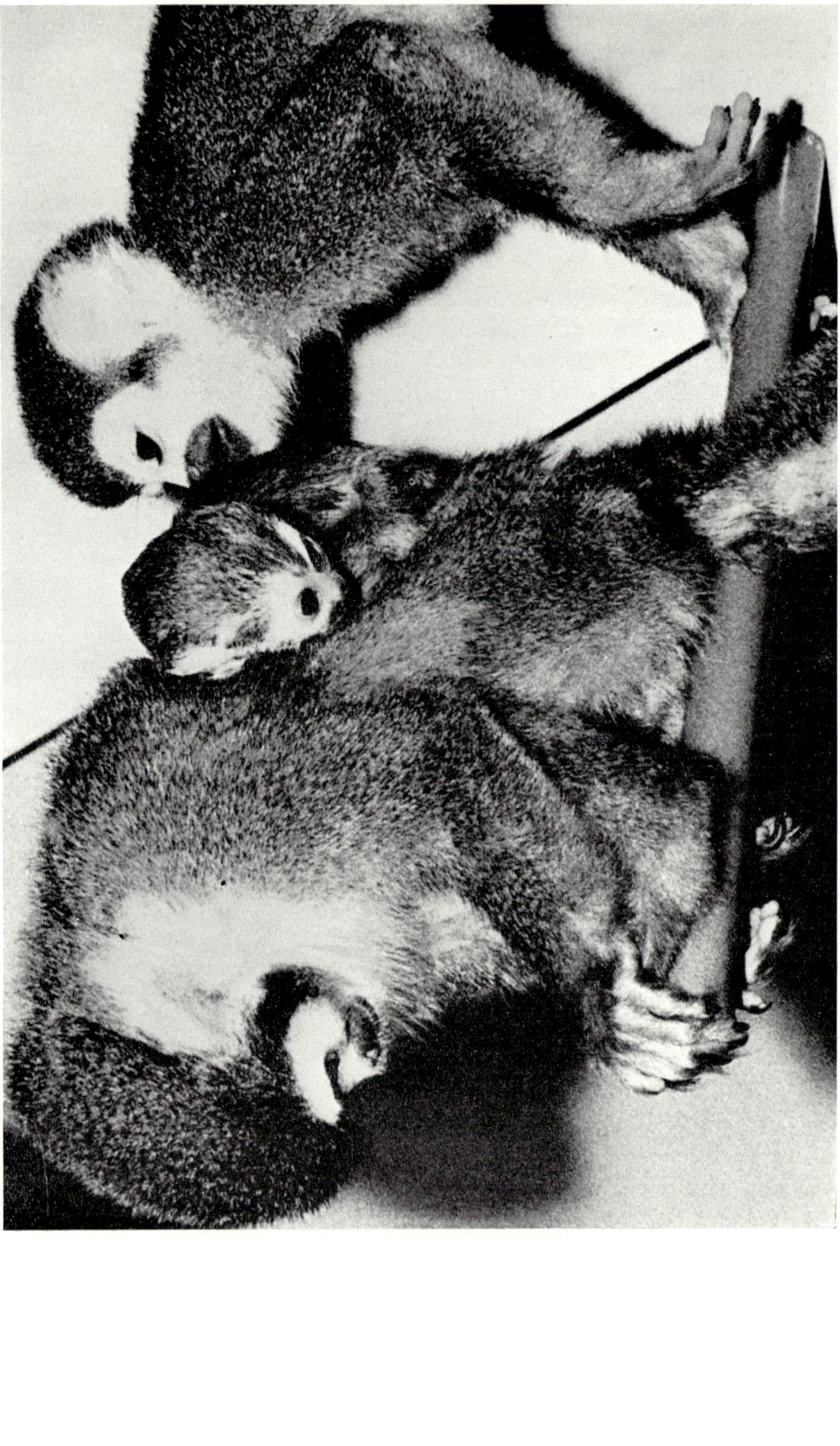

FIG. 6. A female group mate nuzzles the newborn. (Ploog *et al*. 1967.) Reproduced by permission of Springer Verlag, Berlin.

of the animal in the group. An infant employs this signal differently from adolescents and adults.

Genital display is always directed towards one partner and consists of several components: laterally positioned leg with hip and knee bent and marked supination of the foot, abduction of the big toe and, according to the sex of the animal, an erection of the penis, or enlarge-

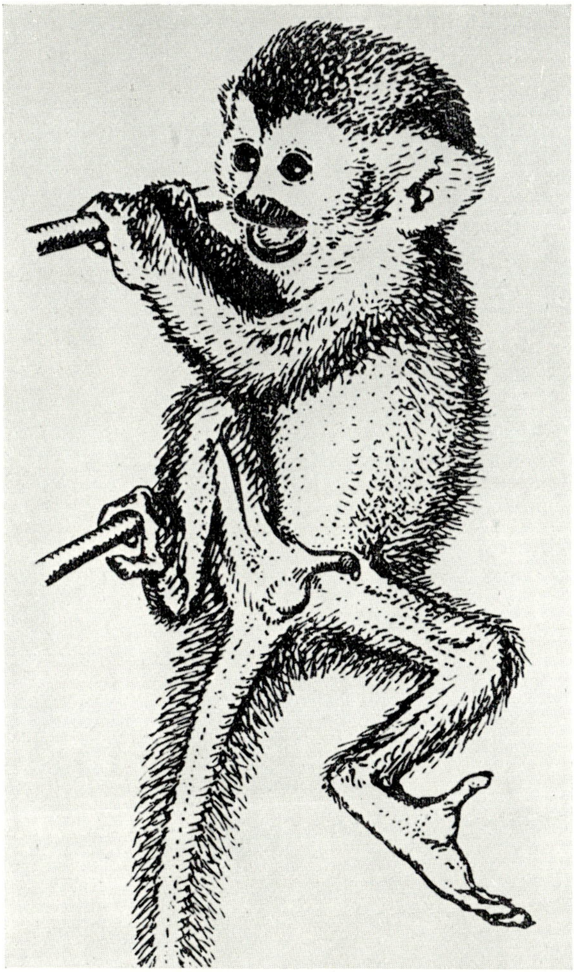

FIG. 7. Genital display of a 49-day-old infant: flexed leg, supine foot, abducted big toe, growing penile erection (with a drop of urine), mouth open for vocalization. Fur on ventral surface still very sparse. (Ploog *et al.* 1967. Drawing by H. Kacher after photographs.) Reproduced by permission of Springer Verlag, Berlin.

ment of the clitoris. The display is frequently accompanied by vocalizations and occasionally, especially in the young, by a few spurts of urine, as can be seen in the picture of an infant of 7 weeks (Fig. 7).

The modes of social communication which have been discussed so far are somewhat unspecific, reflex-like, or fragmental, but genital display seems to be a highly integrated pattern which includes visual orientation and recognition, partner-directed relations, and co-ordination of motor and autonomic functions. This social signal may be used as early as the second day of life. Figure 8 shows a $1\frac{1}{2}$-day-old female display-

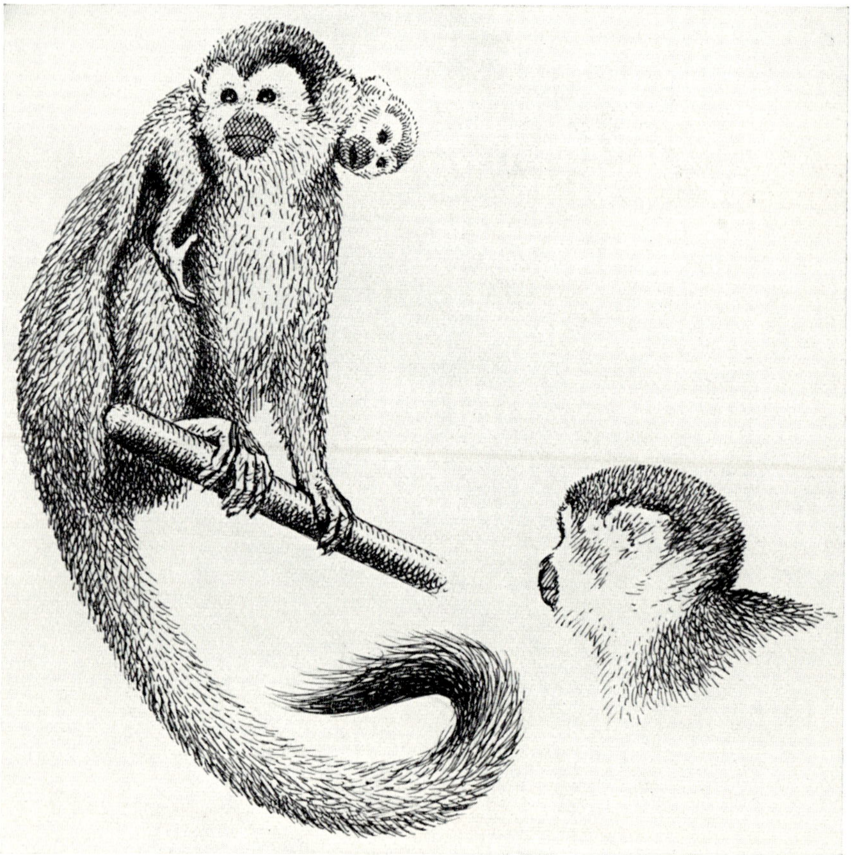

FIG. 8. Genital display of a $1\frac{1}{2}$-day-old female infant towards a group mate. Infant's mouth is slightly open for vocalization as revealed by the original motion picture frames. (Ploog *et al.* 1967. Drawing by H. Kacher.) Note the flexed leg and the abducted big toe, both being obligatory and indicative components of genital display. Reproduced by permission of Springer Verlag, Berlin.

ing to a cage mate: the infant's mouth is slightly open for vocalization.

There is a great variation in the age at which this signal first occurs. Up to a certain age the signal, although used more and more often, does not affect the adult partner's behaviour. At the end of the first year and the beginning of the second, which is also the time of final weaning, the situation changes. I will take the example of the alpha animal, that is, the dominant male of the group, and the young (Fig. 9c).

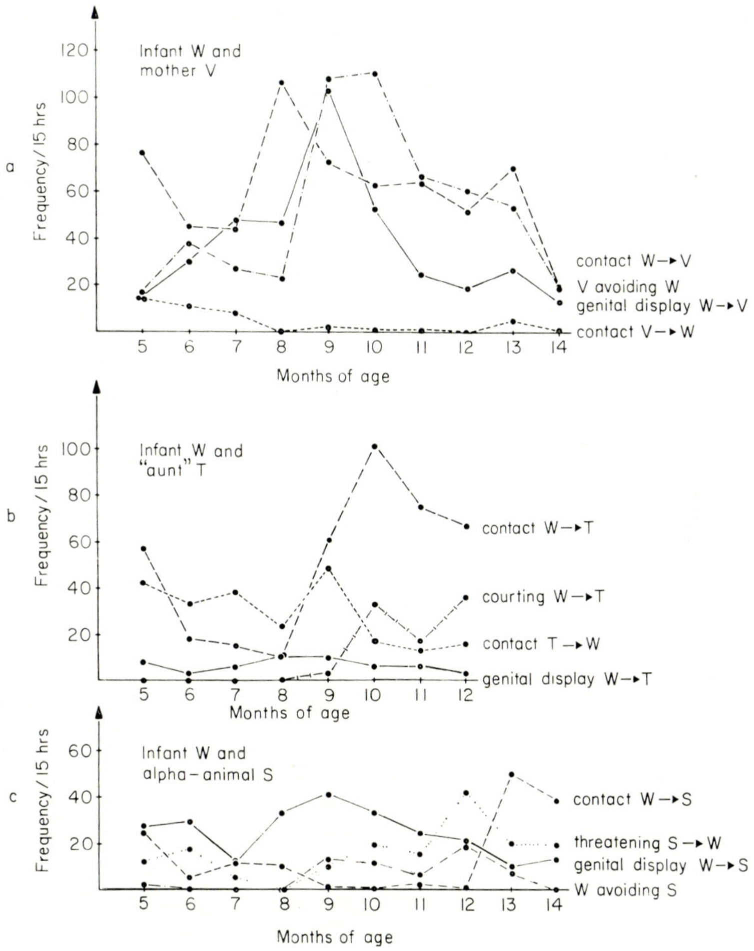

FIG. 9. Typical developmental phases of social interactions from the 5th to the 14th month. (Ploog *et al.* 1967.) Reproduced by permission of Springer Verlag, Berlin.

Up to about 9 months the "boss" of the group threatens only mildly and infrequently when the male young displays towards him, and the young uses this opportunity many times. In fact, as we have shown in sociometric studies, genital display at this age is far more frequently addressed to the boss and the mother than to other members of the group (Fig. 9a). However, the situation with the alpha animal then changes radically. He threatens severely and may attack the young male when it displays towards him. There is an amusing transitional phase during which the young turns away while displaying but glances over his shoulder at the alpha partner—who may already threaten him from time to time. At the beginning of the second year the display behaviour decreases markedly and the young male establishes a new relationship with alpha. Before that age contact between infant and alpha is rarely seen: after it, such contacts are most frequent, consisting mainly of huddling and playing. The play includes a characteristic form, which is no doubt schooling for fighting, a playful but well controlled training by the alpha animal.

Genital display as a social signal shows some features which may be important for all primates, including man. This complex social signal, which expresses self-assertion, is innate. The distributional pattern of the signal shows that the child is fully aware of the hierarchical structure of the group. The signal is used by the infant over and over again, virtually without consequences for either the sender or recipient. Despite this lack of reinforcement it persists up to a predetermined age—after which it is followed by severe consequences and the animal quickly learns the contexts in which it may or may not be used. This protracted maturation process, which coincides with other biological data such as second dentition and final weaning, seems to be characteristic of the social development of primates. It is different from object-related learning processes.

These observations are closely paralleled by Sackett's (1966) findings. He raised Rhesus infants in complete isolation and exposed them to projected slides showing four kinds of situation: Rhesus infants, threatening adult males, other Rhesus monkeys without emotional expressions, and "neutral" pictures, among them a human girl. At the beginning the infants and the threatening males were equally preferred. At 3 months the preference for the male pictures dropped drastically and was suppressed. Of course the "threats" produced no consequences. After the fourth month, preference for the threat pictures increased again and by 5·5 months both infant and threat pictures were preferred to "other monkeys" and "neutral".

Social partners. (a) The Mother as Social Partner. Although the first partner interactions with members of the group already occur during the first 2 weeks of life, the mother gains partner status during the third and fourth weeks when the infant begins to dismount for short periods and for very short distances. Now mother and child begin to unfold a great variety of motor and vocal interactions which are closely linked to four developmental tendencies:

1. The infant tends to move away; the mother guards each step. This 4-week-old infant displays and vocalizes to the animals in the adjacent cage while the mother guards it.
2. Infant and mother exhibit strong ties. As soon as the mother moves away, the child follows; the slightest disturbance in the environment causes fleeing to the mother's back. This is also true of infants with substitute mothers.
3. As part of the maternal protective behaviour, dismounting and mounting, separation and reunification are taught by repetition. All mothers assume the species-specific posture shown in Fig. 10 if they

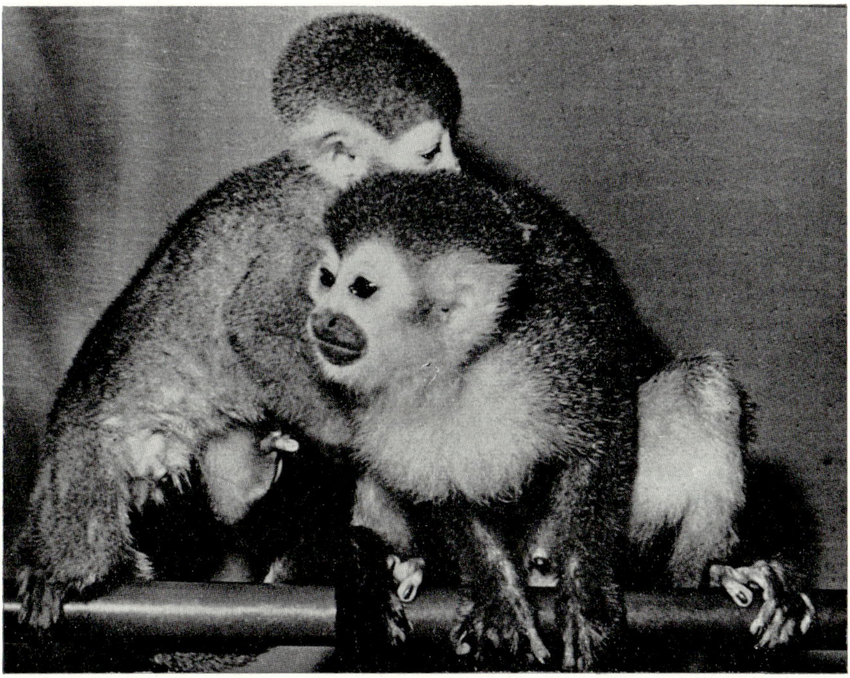

FIG. 10. Infant of 9 weeks mounts mother which offers her back in a typical posture. (Ploog *et al.* 1967.) Reproduced by permission of Springer Verlag, Berlin.

want the child to mount. In exceptional cases if the child does not respond to this signal, the mother becomes uneasy and may, when actual danger threatens, carry the infant away in her arms.

4. The first steps of weaning are taken. When the infant wants to suck, the mother forces it from her back. Both resort to screaming. Precisely at this time the infant begins to display towards the mother. This change of behaviour is associated with the acquisition of fur on the naked ventral side. From now on the prolonged and progressive weaning is one of the major factors which influence the maturation of the infant's social behaviour. In fact, weaning is a continuously increasing withdrawal of the main reward that the mother has to offer to the infant. By the time this process comes to an end, at 13 months, the relations between mother and child are indistinguishable from the relations between any adult female and other 13-month-old members of the group.

(b) The "Aunt" as Social Partner. The so-called aunt is the female in a group which takes special interest in a particular infant. The aunt-infant relationship begins to form as early as 2 weeks after birth. The mother gradually tolerates these contacts with the infant. The aunt becomes the huddling partner for mother and child. She protects the infant and may even be its wet nurse. She carries the infant on her back and it may resort to her when temporarily rejected by its mother. Unlike the mother the aunt engages in play with the infant, which directs its first courtship to her (Fig. 9b).

(c) Peers as Social Partners. The predominant activity with peers of both sexes is play, which begins at 8 weeks and continues throughout development. The most intense play period occurs between the fifth and eighth months. It decreases gradually in the second and more so the third year of life.

The essential point here is that the social roles (which later on become stereotyped and much more rigid) are incredibly flexible and, indeed, for quite a time they are more or less independent of the sex of the animal. In play the "attacking" and the "fleeing", the "dominant" and the "submissive", the "male" and the "female" may easily and at any time exchange their roles. The play gradually includes sexual elements (Latta *et al.*, 1967). The active male role appears first and earliest at 5 months; the active female role appears earliest at 6 months. Juveniles also play mother and child, riding the back and trying to suckle the nipples. The alpha animal may be playfully approached by a male juvenile in the female as in the male role. A mature female whose be-

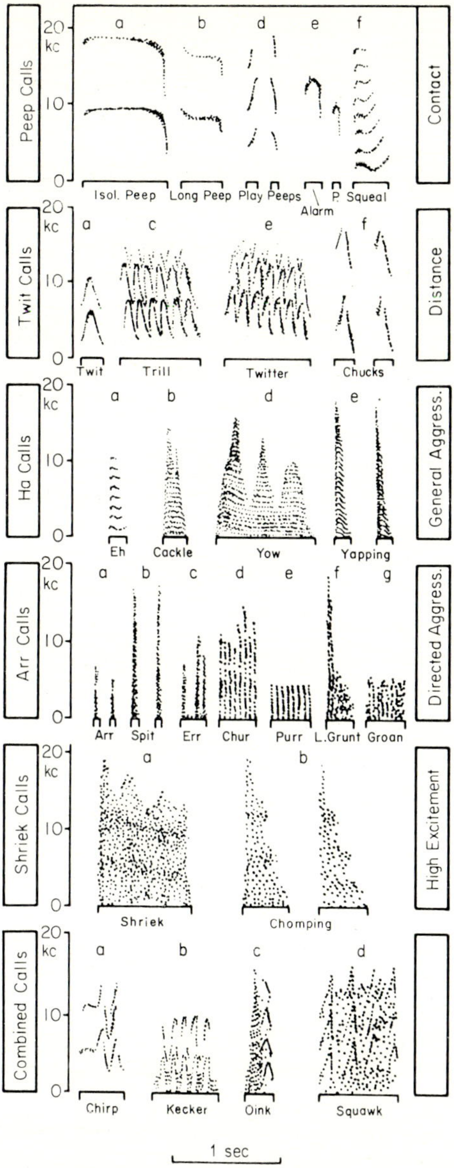

FIG. 11. Schematic presentation of the vocal repertoire: drawings made from sound spectrograms. The recorded sounds were systematically arranged according to their physical characteristics (e.g. frequencies in KC and time course in sec) as determined by spectrographic analysis, and divided up into six groups. For the designation of calls a characteristic property of a call or an onomatopoeic description was used. The groups were designated by a descriptive name (e.g. peep calls) and a name which refers to the behavioural function (e.g. contact). agress. = aggression; Alarm p. = alarm peep; L. grunt = labour grunt. (Winter *et al.* 1966.) Reproduced by permission of Springer Verlag, Berlin.

haviour towards alpha is always purely female responds to the female courtship of a male juvenile with male copulatory movements.

Vocalization. Vocalizations are the most important signals in squirrel monkey communication. The first shrieks may be heard immediately after birth. Rooting and sucking are accompanied by the so-called milk purring which occurs within the first hours of life. In later life it may be heard during huddling and short interruptions of play and in connection with genital display. When a female begins smelling or touching an infant on its mother's back, the female may utter a series of purrs. The low intensity of this call suggests that it is directed towards an animal close by. In certain contexts purrs indicate a slightly aggressive motivation. Otherwise, the signal content is not yet fully understood. Peeps as well as trills are heard during the first days, and several other calls can be recorded during the first week. The total repertoire of the adult consists of about 26 distinguishable calls (Fig. 11). Because of technical difficulties we do not yet know how many of them are present in the period immediately after birth. At least some of them occur only later—during maturation—for they are linked to behavioural stages, such as play, which appear sequentially. There is a great variability in baby calls, with continuous intermediates occurring between all the basic five groups. Within the first 6 months of life these transitions are gradually replaced by more discrete call types (Ploog *et al.*, 1967; Winter *et al.*, 1966).

As far as we know, squirrel monkeys are not capable of imitating sounds (Winter *et al.*, 1966). It is very unlikely that even the simplest call can be learned. In general, the physical characteristics of the infant's calls are more irregular and show a greater variability than the adult calls. The course of this maturation process of calls remains to be investigated (Winter, 1969).

The early calls of an infant elicit far greater attention from the group than do visual signals. The infants respond very early to alarm calls, which signal an aerial predator, or to yapping which is comparable to the mobbing response of songbirds.

The following example shows one of several methods for analysing signal content (Fig. 12). Before play, call 2 is not present. During play between two juveniles this call appears. Since its physical characteristics fit into the group of peeps and it occurs only during play, and especially during play fighting, it is called play peeping. It conveys a non-aggressive intention on the part of the emitter. If play becomes too rough, peeping stops and play breaks off.

As in the case of genital display or other motor signals, vocal signals

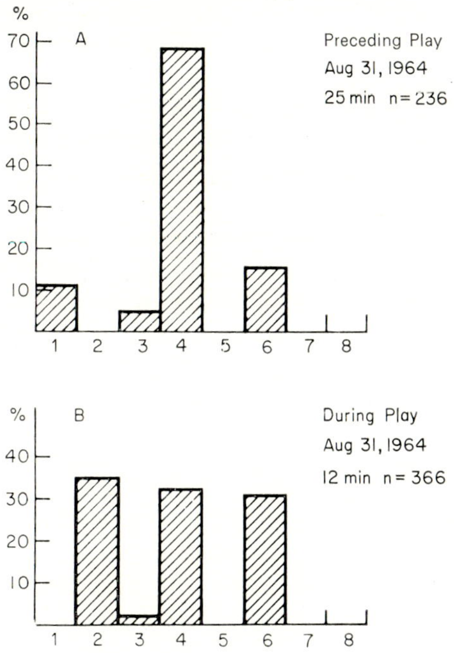

FIG. 12. Changes of vocalization pattern in a group of four monkeys before and during play. (Winter *et al.* 1966.) Call types 1—8 according to Fig. 1. Reproduced by permission of Springer Verlag, Berlin.

must also be related to the behavioural situation in which they occur and to the current social status of the animals involved. For instance, the reaction of a mother to an infant's purring varies according to the infant's age. Some calls are heard only if at least four animals of different ages and including both sexes form the group. Other calls are heard only in the presence of babies and young animals.

Motor patterns and vocalizations combined form an early communication system which is fairly complex and multiform. The maturation process of the communication system is correlated with developments such as teething, weaning, and increase in weight. Spermatogenesis is complete at 2 years 9 months. But it takes the animal, at least the male, 1 or probably 2 more years to become fully adult and socially mature.

It must be stressed that very little of the multiform communication system is object-related. In the case of calls only the alarm and the mobbing call are strictly object-related; they are in fact enemy-related. There are calls related to food but they are used also in a non-food, partner-related context. The overwhelming majority of the signals are social: that is, either group-directed in that the whole group is addressed or partner-directed where a specific individual is addressed. The group calls are fairly stereotyped and invariable but the partner-directed calls show many shades and great variability. Nevertheless, there is little doubt that the total communication system, as far as the single signals are concerned, is innate or, to say it even more provocatively, genetically determined. Subspecies appear to deviate slightly in their "dialects" (Winter, 1969). But the use of the communication system, the distributional patterns of the signals within the group, the sequences in which they occur, and the rituals which develop are all subject to change as time passes. Much social learning is involved and it is impossible at this point to make sharp distinctions between maturation and learning processes. One of the astonishing findings is the timing in these long-term processes, particularly since it seems to be largely independent of all external variables, social ones included, provided there is a structured environment at all. There is only one factor which has a strong influence on the otherwise well-timed developmental processes, and that is an intact brain. Through early brain damage the course of the development can be considerably retarded and altered in various respects.

BRAIN MECHANISMS UNDERLYING COMMUNICATION PROCESSES

It has been shown that complex motor patterns (such as genital display), combined with autonomic functions (such as penile erection), as well as a variety of vocal patterns—which may also be considered as motor patterns—are already present at birth or very shortly thereafter. It has also been shown that cognitive functions such as addressing a partner or responding to calls are present in part during the first few days of life. This means that the brain structures which mediate these performances must be functioning at birth.

Since we still lack neuroanatomical data on squirrel monkey fetuses and neonates, and neurophysiological data on early brain functions, we have to draw conclusions by inference. That is to say, we must confine ourselves to considering data on electrical brain stimulation of adult animals. Those structures from which responses can be elicited in the adult and which are already present in the infant must be the structures which are involved in infant behaviour.

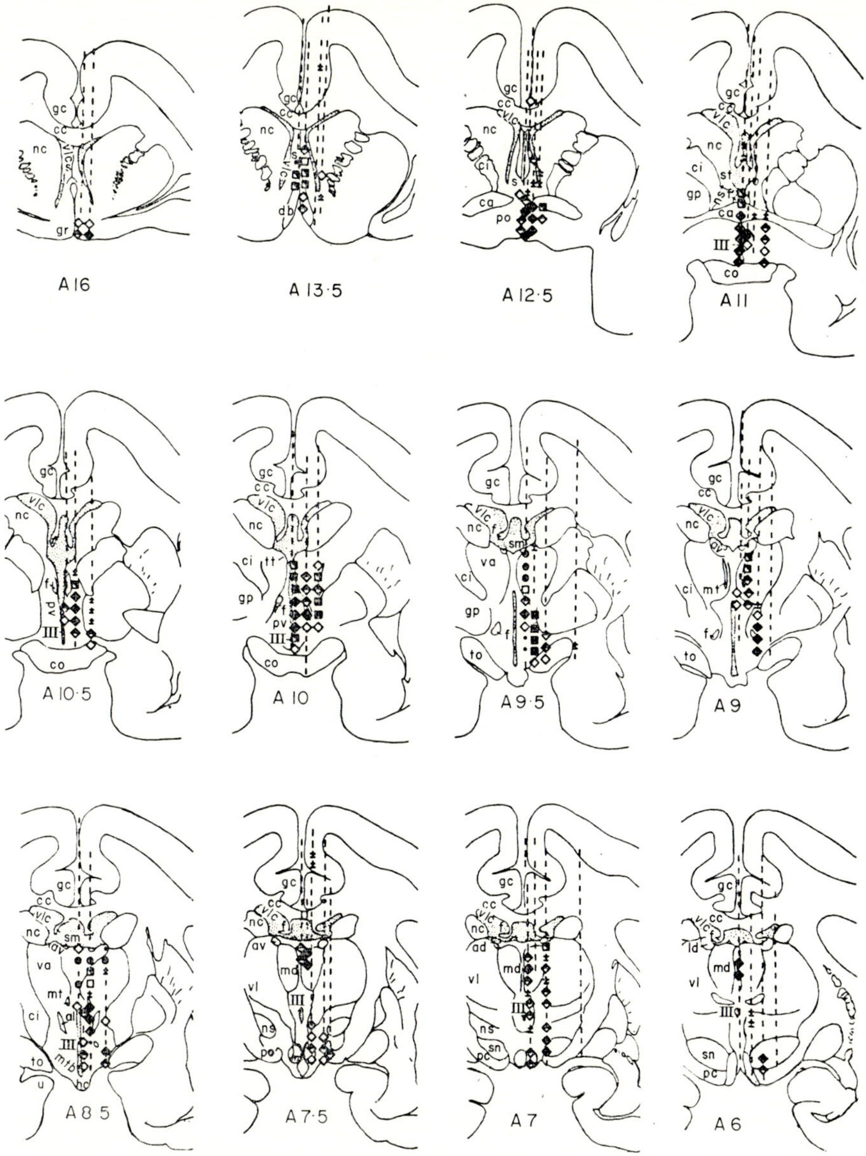

FIG. 13. Cerebral representation of genital function in male squirrel monkeys. Positive and negative points with respect to penile erection are plotted on brain diagrams of a stereotaxic atlas (Gergen and MacLean) at representative frontal planes from A 16 to A 6. (Ploog. *Psychiatrie der Gegenwart*. Vol. I/1B. 1964.) Reproduced by permission of Springer Verlag, Berlin. |: points explored with negative results. ◇ ⬘ ◆ small, medium or large (left to right) erections elicited without hippocampal after-discharges. □ ◪ ■ small, medium or large (left to right) erections elicited, with the stimulations accompanied or followed by hippocampal after-discharges. (For further details *see* MacLean and Ploog, 1962.)

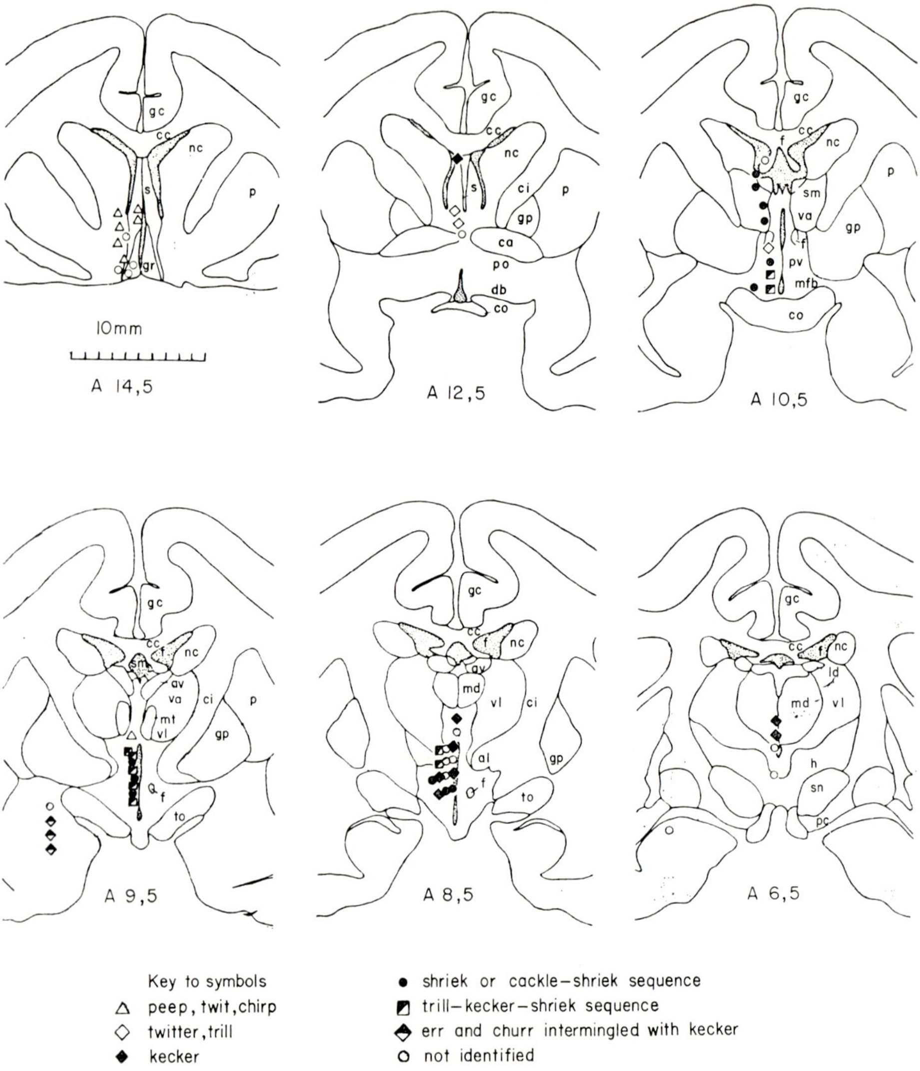

FIG. 14. Brain diagrams with loci for vocal responses. Representative frontal planes of a stereotaxic atlas from A 14·5—A 6·5. The brain area explored encompasses a medial section 2 mm wide on either side of the midline. The amygdala and hippocamus were supplementarily included. (Jürgens *et al.*, 1967.) Reproduced by permission of Springer Verlag, Berlin.

We have two sets of data. The first is the cerebral representation of penile erection (Fig. 13) which was worked out by MacLean and his co-workers including this author, and the cerebral representation of the clitoris, worked out in our laboratory (MacLean and Ploog, 1962; Maurus *et al.*, 1965). The male and the female systems do not differ with

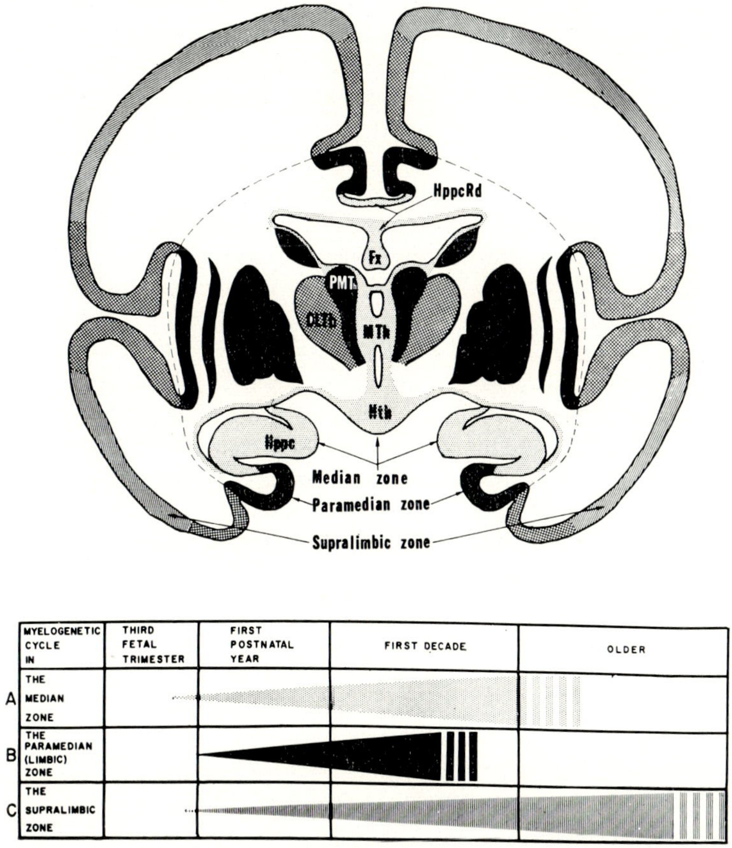

FIG. 15. *Top*: Three zones of the cerebral wall of the human brain. *Median zone*: grey. *Paramedian zone*: black. *Dorsolateral zone*: diagonal hatching—the supralimbic association areas; cross-hatching—the opercular and paralimbic areas. *Bottom*: Graphs A, B, C represent comparatively the cycles of myelination of the respective myeloarchitectonic zones in the brain wall.

Key to abbreviations:

Mth = Median thalamic zone; PMTh = Paramedian thalamic zone; DLTh = Dorsolateral (and posterior) thalamic zone; Fx = Fornix; Hppc = Hippocampus; HppcRd = Hippocampus Rudiment; HTh = Hypothalamus.

(Reproduced with permission from Yakovlev and Lecours, 1967, and Blackwell, Oxford.)

respect to localization. The second set of data is concerned with the cerebral representation of vocalization of which we have a pilot study (Fig. 14). A much more elaborate study is under way (Jürgens, 1968; Jürgens *et al.*, 1967).

Both systems, that for genital function as well as that for vocal function, are located in parts of the limbic system, the midline structures of the thalamus, the hypothalamus, and midline structures of the mid-brain. With respect to the vocalizations, it is worth mentioning that there is a rough subdivision: the points for aggressive calls cluster in the lower, and the points for communal calls in the higher, levels of the brain. It should also be noted that other investigators have never found points for vocal responses in the neocortex of non-human primates.

It is not my intention to go into anatomical details here. But it is important to refer to studies by Yakovlev and André-Roch Lecours (1967) on regional development of the brain in the early life of humans (Fig. 15). Unfortunately, no equivalent comparative data on non-human primates are available. The figure shows three zones of myelination. The median zone matches the locations just mentioned in parts of the limbic system and the midline structures. Parts of the paramedian limbic zones may also be included. The figure (graphs A, B, and C) shows that the myelination of the median zone starts during the last third of the gestation time and stretches over a long period of human life. We may speculate that comparative data on the squirrel monkey's median zone would be likely to show a relatively faster and more intense myelination of the median zone.

SIGNIFICANCE OF SOCIAL COMMUNICATION

In conclusion I would like to raise three questions. Firstly, why is it that all primates have to devote so much of their lives to developing a social communication system, albeit one that is highly complex? In monkeys this is less so than in apes, in apes less so than in man. Secondly, is the social communication system of non-human primates a phyletic prerequisite for the acquisition of language, although human language seems to be predominantly object-related whereas the non-verbal communication system is partner-related? Thirdly, if the social communication system is a prerequisite for language, what role has the non-verbal vocal system—undoubtedly still present in man—within the functioning of human speech?

SUMMARY

The behavioural ontogeny and early communication processes in 15 infant squirrel monkeys raised in mixed groups were studied from birth to the third year. The complete development is divided into seven phases.

For the first week of life the mother appears to be merely a composite of objects for the child. During the first 2 weeks of life interactions between mother and child which resemble specific features of social behaviour, that is, partner-directed interactions, are rare. The mother fully gains partner status during the third and fourth weeks when the infant begins to dismount for short periods.

Tactile, acoustic and visual communication with group mates starts as early as the first day of life. Examples of early social signals are given. From about 2 weeks onwards a strong social bond is established between the infant and a female group mate, the so-called aunt. Aunt-infant interactions show greater variation than mother-infant interactions.

As the infant gains motor independence during its second month mother-infant visual communication increases and weaning starts. Most of the species-specific behaviour elements are already present. Between the fifth and ninth months new behaviour patterns develop and others change in frequency and in the context of their occurrence.

The behaviour, based on innate elements, is developed further through learning during stage-specific interaction with group mates. Prolonged and progressive weaning until the beginning of the second year, social play, and various forms of rejective and suppressive behaviour shape the mode of social communication.

From brain stimulation experiments on adult squirrel monkeys and from neuroanatomical data on brain maturation it can be inferred that brain structures important for complex communication processes are already fulfilling their function at birth. Specific characteristics of early social communication in primates are discussed.

REFERENCES

Bowden, D., Winter, P. and Ploog, D. 1967. Pregnancy and delivery behaviour in the squirrel monkey (*Saimiri sciureus*) and other primates. *Folia Primat., Basel* **5,** 1–42.

Castell, R. and Ploog, D. 1967. Zum Sozialverhalten der Totenkopfaffen (*Saimiri sciureus*): Auseinandersetzung zwischen zwei Kolonien. *Z. Tierpsychol.* **24,** 625–641.

CASTELL, R., KROHN, H. and PLOOG, D. 1969. Rückenwälzen bei Totenkopfaffen (*Saimiri sciureus*): Körperpflege und soziale Funktion. *Z. Tierpsychol.* **26,** 488–497.

HOPF, S. 1967. Notes on pregnancy, delivery, and infant survival in captive squirrel monkeys. *Primates* **8,** 323–332.

HOPF, S. 1970. Report on a hand-reared squirrel monkey (*Saimiri sciureus*). *Z. Tierpsychol.* (in press).

JÜRGENS, U. 1968. Correlation between brain structure and vocalization type elicited in the squirrel monkey. In G. H. Bourne (Ed.). *Proc. 2nd International Congress of Primatology.* S. Karger: Basel, Freiburg, New York (in press).

JÜRGENS, U., MAURUS, M., PLOOG, D. and WINTER, P. 1967. Vocalization in the squirrel monkey (*Saimiri sciureus*) elicited by brain stimulation. *Expl Brain Res.* **4,** 114–117.

LATTA, J., HOPF, S. and PLOOG, D. 1967. Observations on mating behaviour and sexual play in the squirrel monkey (*Saimiri sciureus*). *Primates* **8,** 229–246.

LORENZ, K. 1932. Betrachtungen über das Erkennen der arteigenen Triebhandlungen der Vögel. *J. Orn., Berlin* **80,** 50–98.

LORENZ, K. 1935. Der Kumpan in der Umwelt des Vogels. *J. Orn., Berlin* **83,** 137–413.

MACLEAN, P. D. and PLOOG, D. W. 1962. Cerebral representation of penile erection. *J. Neurophysiol.* **25,** 29–55.

MAURUS, M. and PLOOG, D. 1968. Motor and vocal interactions in groups of squirrel monkeys, elicited by remote-controlled electrical brain stimulation. In G. H. Bourne (Ed.). *Proc. 2nd International Congress of Primatology.* S. Karger: Basel, Freiburg, New York (in press).

MAURUS, M., MITRA, J. and PLOOG, D. 1965. Cerebral representation of the clitoris in ovariectomized squirrel monkeys. *Expl Neurol.* **13,** 283–288.

PLOOG, D. 1966. Biological bases for instinct and behaviour: studies on the development of social behaviour in squirrel monkeys. In J. Wortis (Ed.), *Recent advances in biological psychiatry* **8,** 199–223. Plenum Press, New York.

PLOOG, D. 1967. The behaviour of squirrel monkeys (*Saimiri sciureus*) as revealed by sociometry, bioacoustics, and brain stimulation. In S. A. Altmann (Ed.), *Social communication among primates.* Univ. of Chicago Press, Chicago, Ill. Pp. 149–184.

PLOOG, D., BLITZ, J., and PLOOG, F. 1963. Studies on social and sexual behaviour of the squirrel monkey (*Saimiri sciureus*). *Folia Primat. Basel* **1,** 29–66.

PLOOG, D., HOPF, S. and WINTER, P. 1967. Ontogenese des Verhaltens von Totenkopfaffen (*Saimiri sciureus*). *Psychol. Forsch.* **31,** 1–41.

SACKETT, G. P. 1966. Monkeys reared in isolation with pictures as visual input: evidence for an innate releasing mechanism. *Science* **154,** 1468–1472.

WINTER, P. 1969. Dialects in squirrel monkeys: vocalization of the Roman arch type. *Folia Primat. Basel,* **10,** 216–229

WINTER, P., PLOOG, D. and LATTA, J. 1966. Vocal repertoire of the squirrel monkey (*Saimiri sciureus*), its analysis and significance. *Expl Brain Res.* **1,** 259–384.

YAKOVLEV, P. I. and LECOURS, A.-R. 1967. The myelogenetic cycles of regional maturation of the brain. In A. Minkowski (Ed.), *Regional development of the brain in early life.* Blackwell, Oxford. Pp. 3–70.

Discussion

Orientation and Exploration

LIPSITT: My question has general implications concerning the way in which we determine causes of behaviour. You said that at 12 days of age the squirrel monkey often became disoriented and climbed around the back of the mother, rather than orienting himself towards the nipple. Were you assuming that the proper orientation for a 12-day-old squirrel monkey would always be at the nipple?

PLOOG: No, ordinarily the monkey is on the back of the mother in a tail-to-tail and head-to-head position. The position for feeding is rare but if the monkey tries to get in that position and becomes disoriented, this certainly causes great confusion to the mother (*see* p. 273).

LIPSITT: My point remains the same. You are assuming that there is some proper orientation on the back even when the animal is not attempting to feed. Might not one aspect of proper orientation in this young animal be that which maximizes exploratory behaviour? After all, the entire body surface of the mother is part of the world of the 12-day-old organism, which he sees and feels very well. Perhaps when he is upside down, as he was, he is in the best position for seeing the world?

PLOOG: There is a "proper" orientation immediately after birth. This is clearly demonstrated in our movies on birth and the early postpartum period. But it is only up to 12 days that the infant may become disoriented. From then on it uses the mother as a walking place and it does exactly what you say, it tries to discover the world. But until the twelfth day, if it is not in the position which is maintained 90 per cent of the time, the mother becomes uneasy and tries to get it back in the right position. So there is a point where discovery of the world starts—it is not there right from the beginning, at least with respect to the mother's body.

Male and Female Roles

WOLFF: In the first year or so there was no sexual dimorphism in the play of these monkeys?

PLOOG: The male role appears at 5 months and the female role—the characteristic courtship behaviour in which the animal looks over its shoulder and darts about—appears not earlier than at 6 months. But at this stage either sex can adopt either role. Only after the first year does each sex assume mostly its own role. For example, only the male is engaged in play fighting and schooling by the alpha animal—not the female.

WOLFF: Does that represent a species difference from what Harlow described in Rhesus monkeys? He seemed to find a clear difference in their kind of play according to their sex.

PLOOG: I have never observed Rhesus monkeys so closely but I think they too have this intermediate stage where they can play both roles, the male or the female.

KAUFMAN: Don't Harlow's data on the Rhesus, and Jensen's on the pigtail, clearly indicate that already in the first year of life the male infants are far more active in the vigorous types of play—rough-and-tumble and chasing—which then in the second year become more clearly aggressive behaviour?

PLOOG: Yes. This sex difference is seen in the case of the squirrel monkey from 9 months on, but from the fifth month to about the eighth month it is very hard to detect, though the females are a little less active in playing.

KAUFMAN: Androgens and oestrogens now appear important in the emergence of female and male behaviour. They do not simply have their effect fairly late in the life of the organism; they play a very significant role in the development of the kind of nervous system, whether the male or the female. Have you any data on the early appearance of androgens and oestrogens?

PLOOG: The only hard data concern spermatogenesis which is fully developed at 2 years 9 months. The few drops of urine we can get are not sufficient to measure steroids. The problem is especially difficult because the animals are moving, and if you put them in single cages in order to collect urine, then their behaviour changes so greatly that this may influence steroid output.

SCHULTE: In human subjects the output of 17 ketosteroids is almost independent of the conditions under which urine is collected.

PLOOG: A squirrel monkey in isolation is not the same squirrel monkey.

Structure Function Relations

SCHULTE: You showed a picture of myelination in the hypothalamic area. Myelination is only one aspect of structural development. Have you any data on dendritic arborization or the development of Nissl substance?

PLOOG: No, and such studies are difficult to perform on the hypothalamus. The new Nauta method which stains the boutons may soon provide much better information on presynaptic functions.

PRECHTL: Can Ploog describe the circuits involved in the behaviour patterns he has described?

PLOOG: There seem to be three or four areas which are interconnected and which play an important role in social as well as sexual behaviour. "Pure" sexual function, that is, penile erection without visible social implications, is most readily elicited by stimulation of the hypothalamus. If you go higher up the septum and other limbic structure and to the frontal area, for example, the gyrus rectus, electrical stimulation takes longer to produce an erection, which then may outlast the stimulus. And the same is true of the medial dorsal nucleus of the thalamus, which seems to be an important interconnecting place for all kinds of social behaviour. By stimulating that region we can obtain vocalizations, erections, and sometimes a long built-up fight. Of course, the medial dorsal nucleus of the thalamus is the nucleus that is greatly developed in primates and especially in man, compared with other thalamic nuclei.

BERGSTRÖM: You said that at the beginning there is a lack of feedback mechanisms. Since the development of feedback mechanisms could be important for a higher degree of organization in the CNS, what kind of feedback mechanisms appear later?

PLOOG: I have no anatomical data—just the observation that for the first few days, but never later, the monkey may scratch the mother's back or in the air. I think this means that the monkey does not get a feedback if he scratches himself. You can touch him anywhere and he starts scratching so it takes time to interlock the localization of the itching exteroceptive stimulus with the scratching mechanism.

Effect of Separation from the Mother

SANDER: You say the separation of the infant and the mother begins around 3 to 4 weeks and progresses. Have you timed the duration of this separation, and is the appearance of threat behaviour related to it?

PLOOG: The infant does not like the separation. The mother forces it off the back—she screams and the infant either learns, or has to be forced, to walk away. This of course differs in different animals. Sometimes mothers are very quiet and wait, and then one day the infant steps off and walks, 5 or 6 centimetres at first, and the next day 10 centimetres and maybe after a week 30 centimetres and so forth.

SANDER: I am thinking of the time duration of the separation. How far has it advanced from the age of 3 to 4 weeks, when it starts, to the age of 1 year when threatening behaviour appears?

PLOOG: Separation proceeds gradually and more or less linearly until most of the time is spent away from the mother. The final period is when the child sleeps on the mother's back only during the night. This continues up to 14 months.

WOLFF: What mechanism starts the mother pushing the baby off?

PLOOG: It depends very much on the external situation. Any kind of disturbance in the environment may make the mother start the separation process very early or even reject the child completely. But the process certainly starts by 6 weeks if the child does not decide to walk off by itself.

WOLFF: Is there something in the species which makes it start at some particular time, though with some variations due to external factors?

PLOOG: Yes.

WOLFF: Is it hormonal?

PLOOG: We don't have measurements, but we know at least that the lactation of a squirrel monkey can go on for as long as 2 years. The timing of separation cannot be explained by hormonal factors alone.

Significance of Prolonged Developmental Period in Primates

PRECHTL: Mammals have found four solutions for bringing up their offspring. One is the method used by the marsupials and the second is to bring them up in a nest. The third is for the newborn to be so mature that they walk soon after birth. The fourth is for the young to be carried around on the mother's body, as in bats and primates. Many years ago Portman stated, from comparative morphological data on the brain, that the human infant is, so to speak, a physiological premature. I think it is better to regard the human species as having another specific way of raising and nursing the offspring.

PLOOG: Yes, but why does it take a primate, whether non-human or human, so many years to develop an elaborate social communication system? I agree with Portman and with Bolk that a primate is premature at birth. That is so with squirrel monkeys: the newborn is absolutely helpless and without the mother it would die in a day.

PRECHTL: I always wonder about this concept of the helpless newborn infant; as you have shown us, the repertoire of the infant monkey, for example, is so marvellously developed.

PLOOG: It is helpless only in the case of separation from the mother. The mother-child dyad is absolutely necessary for survival, but my point is that the mother-child dyad is not the place where social communication first occurs. It takes place with partners. The mother becomes a partner after the first separation, but before that she is treated as an object.

KAUFMAN: Your question of why development takes so long is a sort of value judgement as to how long is so long, but it is generally believed that the scheme which evolved with the higher primates—of the helpless infant and the mother who had to be properly motivated to take care of this helpless infant—had one great advantage, namely it provided a longer, more leisurely time for the organism to reach maturity and to learn all the important behaviours. For example, before young females reach sexual maturity they become involved in junior maternal behaviours and begin to acquire the knowledge of how a mother behaves from observation, imitation, and actual participation.

PLOOG: Only primates develop such a repertoire of communication means. More than 30 motor signals and 26 separate vocal signals are important for the squirrel monkey. Imagine how complicated this is, if you remember that the vocal signals directed to a partner are shaded and graded, and that visual and vocal cues have to occur together in order to give the right message. Discussion of human communication usually neglects the non-verbal communication system. In all the language research it has never been considered that there is a vocal system, separate from any language, which has a cerebral representation that might depend on something other than the temporal lobe and the third convolution of the frontal lobe.

BRONSON: People with damage to those areas who are unable to speak can, if they are sufficiently emotionally disturbed, make an emotional sound—which indicates that a more primitive vocalization centre remains, but not under volitional control.

Attempts at Synthesis:
organization in the development of behaviour

"Organization" in Behaviour

GENERAL DISCUSSION

PLOOG: May I draw your attention to two papers by Lashley. One is devoted to the problem of organization (1958. *Proc. Ass. Res. nerv. ment. Dis.* **36,** 1); and the other to the sequential order of behaviour (1951. In L. A. Jeffress (Ed.), *Cerebral Mechanisms in Behaviour*, p. 112. Wiley, New York). He argued that one cannot explain the whole of behaviour with either of these terms: one has to consider at all times the various levels and the order and disorder in terms of the sequential order. To tackle this problem by talking in general about organization of sequential behaviour is unhelpful. One should rather talk about specific areas. With respect to environment and development, regardless of whether the environment is rich or poor, the animal will search for its reinforcers and if it does not find primary reinforcers in its environment, then its behaviour will be distorted. That is just the opposite from what most psychologists think.

LIPSITT: Can you give us an example in the squirrel monkey?

PLOOG: Yes, if you change the stimulus properties for riding on the back, for searching for the nipples, or for reaching for food then the animal will perform perfectly well until a certain poverty of the environment is reached where it has no means of obtaining the primary reinforcers. The total behaviour is organized in such a way as to search for a small bit of reinforcer, and this promotes learning in a very rapid manner—as compared with lower animals where the stimulus property has to be much more specific in order to elicit an appropriate behaviour.

LIPSITT: Do you see disordered, distorted behaviour in your monkeys on the stuffed woollen sock?

PLOOG: No, not at all. Even the call which the baby normally emits when it returns to the mother's back, that is a certain trill, is emitted at exactly the same time on the sock.

BRONSON: What about the range of stimuli which a newborn squirrel monkey requires? You mentioned tactile stimulation and sucking.

PLOOG: A certain amount of sucking and a certain amount of milk are necessary to satisfy the animal. If you separate the two then the one can supplement the other to a certain degree; for example, if you give a longer sucking time, the animal is faster satiated with less food. I tried this in human infants, too, with bigger and smaller holes in the nipple, and found the same thing.

BRONSON: If you deprive the monkey of sucking, can this be compensated by more clinging or are these fairly discrete systems?

PLOOG: I don't know. My main point is that impoverishment of the external stimuli—which are the set of primary reinforcers—causes distortion of the organization of the behaviour. Up to a certain point it doesn't matter how the world is organized; all you need is that all these little bits of primary reinforcers be available.

SANDER: Do they have to be used in any particular state of the infant monkey, so that their value as reinforcers has some connection with the basic programme of periodic functions like sleep and hunger?

PLOOG: We haven't the measurements by which we agreed to define "state" in Prechtl's sense.

BERGSTRÖM: Can you define "organization"? Can the concept of organization—higher organization, lower organization— be replaced by the concept of order and disorder? It would then be possible to connect the concept of organization with the concept of order, then with probability functions, and also with the concept of entropy.

WOLFF: I can try to define organization by using an illustration borrowed from Weiss (unpublished). Imagine a system (do not ask me what I mean by a system, that becomes an infinite regress) of more than two parts, in which the parts are not freely interchangeable and are in a particular relationship to each other, such that if you disordered them you would change the whole system. In a bucket of sand there are millions of grains but there is certainly no organization. On the other hand, if you have elements:

A A A A
B B B B
C C C C

you have a certain level of order, but if the arrangement is:

A B C A
B C A B
C A B C

then you have a higher degree of organization. In the first case a certain amount of rearrangement is possible without disturbing the system, but you no longer have the same latitude for rearrangement in the second case. And it is the degree of inter-dependence of the parts on each other in the whole system that I would define as organization.

BERGSTRÖM: Dependency is order, independency is disorder. We can now go futher in the analysis of the unit activity in the brain using the concept of order, and relate this analysis to the problems in the development of behaviour.

BRONSON: I have been trying to fit Wolff's notion into a developmental framework. His definition of order implies an observer who knows the symbols; the bucket of sand could conceivably be ordered to someone who knew about sand grains and the way they distribute themselves. But what is the standard which might be applied to order in the nervous system? It may be that we have two types of criterion of order. In the adult what is ordered is partly a product of our past experience. But in the newborn or the very young, what is the criterion as to whether its central state is an ordered one? Perhaps there is an inherent criterion as to whether it is ordered. For example, rhythmicity or general level of excitation might be the criterion of order.

LIPSITT: Order or organization to me are something like the patterns of behaviour in response to a facial stimulus that Humphrey showed in the fetus. It seemed that the baby was executing a pattern of behaviour, a constellation of responses which were integrated with considerable grace. The full pattern of behaviour from beginning to end in response to that particular stimulus isn't a mere head withdrawal or a mere head turn. The stimulus Humphrey applied triggered a succession of responses. Should we discuss patterns or organization of behaviour of that sort?

WOLFF: What you call "grace" is exactly this problem. When you talk of a pattern of behaviour, you are talking about organization—it is exactly the same.

HUMPHREY: I know nothing about grace in the fetus, except that according to Hooker (1952. *The Prenatal Origin of Behaviour*. Univ. of Kansas Press, Laurence) at about 14 weeks the reflexes become variable and "graceful" rather than stereotyped as in earlier development. However, I believe that there is organization and integration from the very first reflex movement in that, I am following the views of the great English physiologist, Sir Charles Sherrington.

KAUFMAN: Organization and patterning have to be looked at in the living organism in terms of level of organization. I don't mean only such things as the difference between a monosynaptic reflex and a very complicated pattern in the central nervous system, but also level in the sense, for example, of the organismic level as compared to the organ system level. Let's go back to the patterns of behaviour that come out of the nervous system. You can, for example, discover where to stimulate the brain in a squirrel monkey to produce a genital display. Delgado and many others know where to stimulate it to produce a burst of aggressive behaviour. But in neither case, unless you know something more than the site you are stimulating, can you predict at whom the display or the aggressive behaviour will be directed. So there is a different level of organization, namely the social level of organization which, so far as we know, cannot really be predicted from the operation of discrete organization within the nervous system.

LIPSITT: So in order to know about organization in the fetus, or in the newborn, or in any organism, we have to take into consideration experiential factors and environmental determinants of behaviour, as well as the kinds of things that Dr. Humphrey has pointed to.

MACKEITH: Once you introduce the term "levels", you are really introducing about a hundred different terms. There is a level, if you like, of complexity and simplicity. There is a level where a response may be dominant over all other responses, or not very dominant, and so on. This is not one concept, but a whole number of dimensions.

Regulation and Organization in the Early Infant-caretaker System[1]

LOUIS W. SANDER[2]
Boston University

ALTHOUGH AT THIS point in the conference we have come to the task of synthesis and to the subject of "organization", my remarks are not intended as any treatment in depth of a subject so central to the whole conceptual framework of biology. It seems more appropriate to illustrate the way we have tried to apply certain notions about organization to studies of infant-environment exchange. Since in living systems, exchange is inseparable from regulation and regulation is inseparable from organization, the expectation is that discussion of one will of necessity involve the others.

My associates and I became interested in the initial organization of infant-caretaker interaction as a result of a longitudinal study of 30 first-born infants, in which the progress of the mother-child relationship was followed in detail over the first 3 years of life (Sander, 1969). At the outset, the organization of functions in the mother and in the child, as reflected by their characteristic tendencies to activity, is quite disparate, even dissonate, in timing, intensity, modality, etc. We can assume that engagement in interaction begins as part and parcel of the problem of regulation. In the adaptive interaction between the two participants mutual modification of the organization of activity in each proceeds until harmony of coordination (and relative stability) endures between the participants. The specific configuration of such coordination reflects the particular contribution to regulation and the particular capacities for modification, or resistance to modification, which characterize each of the partners, and, in unique profile, each of their various functions.

[1] This research is being supported by USPHS Grants: 1 KO5 MH 20505–06, 5 RO1 HD01766–04, 5 K2 MH 18521–07, and 3 RO1 HD 01766–04s2.

[2] Authorship of this paper is shared with Harry Julia, Gerald Stechler, and Padraic Burns.

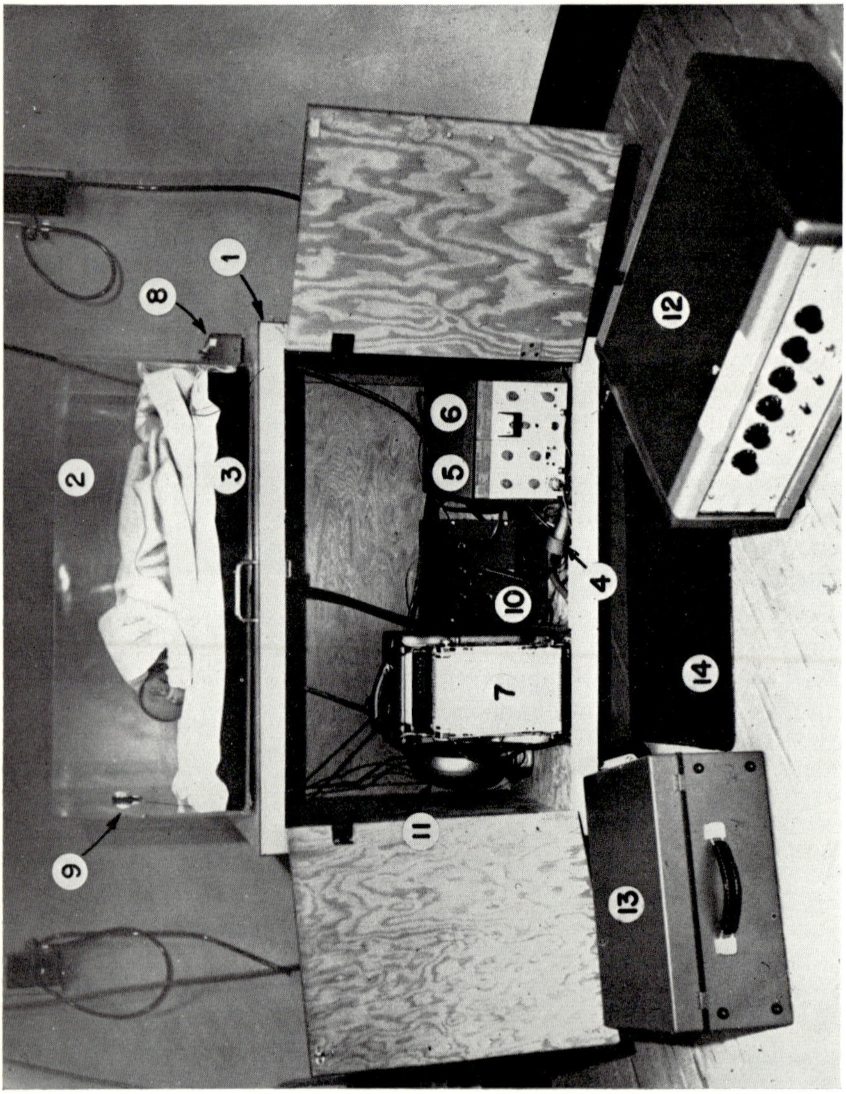

FIG. 1. Activity and Interactional Monitor. (1) Formica covered plywood cabinet on large 4″ roller-bearing castors: height = 20″, length = 36″, width = 20″; (2) Clear $\frac{1}{2}$″ plastic bassinet, 15″ × 30″ × 13″; (3) Air mattress, 15″ × 30″ × 3″; (4) Pressure transducer; (5) Pressure amplifier; (6) Integrator; (7) Event recorder; (8) Caretaker-operation buttons; (9) Crystal microphone; (10) Voice-activated timer and junction box; (11) Automatic take-up reel for 25′ power cord; (12) Magnetic tape controller and addressor; (13) Digital stepping magnetic tape recorder; (14) Tapeswitch signal mat.

To pursue the argument further, in the growing infant each new thrust of activity of which he becomes capable requires a new period of interactional adjustment with the caretaking environment to reach stable coordination on the basis of new exchanges. Our experience in comparing the longitudinal interactional picture of different mother-child pairs in our sample led to evidence that the manner in which the *first* adaptive issue is negotiated over the first 2 or 3 months of life predicts certain later characteristics of interaction as the pair struggles to achieve coordination in subsequent adaptations.

Thus our attention became focused on the problem of initial regulation in the infant and its relation to his interaction with his environment. Since regulation implies a continuous round-the-clock-process, it seemed to us that a useful approach would be a 24-hour surveillance of infant, of mother, and of interaction between them.

I should like now to describe our method and to illustrate the kind of information which is emerging; at the end I shall return to possible relations to organization and brain mechanisms.

Three groups of normal neonates, each group reared under somewhat different caretaking conditions, are being compared in respect of continuously monitored variables related to infant activity, quiescence, and crying, along with the occurrence, duration, and nature of caretaking interventions. The 24-hour records are obtained by a specially designed monitoring bassinet (Fig. 1), which utilizes a multichannel Esterline-Angus event recorder to combine a continuous record of motility and crying from the infant with a parallel caretaking record, in real time, of approach, removal of infant from bassinet, return to bassinet, plus coded input of type of procedure. The motility record is obtained from a specially constructed air mattress in the bassinet coupled to a strain-gauge-amplifier-integrator combination. This gives a digital output, each blip occurring after small cumulations of infant movement by the integrator have triggered a pen on the event recorder. Similarly 15-second cumulations of crying time, obtained by a microphone in the crib coupled to a voice-activated timer, are recorded as a digital crying output by a pen in parallel.

The Esterline-Angus record of an infant's brief nocturnal awakening on the fifteenth day of life (Fig. 2) illustrates the type of data provided, and the operational measure which can be derived from it. The tape, running at 12 inches per hour, shows that the widely spaced motility blips in the sleeping state (segment A) become denser as the infant awakens, and finally begins to cry (segment B). Caretaker approach and removal from bassinet (segment C) follow after a period of delay, with

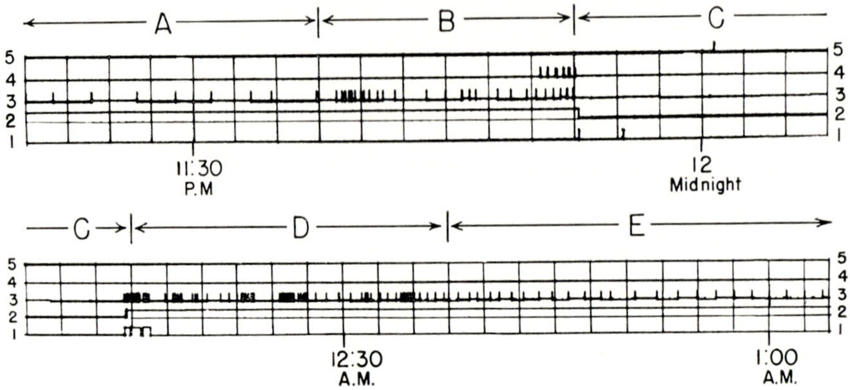

FIG. 2. Episode of nocturnal awakening in 15-day-old male infant. Numbered pen channels are as follows: 1. Switchmat; 2. Lift switch; 3. Motility; 4. Crying; 5. Caretaker operation (feeding). Event sequence is represented in the following segments: (A) sleep; (B) arousal with crying; (C) removal from bassinet and feeding; (D) return with episodes of vigorous motility but without crying; (E) quiescence and return to sleep.

a feeding indicated by a blip on the caretaking operations channel. Segment C ends with the return of the infant to the bassinet. Episodic and rather intense motility ensues (segment D), but without further crying or any further interaction, and eventually the infant goes to sleep spontaneously (segment E).

This fragment of a record indicates that even a brief nocturnal awakening takes a certain period of time and involves a certain sequence of events, with time required for transition from one state to the other and for the necessary environmental interaction—in this case, feeding. Usually the infant does not just suddenly pop open his eyes and remain awake without other concurrent evidence of state change. Quiescent and active epochs alternate with each other in cyclic fashion over the 24 hours of the day, showing interesting changes in character and distribution over the 24 hours, and, as one follows the infant, over the first 10 or 20 days of life.

A number of operational definitions which can be derived from the monitor record tell us something about the baby, about the caretaker, and about their interaction.

1. Motility and crying counts can be obtained in daily totals or summed over smaller periods of 1, 4, 6, or 12 hours. Trends obtained in this way show a close correlation between motility and crying in time of occurrence, duration, and intensity.

2. The duration of the "waking up" and "going to sleep" segments can be used to study individual differences between babies in negotiating state transitions and the changes which take place in these over the first two weeks of life.

3. Interactions by the caretaker can be measured in terms of their frequency, duration, timing and relation to cycles of infant activity. The pattern of interactions and the distribution of between-intervention intervals reveal distinguishing characteristics of caretaking environments.

4. An operational measure of great interest to us, to be touched upon further below, is that of "delay time": the time which elapses between the onset of crying and the caretaker's removal of the baby from the bassinet.

5. When the caretaker's first intervention has not been successful in quieting the baby, one or more interventions follow before a lengthy quiescent epoch appears on the record. Criteria have been set up to identify such "fussy periods". We construe these repetitive sequences of crying and response to be important episodes during which consistent caretaking response characteristics are becoming established as part of the infant's expectancy. The frequency and distribution of "fussy periods" are being studied as an indication of the progress of the adaptation and of the stability of regulation accompanying it.

6. One further useful monitor measure is the "activity period" by which the duration of an episode such as is illustrated in Fig. 2 can be defined, and distinguished from the ensuing and preceding "quiescent periods". These approximate closely to the observed periods of sleep and waking.

The concurrent data from both infant and caretaker, obtained as a continuous record by this method, suggested the possibility that we might have here a means of studying 24-hour rhythmicity and its relationship to interactional patterns from which investigation of regulation might proceed.

In displaying the data we have adopted the custom of identifying a 24-hour "day" as extending from 6 a.m. to 6 a.m. with the 12-hour diurnal epoch between 6 a.m. and 6 p.m. and the nocturnal epoch between 6 p.m. and 6 a.m. Figure 3 illustrates such a display of motility data during the sixth day of life of a normal infant in a lying-in nursery situation with 4-hourly scheduled feeding. This illustrates the cyclic character of infant activity peaks over the course of a day, six peaks having occurred in this instance. When the timing of interventions, also

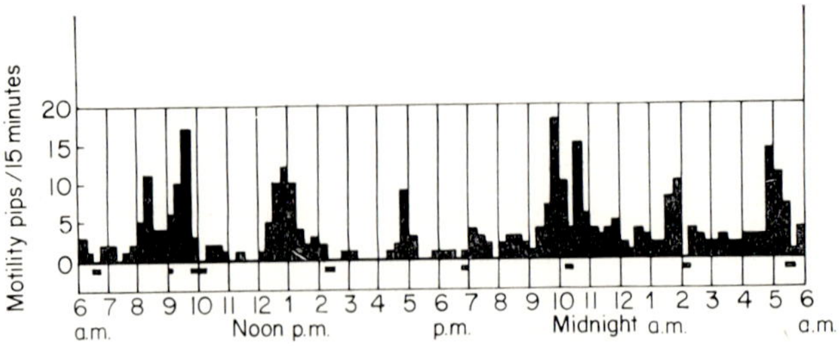

FIG. 3. Motility counts per 15-minute-period during the sixth day of life in nursery situation. Six peaks of activity can be seen. Small rectangles beneath bar graph indicate time and duration of intervention periods.

recorded by the monitor, is compared with the timing of activity periods, an inconstant relation is at once apparent. Feedings are noted here to occur in the midst of quiescence or at the peak of activity, with "delay time" varying widely from intervention to intervention. It is readily apparent from this illustration that if one were selecting infants from a neonatal nursery for psychophysiological experiments in a standardized way, so that subjects were obtained half an hour after ending a feeding and in a relatively quiet state, he might have chosen this infant at 7.30 a.m. or at 3 p.m. However, the position of the infant in respect to his natural 24-hour activity cycling would show these timings to be strikingly different. At 7.30 a.m. the infant would be beginning a period of activity, at 3 p.m. a period of quiescence. It is also worth pointing out that some of the activity periods appear to end at or near the time of an intervention, such as at 2 p.m. Others appear to end independently of intervention, as at 5.10 p.m.

When we were first exploring the usefulness of continuous monitoring, we had hoped to define infant activity types from the motility data. However, when we had followed infants through a change from the nursery environment at 5 days of life, it became obvious at once that the caretaking environment had to be comparable before infants could be reliably compared by the monitor in respect of their activity. Figure 4 represents one of our earliest studies, showing a striking reduction in 4-hour summations of motility in the home situation as compared with the nursery. It was this experience that led us to add a lift switch to the monitor, which would register the removal of the infant in order to correct motility records for length of time out of the bassinet when records from different environments were being compared. In the instance illustrated in Fig. 4, time out of the bassinet amounted to approximately 5 hours in the nursery situation as compared to 4·5 hours per 24-hour day in the home

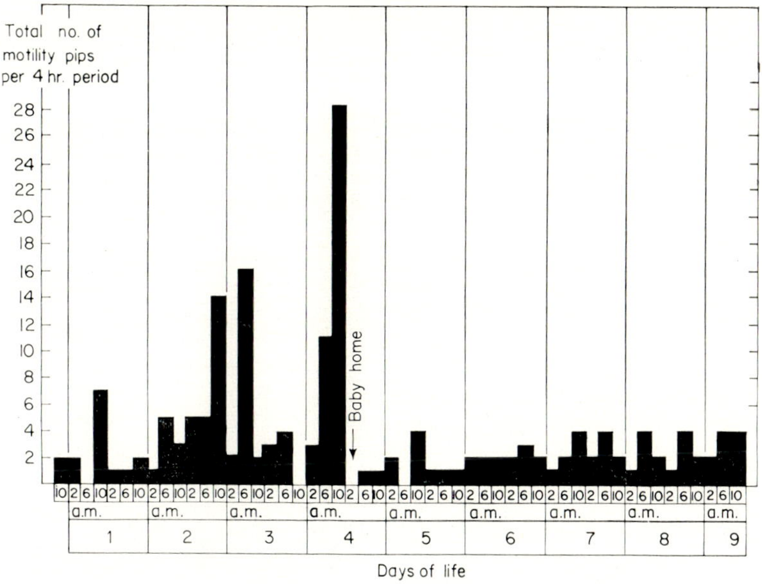

FIG. 4. Frequency and distribution of motility pips for the same baby in two different environments: Hospital nursery (Days 1—4) and Home (Days 5—9).

situation. This suggested that the immediate change in motility output which began at once in the home situation might be related to pattern difference in the occurrence of interventions rather than in the duration of interventions. It also suggested that the monitor with the intervention record might be more useful in studies of infant-caretaker interaction than in attempts to distinguish activity types in a sample of infants. The present study, therefore, was designed to compare this interaction in three different caretaking environments.

Table I outlines the design of the groups and their differences. Data collection is about half-finished at present, data from Group I and from about the first half of the subjects from Group II being drawn upon for the ensuing illustrations. The development of visual perceptual behaviour in these infants reared under different circumstances is an important aspect of this study but data relating to it are not included in the present account.

The first two groups consisted of infants awaiting adoption, whereas the third group will remain with their natural mothers, all of whom will be multiparous. A special effort is being made to ensure that the infants in the sample are "normal".

TABLE I

	N	0—10 *days*	11—28 *days*	29—56 *days*
Group I	9	Nursery	Single care-taker (A or B), rooming-in	Foster home
Group II	9	Single care-taker A, rooming-in	Single care-taker B, rooming-in	Foster home
Group III	10, still to be selected	Natural mother rooming-in	Natural mother at home	Natural mother at home

"Nursery" represents a routine lying-in nursery situation in a general hospital with scheduled 4-hourly feedings and a three-shift nursing day. The schedules for days off, illness and holidays are so arranged that variability in personnel over one baby's experience is roughly comparable to that of another.

"Single caretaker rooming-in" represents the care given by one or the other of two registered private duty nurses, A and B, who room-in with the infants, each nurse for a designated 10- or 18-day period. These are women who have each reared two or more of their own children, who have had prior paediatric nursing experience, and who are highly motivated to participate in the study. Their only instructions from us are that they shall provide their optimal care to these infants, each as if this were her own offspring. In Group II the caretakers alternate for each infant in respect of time period, whether 0-10 or 11-28 days. Foster home represents the usual foster care placement provided for Group I and II infants by agencies during the period when they are awaiting placement for adoption. Obviously infants who are directly placed for adoption cannot be included in the study.

The study was designed to permit examination of data according to infants, time periods, and caretaking environment.

It is evident that continuous monitoring provides a different category of data from that obtained in the acute experiment. One of the difficult tasks in presenting such data is that of display, whereby relationships between longer term variables in complex interaction can be depicted in a single visual array.

Figure 5 represents an initial effort in this direction. It compares the monitoring record over the first 10 days of life from an infant in the nursery situation with that from an infant cared for by a single caretaker rooming-in with the baby. In the nursery situation, the periodic peaks of infant activity and quiescence are again evident, as in Fig. 3, with a clear asynchrony in relation to the timing of the 4-hourly caretaking interventions. This discrepant timing can be expressed also as prolonged delay time. Motility and crying closely parallel each other in

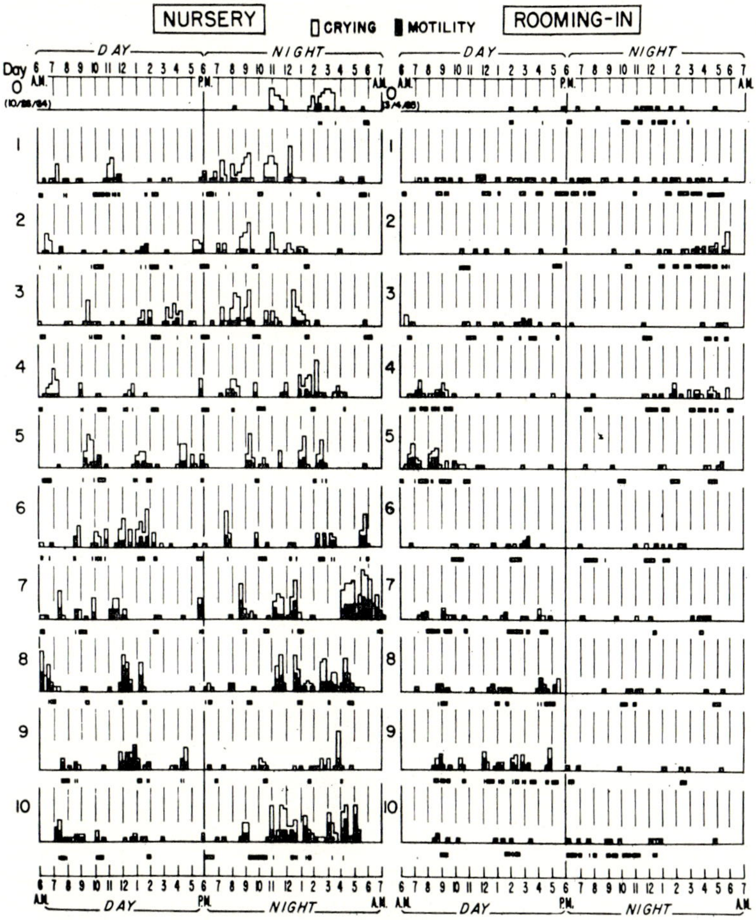

FIG. 5. Relative frequency, duration, and distribution, of motility, crying, and caretaking pips as measured by monitor for a nursery and a rooming-in baby for the first 10 days of life. Caretaker intervention pips for each baby and for each day of life are represented by black marks directly below solid lines indicating day of life.

the record, output gradually rising over the course of the 10 days, showing increasing hour-to-hour variability (Sander and Julia, 1966). One notices also that the predominant motility and crying output over a 24-hour period remains in the 12-hour nocturnal segment. The rooming-in picture shows, by contrast, a greatly reduced activity and crying output in general. On the second day of life there is a high frequency of interventions scattered over the entire 24 hours. There is, however, increasing clustering on subsequent days in which a coincidence becomes clear between periods of infant activity and of caretaking activity. There is not only a much reduced delay time but an intermittent occurrence of caretaker response over the entire duration of an activity epoch of the infant. In other words, activity epoch of caretaker matches activity epoch of infant in duration, as well as in onset. One then sees a very interesting phenomenon. A qualitative difference from the nursery record appears in the rooming-in record; between the fourth and sixth day the predominance of activity shifts to the daytime segment. This tendency towards an early establishment of a day-night organization of activity in the rooming-in situation is being studied in detail in comparisons between the three groups. Day-night organization appears to be sensitive to very subtle influences which come into play during the first 10 days of life.

The pragmatic question we have been tackling has concerned the usefulness of this kind of data in studying adaptive processes. Since we have assumed that the initial adaptation (or "fitting together") centres about the achievement of a relative regulatory stability, we are confronted by the difficulty first of conceptualizing "regulation" in the infant-environment interactional field and, then, measuring something like stability or instability in the field. The pattern of exchanges which mediates such "regulation" is itself an interaction of infant factors and caretaking factors, so stability is something that must reside between the participants rather than in one or the other.

Crying suggested itself to us, at the outset, as a behavioural indicator of comfort or discomfort in the infant and consequently a possible indicator over days or weeks of the stability of regulation in the system of which the infant was a part. However, we soon found that crying is not a simple behaviour and that it can have different meanings in different infants and in the same infant at different times. For example, in some of our infants crying has been encountered as a regular feature of certain sleep states, which are also characterized by rapid eye movements.

In these infants it may appear with striking consistency, whereas in others it never appears at such times. Crying at the point of wakening also has an idiosyncratic occurrence and infants customarily showing this behaviour can be distinguished from infants who awaken first and then begin to cry. In this sense, therefore, crying behaviour as a characteristic of state or change of state appears as an individual difference between infants, and something more difficult to relate to regulation than is crying observed, for example, during a delay in arrival of the caretaker. Furthermore, changes with age in crying behaviour may occur rapidly over the first month of life in one infant and less rapidly in another, both of whom may have been cared for by the same nurse in the same caretaking situation.

Continuous monitoring of crying shows both the wide range of individual differences between infants reared in the same caretaking environment as well as wide group differences between groups of infants reared in different caretaking environments. The left hand part of Fig. 6

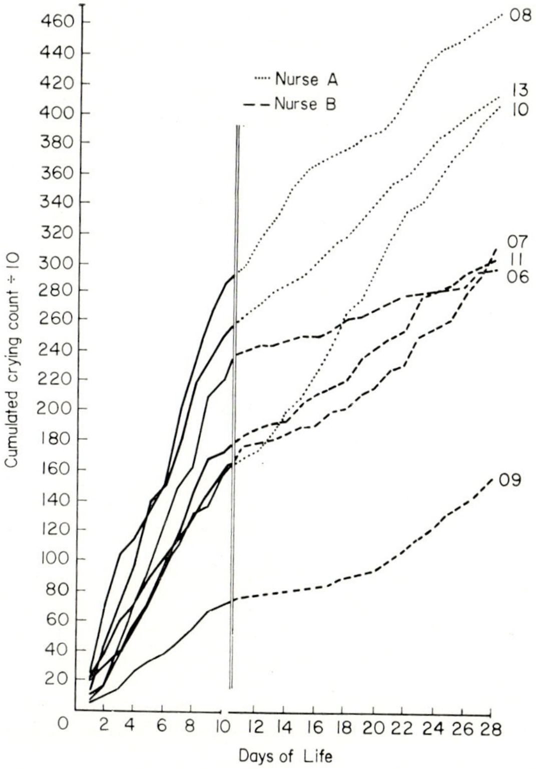

FIG. 6. Cumulative crying counts in seven babies reared in the nursery during the first 10 days of life and then cared for either by Nurse A or Nurse B on days 11 to 28.

TABLE II. MONITORED RECORD OF INTERVENTION VARIABLES FOR 3 ENVIRONMENTS (NURSERY, SURROGATE A, SURROGATE B) GIVEN AS VALUES FOR 5 DAY EPOCHS FROM DAY 0 TO DAY 25.*

Variable	*Infant*	*Lying in nursery*		*Days cared for by Nurse A*			*Days cared for by Nurse B*		
		1—5	6—10	11—15	16—20	21—25	11—15	16—20	21—25
Mean delay time (mins)	06	30·9	32·0				18·1	10·8	14·9
	07	29·9	29·3				20·2	19·2	18·2
	09	26·50	34·4				16·3	12·6	14·3
	11	44·2	48·2				21·3	15·4	21·4
	08	60·6	44·9	14·1	9·3	11·9			
	10	41·3	29·6	16·1	14·4	12·8			
	13	44·2	32·4	14·0	16·4	11·9			
Frequency of removal from bassinet	06	39	32				43	48	40
	07	41	32				50	51	48
	09	40	43				41	52	59
	11	47	44				50	63	59
	08	41	50	89	83	88			
	10	38	36	38	64	76			
	13	39	34	63	62	75			

Average time out of bassinet per removal (mins)	06	29·6	15·3				28·6	25·9	34·7
	07	34·2	15·0				25·9	24·4	22·7
	09	27·8	15·4				33·9	28·7	28·5
	11	23·6	16·4				25·7	20·2	23·1
	08	19·1	15·8	14·8	20·6	18·7			
	10	30·1	22·4	20·5	18·7	17·9			
	13	30·5	16·8	15·8	20·4	17·2			
Total time out of bassinet (mins)	06	1152·5	490·0				1230·0	1247·5	1387·5
	07	1402·5	480·0				1292·5	1297·5	1087·5
	09	1112·5	662·5				1390·0	1492·5	1680·0
	11	1107·5	720·0				1282·5	1275·0	1365·0
	08	782·5	787·5	1315·0	1710·0	1647·5			
	10	1145·0	805·0	780·0	1197·5	1357·5			
	13	1187·5	572·5	997·5	1262·5	1292·5			

*The data refer to the Group I babies whose crying is depicted in Fig. 6.

illustrates the cumulated crying counts of seven infants reared over the first 10 days of life in the neonatal nursery. The observer gains the impression that the lying-in nursery is a most stressful experience for neonates with its scheduled four-hourly feedings given by a changing roster of caretakers, yet the range of individual differences in their crying under these circumstances is striking. The continuous record permits the use of each infant as his own control and makes it possible to use the crying measure as a means of studying effects of change in caretaking environment at the 11 and 29 day points. The right-hand part of Fig. 6 illustrates the change in crying output of the nursery group at the eleventh day.

One might expect *all* infants from the stressful, non-specific situation of the neonatal nursery to show an immediate response, once they were with a single caretaker. But here a distinction by caretaker *does* appear: the infants showing the most abrupt reduction in crying had all been transferred to Nurse B's care, while those transferred to Nurse A's care show a much less definite change in crying output between the eleventh day and the twenty-eighth day. Babies cared for by Nurse B showed an immediate flattening of the cumulative curve after the eleventh day, regardless of whether they had initially cried much or little. This suggests the possibility that Nurse B was working harder than Nurse A, giving more attention to her babies and consequently achieving a superior stability.

Here we can turn to the intervention record which the monitor provides, and see what a comparison between the two nurses reveals in respect to some of the grosser dimensions of caretaking (see Table II).

The first variable, delay-time index, is an operational estimate of delay between onset of crying and the beginning of an intervention. We find that Nurse A is actually responding more immediately than Nurse B, having a delay-time index which is significantly shorter. (Using a two-tailed Mann-Whitney U test, $P = {\cdot}028$ for days 11—15 and days 21—25; $P = {\cdot}058$ for all 15 days together. During days 16—20 the difference does not reach significance.)

As would be expected, the value for delay time in the nursery environment (days 1—10) is two to three times that in the rooming-in situation and probably contributes in a major way to the differences between Group I (nursery) and Group II (rooming-in) babies in respect of crying behaviour over the first 10 days (Fig. 7). As might be expected there is much less crying in the rooming-in group and with one exception Group I shows no overlap with Group II. A second important contribution to the nursery crying picture in the second 5 days of life is the striking decrease in total intervention time during this period. After

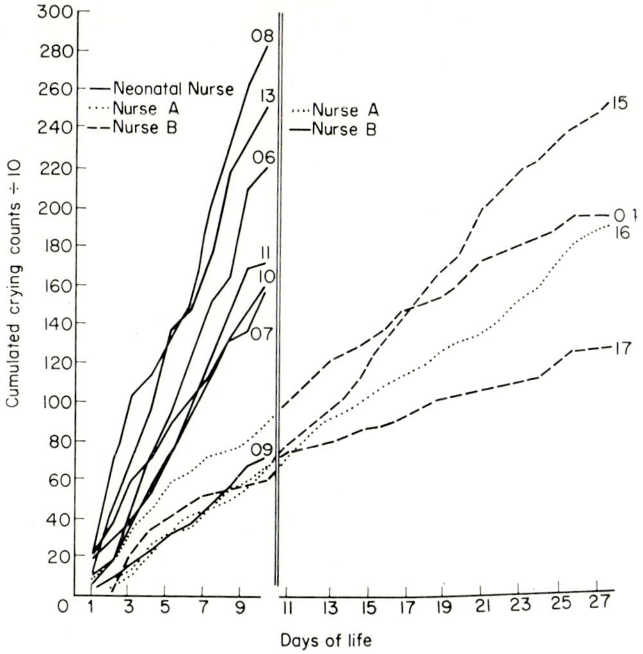

FIG. 7. Cumulative crying counts in seven Group I babies reared in the nursery during the first 10 days (solid lines) and in four Group II babies roomed-in during the first 10 days and then transferred from Nurse A to B or from Nurse B to A.

the mothers have been discharged on day 5 the infants are fed by nurses in the nursery, not taken out to a ward for feeding.

A second comparison revealed by the intervention record is that Nurse A could be considered, in fact, to be working harder than Nurse B also in that the *frequency* of her responses is higher ($P = \cdot 056$, combining all 15 days, Mann-Whitney U test, two-tailed). The average duration of each removal from the bassinet indicates that, while Nurse A intervenes oftener and for briefer periods, Nurse B spends a longer time in each of her fewer interventions. Values for total intervention are not significantly different and indicate that both nurses are giving approximately the same duration of care. Interestingly enough there is also no significant difference in total intervention time between the first 5 days in the nursery and the first 5 days in which the babies are rooming-in with either Nurse A or B. One might have supposed that, with nothing else to do in the rooming-in situation, the surrogate mothers would have greatly increased caretaking time. At least we might have expected that an increased total caretaking time would have been a factor operating to produce the immediate flattening of crying curves of the babies cared for by Nurse B.

These data point to a role for both quantity and quality in the exchange picture. We can look now with a better focus at the question of how Nurse B achieves something in her fewer, longer interventions that Nurse A does not in her briefer, more frequent ones. Thus far the material suggests that the essential mechanism is concerned with a key factor, which we designate as "specificity", something which we hope to elaborate at a future time.

A point which seems important to include here is that Group I babies were taken on their eleventh day by the Nurses A and B after the relatively stressful 10-day experience in the neonatal nursery. What do we find when comparing the crying records of the babies who were roomed-in with Nurse A or Nurse B from the first day of life? The experimental design is such that Group II babies will go as often at 11 days from Nurse A to B as from B to A. Figure 7 covering the first month of life allows us to compare infants who have been transferred at the 11-day point from one of the two nurses to the other. Here we find that with three infants cared for by Nurse A in 1—10 days there is no appreciable change in the slope of the curves when Nurse B takes the baby. At the moment it is an attractive hypothesis to consider that, if there is an optimal time in the first 10 days for the establishment of initial regulatory coordination with the caretaking environment, even a less effective mother might get along very well with her baby if she could provide its caretaking from birth; whereas this same mother might have a relatively greater difficulty if she took the same baby after its initial 10 days had been spent in a busy lying-in nursery.

The crying data have been included as an illustration of the complex interaction of infant differences, caretaking influences, and age effects in respect of a single measure. Since in assessing regulation one is dealing with the subject of both the variability and the relative stability of functions, one cannot escape the fact that oscillation, or periodic variation over the 24 hours, is an essential characteristic of organic functions. The investigator of "regulation" should begin with an appreciation of "natural" cyclic characteristics. However, as one attempts to assess the "natural" condition under which the cycling will be investigated, one is again confronted by the interaction of caretaking effects, infant effects, and age effects. Since we have a number of infants being roomed-in with the same surrogate mother over the same age period, as well as the possibility of comparing groups of infants in the different

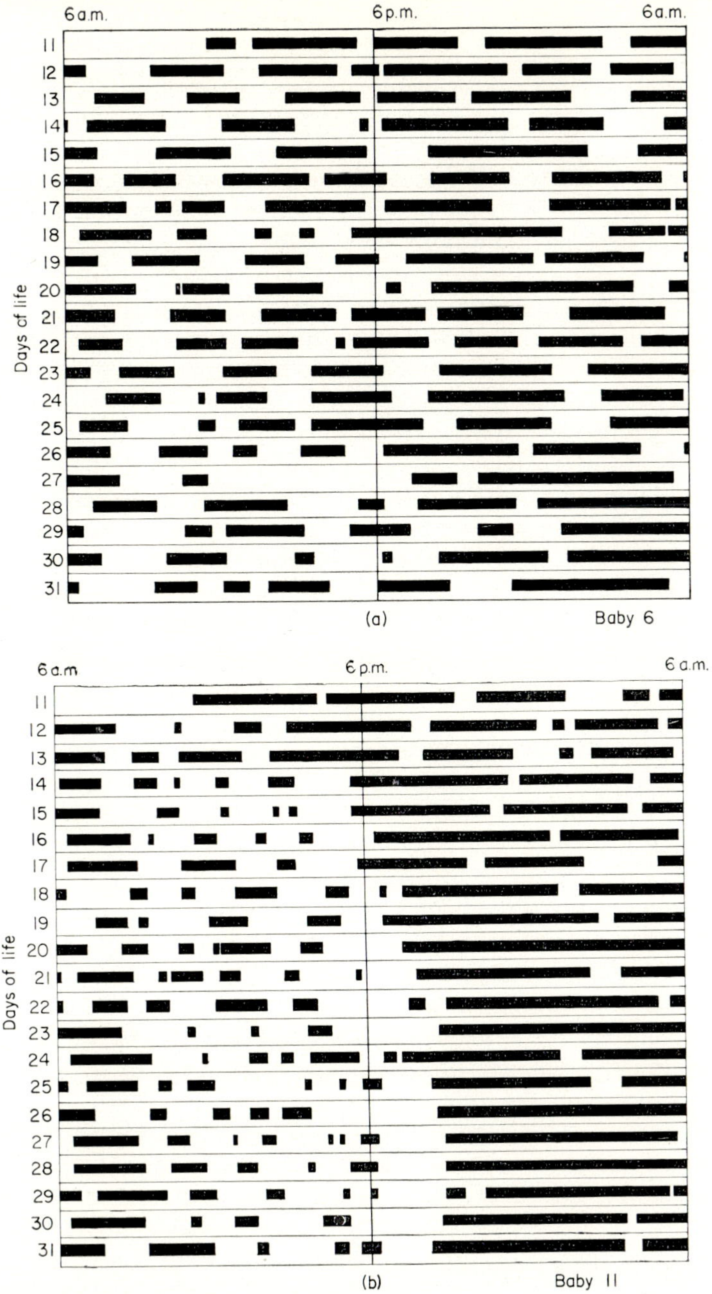

FIG. 8. (a and b). Sequence of sleeping and waking between 11 and 28 days of life in two female infants both cared for by Nurse B after an initial 10 days in neonatal nursery. The solid bars represent periods asleep and the intervals between the solid bars periods awake.

caretaking environments, a beginning can be made in separating the contribution of these different influences on cyclic or period characteristics.

The 24-hour record of the onset of sleep and wakefulness kept by the surrogate mother nurses illustrates individual differences (Fig. 8). The sequence of sleeping and waking states in the two female infants between the ages of 11 and 31 days of life is shown. Both infants were cared for by Nurse B during this time, after an initial 10 days in the same lying-in nursery situation. It is evident that in the caretaking task not only would the timing and nature of the interventions required be strikingly different for these two infants, but that the mechanics of regulation in the two infants might become based on quite different mechanisms, for example, in respect of the degree to which intrinsic or extrinsic factors might govern the pattern. Thus far it does appear that some babies fall asleep regularly, as though largely governed by inner regulation of sleep-wake cycling, with little regard for environmental conditions; others, even by the eighth day of life, appear most sensitive to any substitution for the familiar caretaker in respect of their ability to fall asleep. Almost from the outset, in other words, individual differences can give rise to a different organization in the interactional field which mediates regulation.

Caretaking also affects the sleep-wake cycling. We used the term "major" sleep period to include all brief awakenings of less than 1 hour in length; and "major" awake period to include all brief naps of less than 1 hour in length. The major sleep-wake cycle, which extends from the onset of one major sleep period to the onset of the next, was significantly longer in the three babies cared for by Nurse B than in the four babies cared for by Nurse A between days 11 and 28.

Our infants appear to range along a continuum of diurnal-nocturnal differentiation in respect to placement of sleep and wakefulness, and to the stability of this differentiation. A frequent occurrence is the loss of an established daytime predominance of awake time for 1 or more days at or just after the time of the change of caretaking environment. This loss may be for a day or two in some cases as in Fig. 9b, or it may last a week or more in others. Figure 9b represents an infant who was easy to care for. The record depicted in Fig. 9c is that of the most difficult of any of the study infants to stabilize and regulate; Fig. 9d represents the record of one of the few abnormal infants we have followed. Both show the emergence of some differentiation between 12 and 27 days followed by the loss of differentiation between 29 and 39 days.

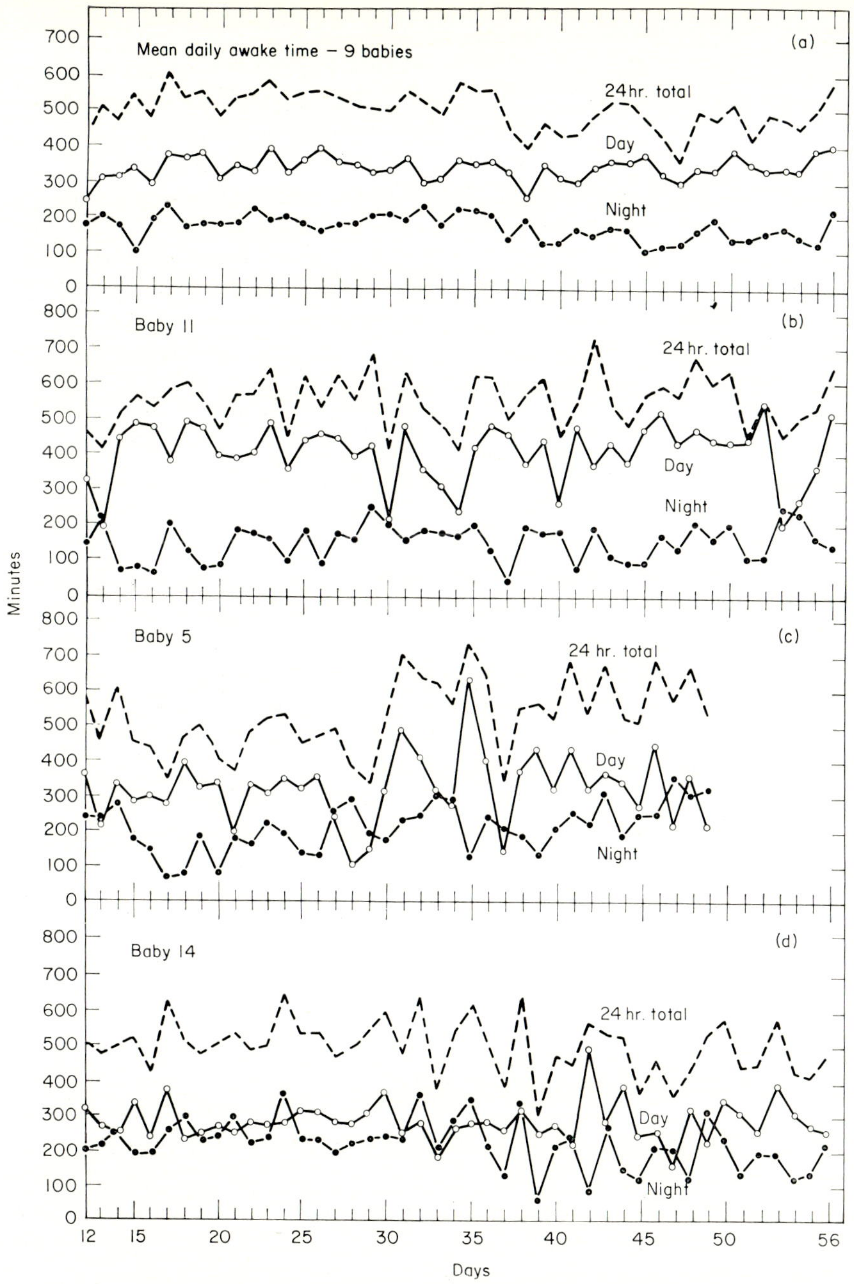

FIG. 9 (a, b, c, and d). Total awake time per 24 hours showing partitions of total 24 hour awake time occurring in diurnal (6 a.m.—6 p.m.) and in nocturnal (6 p.m.—6 a.m.) periods.

a. Represents mean values for nine nursery babies between 11 and 56 days of life; b. Represents daily values for baby 11; c. Daily total, diurnal and nocturnal awake time in baby 5—a very difficult infant; d. Baby 14—one of the few abnormal babies followed (having developed neonatal tetany by the 7th postnatal day).

CONCLUSION

I have reported an approach to early postnatal development centring about the collection of continuous data for several functional systems of the infant. In such data, cyclic characteristics of the functions are encountered. The design of subject groups and caretaking experience in the study has encouraged the attempt to distinguish infant, caretaking, and age effects on the measures used. Data on modification or stability of the functions at points of caretaking (interactional) change open an approach to investigation of mechanisms of the adaptive process in early infancy.

The concept of adaptation has been employed to explain, in part at least, the gain in order over time shown by open (biologic) systems in contrast to the gain in disorder over time shown by closed thermodynamic systems. Furthermore in the biologic system, adaptation bears a direct relation to organization. Piaget (1936) sums up the matter in the following way: "From the biological point of view organization is inseparable from adaptation. They are two complementary processes of a single mechanism, the first being the internal aspect of the cycle of which adaptation constitutes the external aspect". From this standpoint a study of organization requires the consideration of the whole "field" (Weiss, 1967) of which the infant is but one component. In asking which exchanges in the infant-environment interaction are the crucial ones to study, and, in asking how intrinsic functions become connected with, and modified in, the extrinsic encounter, we have followed the hypothesis that it is the requirement for regulation which is the basic determinant of the crucial exchanges.

Regulation is a broad and exceedingly complex concept in biology which can be discussed on many levels from the biochemical to the behavioural. Since the time of Lavoisier, regulation has had the meaning of "governed exchange" (Brobeck, 1965). Cybernetic theory has more recently provided conceptual tools which have clarified the way "governing" or "control" may be effected in biological systems. We have approached regulation in the neonate perhaps in an over-simplified way, by regarding the infant's active functions such as waking, sleeping, feeding, perceptual and motor activity to be semi-separate cybernetic control loops, each a system organized in time with its own circadian pattern of activation, giving the cyclic or oscillatory characteristics of feedback control. Through repetitive interaction with the caretaker each system or function comes to operate around specific inputs which provide key feedback control criteria and which represent, then, the infant's significant connections with its environment. One loop can become biased by another, linking the several systems as one coherent organization. Genetic determinants contribute to individual variation in the functional profile of the component systems and their biases. The problem for regulation posed by any given infant may eventually be assessable in terms of such a profile.

With many infants reared by the same surrogate mother, the semi-independence of the various component systems emerges. We have, for example, encountered infants who have shown unstable, unpredictable feeding behaviour but stable, highly predictable sleep-wake cycling and yet other infants, reared by the same individual, who have shown precisely the reverse. Just as it takes time at the onset of life for some infants to develop smooth coordination between the activities of sucking, breathing, and swallowing, so in other infants, rhythms of waking and sleeping may not be initially coordinated with hunger, feeding, and satiation. It is common experience that a mother will use one of these functions to regulate, control, or "govern" another: for example, feeding to induce sleeping, or perceptual activity to maintain quiescence or to prolong waking. It has been suggested by Halberg (1960) that the nature of adaptation itself may be resolved as a characteristic of biological rhythms and the determinants of their synchrony.

There would exist a possibility for great stability in a system of interlocking feedback loops in synchrony with basic environmental periodicities which provide key inputs (in terms of specific extrinsic perceptual cues) around which the component cyclic or oscillatory functions are regulated. One advantage of such stability at an early point in postnatal life might be to provide the infant with recurrent "free" epochs, during which initiation of exploratory activity (providing contingencies necessary for formation of new perceptual motor schemata) would be free from obligatory bias by the control requirements of the regulatory systems. A possible bridge from such a model to brain mechanisms is already available in Pribram's conceptualization of the organization of the regulatory centres in the brain stem as an ultrastable system consisting of multiple biased homeostats in series (Pribram, 1960).

Needless to say, comparison of the synchrony in multiple functions observed in the normal infant by Dr. Prechtl with the asynchrony of the same functions in his hyperexcitable infants has been of the greatest interest to us—as have his observations of the caretaking difficulties this latter group presents (Prechtl, 1963). Of great interest, too, are the suggestions made by Dr. Petre-Quadens concerning the possibility that the sleep changes occurring in late pregnancy may be in a direction that would set the stage at the outset for a more ready synchrony of the mother's activity cycles with those of her neonate.

A great gap exists between the phenomena of infant-caretaker interaction and brain mechanisms. However, this study of the way a first order derivative of brain function, namely state regulation, influences interactional processes between neonate and environment suggests a possible means of narrowing the gap. Much depends on improving our conceptualization of this initial interaction and its relation to the all too broad concepts of regulation, adaptation, and organization.

REFERENCES

BROBECK, J. R. 1965. Exchange, control and regulation. In W. S. Yamamoto and and J. R. Brobeck (Eds.), *Physiological controls and regulations.* Saunders, Philadelphia, Penn. Pp. 1–14.

HALBERG, F. 1960. Temporal coordination of physiological function. *Cold Spring Harb. Symp. quant. Biol.* **25,** 289–308.

PIAGET, J. 1936. *The origins of intelligence in children.* Transl. by Margaret Cook (1952). International Univ. Press, New York.

PRECHTL, H. F. R. 1963. The mother-child interaction in babies with minimal brain damage. In B. M. Foss (Ed.), *Determinants of infant behaviour II.* Methuen, London; Wiley, New York. Pp. 53–66.

PRIBRAM, K. 1960. A review of theory in physiological psychology. *Am. Rev. Psychol.* **11,** 1–40.

SANDER, L. W. 1969. The longitudinal course of early mother-child interaction—cross-case comparison in a sample of mother-child pairs. In B. M. Foss (Ed.), *Determinants of infant behaviour IV.* Methuen, London; Wiley, New York. Pp. 189–227.

SANDER, L. W. and JULIA, H. L. 1966. Continuous interactional monitoring in the neonate. *Psychosom. Med.* **28,** 822–835.

WEISS, P. A. 1967. $1 + 1 \neq 2$ (When one plus one does not equal two). In C. Gardner, T. M. Quarton, and F. O. Schmitt (Eds.), *Neurosciences, a study program.* Rockefeller Univ. Press, New York. Pp. 801–822.

Discussion

SCHULTE: I am always surprised that more behavioural studies have not been done already in premature nurseries, particularly with preterm infants kept for 2 months in an incubator. We are keeping them under very artificial conditions which may be harmful. There is already such a long list of things we have done wrong with these infants—drugs, oxygen, and temperature—we may be doing something wrong from the behavioural point of view.

ROBINSON: I agree with that. We have no evidence for the assumption that premature babies are too premature for their behaviour to be affected by the way they are handled. This is very artificial compared with conditions in the uterus or compared with the way in which a term baby is handled.

LIPSITT: At Providence we are now doing a comparative study in which some of the babies in the premature nursery are being stimulated auditorily, visually, tactually, and so on, as contrasted with a control group which is just getting routine nursery care. We shall follow these children for at least 3 years to see whether there are different outcomes. Other studies of this sort have recently been begun.

WOLFF: Does the surrogate mother sleep in the same room as the babies at night?

SANDER: Yes, she is with them day and night. They wake her in the morning.

WOLFF: Is the light in the nursery on all the time?

SANDER: Yes, we are doing a study of alternating light and dark. So far we have studied two babies in the rooming-in situation in continuous light, and it hasn't made any difference.

Attempts at Synthesis:

structure-function relationships

Structure-function Relationships in the Spinal Cord

F. J. SCHULTE

University of Göttingen

MYELINATION OF AXONS and arborization of dendrites are the two basic structural changes which occur in the course of development of the nervous system. Both the thickness of the myelin sheath and the quantity of dendrites have important implications for nervous activity.

Axonal myelination is positively related to impulse conduction velocity, to the amplitude of the action potential, to membrane excitability, and sometimes to the maximal frequency of impulses. The slow conduction rate of the immature nerve has little bearing on the functional incapacity of the newborn infant, for the interneuronal and neuromuscular distances are shorter, and that more than compensates for the low speed of conduction. The amplitude of the action potential determines the amount of transmitter which is secreted at the nerve endings. However, as far as I know, we have little information as to whether there is much variation in the thickness of presynaptic endings and whether their thickness is related to the thickness of the myelin sheath. If such a relationship did exist, axonal myelination would have a tremendous effect on synaptic activity, since the amount of transmitter determines the depolarization pressure on the next neurone. Increasing membrane excitability and maximum spike frequency due to a growing thickness of the myelin sheath are not important only for electrophysiological experiments on the exposed nerve in student courses. The thickness of the myelin sheath at the first Ranvier node determines how much depolarization is needed—or, in other words, how many excitatory postsynaptic potentials are needed—to generate a certain number of action potentials. It is at the Ranvier node that the generator potential of the nerve cell or of the receptor is transferred quantitatively by means of frequency modulation into spike potentials. Maximum discharge frequency and its maintenance over a long period of time are severely restricted in the newborn kitten as compared with the adult animal (Skoglund 1960a,b). The absence of both tonic gamma motoneurone and muscle spindle activity may well account for the lack of muscle tone in immature preterm infants. For the same reason, abnormal nervous overactivation due to hypocalcaemia is more easily elicited in the mature nerve and probably not seen in the very immature and unmyelinated axon.

Dendritic arborization with the formation of axodendritic synapses, probably the most important structural change in the cortex during postnatal human development, is already virtually complete in the spinal cord of the fullterm newborn infant. However, exact counts of spinal-nerve-cell dendrites are not to my knowledge available. In fullterm newborn kittens, axodendritic connections seem to be less complex than in adult animals, since a smaller number of motoneurones is reached by a given afferent stimulus. The subliminal fringe is considerably smaller in the immature, than in the mature, animal. If this holds true for human infants as well, preterm or fullterm, the recruitment of motoneurones—and hence the increasing strength of muscle contraction—would probably occur stepwise rather than smoothly.

I am well aware that there are many other aspects of structure-function relations in the spinal cord which need discussion. Parallel to the dendritic arborization, Nissl substance is formed and typical enzymes are accumulated. In a future conference of this kind, the relationships between histochemistry and behaviour might be a more revealing topic than the relationship between structure and function.

REFERENCES

Skoglund, S. 1960a. On the postnatal development of postural mechanisms as revealed by electromyography and myography in decerebrate kittens. *Acta physiol. scand.* **49,** 299–317.

Skoglund, S. 1960b. The spinal transmission of proprioceptive reflexes and the postnatal development of conduction velocity in different hindlimb nerves in the kitten. *Acta physiol. scand.* **49,** 318–329.

Structure-function Relationships: a Classification of Concepts

R. M. BERGSTRÖM

University of Helsinki

DURING SESSIONS OF this study group, I have frequently asked for definitions of concepts, and I have collected the terms and concepts whose definitions were somewhat unclear (Table I). In the left-hand part of the table are those concepts which have to do with structure, and in the right-hand part those to do with function. Those concepts which have to do with order, are in the top part of the table, and those to do with disorder, are in the bottom part. So we have four groups of concepts used throughout this meeting. I believe that for future studies we need clearer definitions, at least if we wish to have more contact between morphologists and physiologists.

Let us look first at the left-hand part of the table, and the concepts concerned with structure. In the "ordered" category we have concepts such as an "anatomically well-localized structure", where we might be talking about, for example, a brain nucleus. The corresponding concept under disorder would be an "anatomically not localized structure". To the ordered structures would also belong "tracts", "circuits", and other well-defined structures. To the corresponding "disordered" structures would belong nets where we cannot discern any orderly connections and which are called "randomly-connected-nets". Another way of expressing this would be as "histological regularity" on the one hand and "histological irregularity" on the other. Finally we have the concepts of "geometrical order" and "disorder", which we could alternatively express as "geometrical non-randomness" and "geometrical randomness."

Now let us look at the concepts on the right-hand side of the table, which are concerned with function. In the "ordered" category at the top, we have those physiological processes which can be explained in a "deterministic" way by means of causal, one-to-one relationships between different stages of the process.

TABLE 1. TERMS USED TO DESCRIBE STRUCTURE-FUNCTION RELATIONSHIPS

STRUCTURE		FUNCTION
	ORDER	
Anatomically well localized structure		Physiologically determined processes
Tracts, circuits, etc.		Regularity of processes
Histological regularity		Organized process (reflexes, servoloops)
Geometrical order		Synchronized processes (coordinated)
Geometrical non-randomness		Inhibitory processes
		Phasic processes
		Time-dependent processes
		Non-random processes
		Low probability
		High negative entropy
		High information-content (signal)
L E V E L S	S T A T E S	
Geometrical randomness		Low information-content (noise)
Geometrical disorder		High entropy
Histological irregularity		High probability
Nets (randomly connected), dendritic masses		Random processes
Anatomically not-localized structure		Time-independent processes
		Tonic processes
		Facilitatory processes
		Unsynchronized processes (non-coordinated)
		Disorganized processes
		Irregularity of processes
		Physiologically stochastic processes
	DISORDER	

The corresponding concept in the "disordered" category would be the "physiologically stochastic" process where we can't use any deterministic concepts. The concepts of "regularity" of processes as against "irregularity", and of "organized" as against "disorganized" processes, are obviously very closely related to the concepts "deterministic" and "stochastic". I have included them all because they have been frequently used. Again, "synchronized" processes are those which exhibit order in time: unsynchronized processes those that do not. "Coordination" can be put in the same category as synchronization if we understand coordination in terms of order among contractions of different muscular groups. "Non-coordination" would correspond closely to "desynchronization".

We can also place the concept of "inhibition" in this framework. If we accept Humphrey's explanation of the role of inhibition in ontogeny, then inhibition belongs on the side of the ordered processes. When there are only facilitatory processes the resulting activity is disordered; there is no local order in the contraction of muscles but instead the generalized type of response which Humphrey described in early fetal life. Inhibitory processes appear later, as can be concluded from the unit studies of cerebral activity in the postnatal rabbit. These inhibitory processes cause order in the time sequence of impulses (Hyvärinen, 1966). This is very closely connected with Humphrey's ideas—that inhibition comes and puts order into the facilitatory function which is the primary one.

Then we have the ideas which we discussed (p. 15 *et seq.*) of "phasic" (disordered) as against "tonic" (ordered); of "time dependency" as against "time independency" and of "non-random" as against "random" processes. The last pair of concepts could also be expressed as "low probability" as against "high probability" or "high negative entropy". This latter is the same as "information", according to Shannon's concepts, and therefore corresponds to "high information content" and "low information content." Corresponding with high information content I have also included "signal" as a kind of order on a noisy background; the converse is "noise"—a random non-signalling process.

There were some concepts which were more difficult to place. The "reflex" is a physiological concept which I think belongs to the "ordered" category because the reflex arc contains tracts and because the reflex process is a regular, highly deterministic physiological process. The feedback loops, or servoloops, are also organized functional things which can become part of deterministic processes.

What I have presented is not a hypothesis but simply a collection of concepts and a possible way of classifying them. In future when such an interdisciplinary conference is held there will be much talk about different concepts, because in different fields terms are used in different ways. So we must consider definitions. For me, at least, it was often impossible to connect the data which I heard at this conference with my own experiments, which are mainly in neurophysiology, and I think this was due to lack of definition.

REFERENCE

HYVÄRINEN, J. 1966. Analysis of spontaneous spike potential activity in developing diencephalon. *Acta physiol. scand.* **68,** Suppl. 278, 1–67.

Cerebral Hemisphere Function in the Newborn

R. J. ROBINSON

Institute of Child Health, London

THREE YEARS AGO I wrote what I now regard as a rather inadequate paper on the subject of cortical function or cerebral function in the newborn (Robinson, 1966). One of the major inadequacies was that I took no account of the kind of evidence on learning in the newborn which we heard yesterday, because I was insufficiently familiar with it. The starting point for this paper was that I had been intrigued by the statement which I repeatedly found in textbooks of paediatrics and of child neurology, that the cerebral hemispheres do not function in the newborn baby. This was a statement which seemed to be passed on from book to book, with increasing authority and decreasing evidence at each passage. I thought I would try to find the arguments on which this statement was originally based and to see if they could be dismantled.

There seemed to be three main arguments. The first was that babies without cerebral hemispheres, that is to say hydranencephalics and surviving anencephalics, behave in exactly the same way as normal newborn babies. The second was that cerebral motor defects, in particular the spastic cerebral palsies, are not apparent in the newborn baby and become apparent only during the course of development. The implication was that these disorders are due to some disturbance in function of the cortex or of the sub-cortical white matter, and that the motor defects are not apparent in the newborn because those structures are not yet functioning. These were the kinds of argument which one found used by Peiper (1963), André-Thomas and Saint-Anne Dargassies (1952), and by Pratt (1954). The third argument, which was used by Ford (1960), was simply that the baby had no volitional activity. Of these arguments, the third seems to be meaningless—it is simply begging the question—and the first two are manifestly untrue. It is not true that babies with no cerebral hemispheres behave in exactly the same way as normal newborns. One has only to look at the accounts on which this statement is based to discover that it is not true. Babies with no cerebral hemispheres do not behave in the same way as normal newborns in respect of sleep cycles, waking, crying, vision, or muscle tone. The second argument, about cerebral motor defects' not being apparent in the newborn, again arises out of lack of observation. Right through the literature, starting with Sarah McNutt (1885), if not earlier, and going through Randolph Byers in 1941 to Heinz Prechtl (1965), who has probably the best documented evidence, it has been made clear that although hemiplegias, for example, need not be apparent in the newborn baby, they often are. So none of these lines of evidence seemed valid.

So far I have not advanced any argument for the belief that the cerebral hemispheres do function in the newborn baby; I have tried to show that the arguments used to support the idea that they do not function were not really valid. Both the arguments and their rebuttal are based on the methods of classical clinical neurology in which one determines which functions are missing when a particular piece of brain is damaged, and then states that those functions must have rested in that particular part of the brain. I think that neither the arguments nor their rebuttal will make very much appeal to members of this study group, because you rightly feel that there are better ways of examining cerebral function than this. Can we then progress to decide whether, in a normal baby with intact cerebral hemispheres, those hemispheres are doing anything?

The two possible lines of evidence that I tried to pursue over this were not entirely satisfactory. The first was concerned with neonatal vision and the possibility that the visual behaviour observed in the newborn baby may involve the cerebral hemispheres. I produced a certain amount of anecdotal evidence to the effect that babies with major lesions or absence of the cerebral hemispheres do not show visual fixation or following or turning towards diffuse light such as one sees in the normal baby. However, this is just anecdotal evidence. Bronson has quoted equally anecdotal evidence which appears to put the reverse view.

The second line of evidence which I put forward even more reluctantly because I felt that the ideas would be regarded as if they were a piece of sentimental whimsy, was that parents do not treat babies as spinal preparations in which nothing functions above that level. After yesterday's papers and discussions, I feel happier about this argument. In their attitudes to newborn babies, parents—and for that matter psychoanalysts—are recognizing that the baby has learning abilities and receptivity to the environmental circumstances of the kind that Lipsitt and Sander presented in their papers (although obviously parents have not formulated them in the same terms).

If anyone feels that parents' evidence about the abilities of newborn babies must be ignored, then I would remind him that no observant mother could possibly have written an account of neonatal vision as uninformative as the chapter in Peiper (1963) on this subject—which is based on the consensus of 137 other authors!

Does discussing cortical function in the newborn help us with the problem of development, when that problem is obviously a dynamic one whereas the idea of the newborn baby on the one hand and the functioning of the cortex on the other, is really a static concept without any movement with time?

I shall attempt a much simpler formulation than Bergström's of how I see the problem of development. It seems to me that we are dealing with something which I will call X, which represents organization, ability or complexity—something we regard as being vaguely "good" that increases in the baby as a function of time:

$$X = f(t) \tag{1}$$

Obviously it is a very complex function of time and a lot of other variables are present. Now in discussing development, we are obviously talking about change, so what we should really be interested in is not this equation, but its first differential. We can't yet differentiate Equation (1) because we don't know the nature of the function, so we have to write the differential as:

$$\frac{dX}{dt} = +f'(t) \tag{2}$$

The one thing we know about this function from Prechtl's definition is that it has a positive sign—that it is something which is increasing with time. Obviously I don't regard this mathematical formulation as having any real mathematical significance. This is just an expression of how I see the problem of development. If we are to progress, and solve these equations, we have to get some coordinates. Two good coordinates with which to start are the time of birth on the time scale and cortical function on the function scale.

REFERENCES

André-Thomas and Saint-Anne Dargassies, S. 1952. *Études neurologiques sur le nouveau-né et le jeune nourrisson.* Masson, Paris.

Byers, R. K. 1941. Evolution of hemiplegias in infancy. *Am. J. Dis. Child.* **61,** 915–927.

Ford, F. R. 1960. *Diseases of the nervous system in infancy, childhood and adolescence.* 4th ed. Thomas, Springfield, Ill. p. 11.

McNutt, S. J. 1885. Apoplexia neonatorum. *Am. J. Obstet. Dis. Wom.* **18,** 73–81.

PEIPER, A. 1963. *Cerebral function in infancy and childhood.* Translation by B. and M. Nagler of 3rd rev. ed. (German). Consultants Bureau, New York.

PRATT, K. C. 1954. The Neonate. In L. Carmichael (Ed.) *Manual of child psychology.* 2nd ed. Wiley, New York, Pp. 215–291.

PRECHTL, H. F. R. 1965. Prognostic value of neurological signs in the newborn infant. *Proc. R. Soc. Med.* **58,** 3–4.

ROBINSON, R. J. 1966. Cerebral function in the newborn. *Devl Med. Child Neurol.* **8,** 561–567.

Discussion

BRONSON: Sometimes you talked about cerebral hemisphere function and sometimes about cortical function.

ROBINSON: In cerebral hemisphere I include the sub-cortical white matter but not the thalamus.

SCHULTE: How much evidence about cerebral hemisphere function in the newborn can we obtain from EEG studies—the evoked responses and the differences in the spontaneous EEG in different behavioural states? If the assumption holds true in the newborn—that what we are recording from the scalp is almost entirely cortical activity—then this would be good evidence that the cortex participates in changes of state even in preterm infants.

ROBINSON: Neonatal focal fits also have EEG concomitants which most electroencephalographers believe come from the cortex. And of course these fits are associated with the kind of peripheral movements that you would expect if they were coming from the cortex. Some children who have had neonatal focal fits will go on to have typical focal fits later in life which clearly do seem to be cortical. However, I am uneasy about arguing from the abnormal situation. Concerning the EEG observations in general, can you be sure that just because electrical activity is going on, it has any function in the sense that we have been discussing? For example, there are evoked potentials to light in the premature baby of 28 weeks' gestation, if not earlier; if we regard them as a manifestation of cortical function, that is going to push cortical function back in development a long time before birth.

WOLFF: Where was the EEG activity coming from in the arrhinencephalic baby?

SCHULTE: Most of it originates in the cerebral cortex, but spontaneous or evoked electrical activity does not imply psychophysiological functions like vision. But EEG changes with a certain type of behaviour or due to stimulation do imply that the cortical neurones participate in these changes, no matter how early in development this occurs.

KAUFMAN: Why does Robinson question the value of the evoked potential as an indication of cortical functions?

ROBINSON: I don't. I simply said that if you argue that the evoked potential is an index of cerebral cortical function, then you have to push cerebral cortical function a long way back before the time of birth, because the evoked potential is there very early on.

KAUFMAN: Then the question really concerns the meaning of the evoked response in terms of cortical function. Earlier, when I asked Schulte about lateral inhibition, I had in mind the kind of experiment Karl Pribram has done, although not in the infant animal (1967. *Am. Psychol.* **22,** 830). He studied the responses evoked by paired flashes of light and paired clicks, with varying intervals, in small cell masses and in single cells. He then noted the effects on the amplitude of the second response of concurrent electrical stimulation to other cortical areas. He found that stimulation of the infero-temporal cortex reduced the second response, whereas stimulation of the frontal cortex enhanced the second response. Pribram's specific interpretation in terms of information processing, redundancy, and image clarity need not concern us except for the demonstration that evoked cortical responses are subject to self-inhibitory and collateral-inhibitory processes, and that these in turn are under corticofugal control. In other words, complex systemic processing of input characterizes the mature brain. If one could show this type of processing going on in the neonate, one would feel more confident that the cortex is really doing something besides "lighting up".

WOLFF: Is anything known about the necessary conditions of architectonics in the cortex that would enable it to function?

ROBINSON: That puts the architectonic argument the wrong way round—to ask whether the cells are sufficiently developed to do something. You surely ought to see if they are doing something and then say, "Well, that seems to correspond with that stage of structural development."

LIPSITT: That went wrong decades ago in the infant-conditioning literature. People assumed that myelination was insufficiently advanced to permit learning in the newborn, and this premature conclusion inhibited functional studies of learning processes.

PRECHTL: Are we right to talk about "the cortex"; shouldn't we break it up? One part of the cortex which one would expect to function early is the rhinencephalon.

PLOOG: Can we get anything out of Yakovlev's studies on myelination in the human brain in terms of neocortical function?

ROBINSON: I question whether we get much out of these studies in terms of any function. The optic nerve and tract are incompletely myelinated at term, but we know perfectly well that the optic nerve is functioning by 28 weeks' gestation. A newborn opossum is quite good at finding its way into the mother's pouch and then finding the nipple, although it has no myelin in the central nervous system at all at the time of birth.

SCHULTE: Some fibres remain unmyelinated throughout life, yet they function quite well. I think dendritic arborization and the elaboration of Nissl substance have more important functional implications than myelination. Rabinowicz (1964. *Prog. Brain Res.* **4,** 39) has shown in a fetus of 8 months' gestation that in the rhinencephalon dendritic arborization is much more advanced than in the motor cortex.

BERGSTRÖM: Myelination may be a very important factor, so are the synapses. Purpura and others (1963. *Expl Neurol.* **7,** 107) showed that, in the kitten cortex at birth, there are axon-dendritic synapses and then 1 week later synapses which are axosomatic. This corresponds to our experiences of unit activity in the kitten cortex. There first appeared long-lasting action potentials with very low frequency and later, in the second week, they became shorter in duration, as in the adult, and their frequency increased.

SCHULTE: Yes, when I talk about dendrites I always imply that I am talking about synapses, since the vast majority of synapses are located on the dendrites although some are located on the soma of the nerve cell and they might have a different function.

LIPSITT: This discussion emphasizes how little we know of a correlative sort, that is of a causative sort, relating structural factors to functional factors. We know a great deal about the development of structural factors with increasing age of the organism, and we know a great deal, I think, about behavioural development as a function of age. But we seriously lack information which will help us to correlate these two areas of knowledge. There are now fairly good data showing that the direction of the causative relationship is not one-sided. While we would all admit that structural factors are important causative agents for function, it has also been shown by Rozenzweig and Krech (1966. *Am. Psychol.* **21,** 321) and others (E. L. Bennett *et al.* 1964. *Science* **146,** 610; E. L. Bennett *et al.* In W. L. Byrne (Ed.), *Molecular approaches to learning and memory.* Academic Press, New York, 1969, in press) that functional factors may affect structure in important ways. These studies show that in rats which are stimulated during early stages of their development, cortical size is enhanced. We also need to know about causes. I believe it is an adequate paraphrase of Schulte's view to say that we don't know about the real role of myelination in the production of behaviour, but at least we know that myelination and behaviour are associated with each other, they go hand in hand. This does not necessarily mean a causal relationship. We know, for example, that eyeball size increases with age, but I do not believe for one minute that eyeball size has any connection, as a causative agent, with the learning properties of the organism. I think there are two ways in which as physiologists, psychologists, and psychiatrists we can ask about causative agents and the production of behaviour. One might have to do with the structural determinants of behaviour, but there is another kind of important causative relationship that is equally of interest to developmental psychologists and developmental physiologists. This has to do with the origins of behaviour as determined by events that occurred to the organism earlier in life. We need to know about behaviour occurring as a function of previous experience as much as we need to know about behaviour as a function of certain structural attributes which are undoubtedly also determinants of behaviour.

KAUFMAN: You repeatedly say "causative". As I tried to make clear yesterday, in trying to analyse phenomena we have to consider levels of organization. The structural is one, the functional is another, and if we find the structural explanation of a particular function we are not thereby finding the cause of it, we are only finding the mechanism whereby it operates. The cause may be something entirely different—it may have to do with the evolutionary determinants of that kind of organism being created in that way to serve a certain function in life.

LIPSITT: I agree that there are levels of explanation, and always in science there is the problem of infinite regress: as soon as you have determined a cause for behaviour you want to know what the precursors of that particular cause of that particular behaviour were. But I think it is important to appreciate that we want to know not only about correlates of behaviour but also about antecedents or determinants of behaviour.

Attempts at Synthesis:

summing up

A Summing-up

PETER H. WOLFF

Harvard Medical School,

CERTAIN COMMON THEMES which recurred throughout our discussions have not been resolved. Nevertheless it may be useful to review these themes as a way of asking contributors to indicate where they think their own future research might lead. Sophisticated work has been presented, but the interaction between disciplines, implied by the title of this study group and proposed by Prechtl in his Introduction, was not always apparent and for the most part it still remains to be worked out. I do not think this failure was a sign of our stupidity: the difficulties are in the nature of the field and in the methods we are using at present. Lack of convergence between the various reports raises the question of whether one should think of brain-behaviour relationships as an interdisciplinary problem to be solved by a team of experts sharing their several skills, or whether it is necessary for persons who have expert knowledge in one aspect of the problem to be familiar with related disciplines as well. Perhaps the chain reaction or "cross-fertilization" so often hoped for at interdisciplinary meetings must take place within one head, which can at least grasp the outlines of the problem from several perspectives. I think it is futile for a student of behaviour, for instance, to hope that somebody else will solve all his neuroanatomical or computer problems; or for a neuroanatomist to hope that somebody else will solve all his problems in behavioural observations. If this is a valid conclusion it means that each of us, as well as being expert in his own specialty, must be at least familiar with other fields. Ploog made this kind of intra-individual synthesis of several disciplines in a remarkable way.

Another difficulty was that, in our attempts to reconcile opposing views, we sometimes got hung up on Platonic concerns about essences. Earlier we discussed the matter of state. Although everybody agreed that state isn't a thing in itself but a concept of mind, our discussions tended to fall back on ontological arguments, and to treat concepts as if they were real things. This applied not only to the definition of state, but also to the problem of learning. Sometimes we spoke of learning as if either this or that instance was the real thing; and as if, once we had demonstrated one instance of learning at one level of complexity, we had somehow captured its essence.

There was also the problem of different methods or strategies of investigation. The need for mathematization of brain-behavioural relationships (or human engineering, as Prechtl called it) became clear. It also became clear that several different mathematical models for studying this relationship in early development are already available. We were given some splendid examples of how models could be applied. The information-theory model, for instance, proved to be very useful, as did the application of stochastic processes. We recognized that particular problems must be solved by particular mathematical models; and that at present we probably do not have a model for solving every concrete problem we might encounter in studying brain-behaviour relationships. I foresee two dangers in this connection. First, having built a model, we might fall into the trap of thinking we had understood what is going on, forgetting that we had merely discovered a technique for formalizing our data in a particular way. In this way, we might begin to substitute the model for the phenomena themselves. The second danger is that, having found one analytic approach which works for certain aspects of our problem, we might be tempted to squeeze a whole class of related problems into the same mould, trying to make the data fit the model rather than selecting the model to fit the phenomena.

In the discussions on development, certain issues came up which will, I think, require further clarification. One problem was whether we can do developmental studies by comparing lower and higher species; or whether, instead, we must treat each species in its own right. The same general question was raised when we made inferences about infant behaviour from studies of adults. Even though there may be a superficial resemblance between certain elements in the behaviour of infants and adults, the neurology of the infant is not simply a primitive copy of that of the adult. Two distinct developmental forms are involved; and even if a particular behaviour pattern seems to be the same in both, it will have a different significance, depending on the context in which it occurs. By the same token, how much can we conclude about normal behaviour from our study of the abnormal? At this meeting we did not supply concrete answers to these questions. It became clear, however, that in some respects, and at some levels of analysis, we must treat each system in its own context. It would be a useful exercise to study a particular developmental process—or indeed several such processes—

in different species, and then to compare *processes of change* rather than isolated segments of behaviour in different species.

I will not discuss the problems that surrounded the question of onset of function—that is, how we decide at what point in development a structure becomes functional. This question was adequately summarized this morning. One of the issues under the general heading of development which we must watch in the future is the organism's "pre-functional adaptation"—as Paul Weiss (1939) called it—to its environment. To what degree is the naive organism at birth already prepared to organize, and respond adaptively to, the objects in the world before it has "learned" about those objects? Bower's and Papoušek's papers suggest that the naive infant is programmed to structure his world in remarkably complex "given" forms before he ever encounters the extra-uterine environment. Thus Euclidian rather than another geometry might for instance be man's biologically "given" way of organizing space. Perhaps the ethologists have overplayed this theme at times. Nevertheless, it came out clearly from several of the discussions that such an inherent coordination between organism and environment does exist at birth.

In the future it will be important for us to specify this relationship further in terms of "pre-functional" neuronal networks using refined methods, some of which were brought up at this meeting.

I would like to review briefly some of the reports in order to ask, perhaps rhetorically, where we should go from here. With Humphrey's marvellous material in mind, I would like to ask her whether she believes that her particular investigations have been completed, or whether more fetuses should be studied. If so, in what particular direction would she like such studies to go, in order further to clarify the problem of brain-behavioural relations, which was our assignment?

Bergström's and Schulte's presentations clearly indicated the usefulness of the analytic-mathematical approach to the study of brain function, but the relevance of their results to observable behaviour did not emerge clearly from the presentations or the discussion. I understand that both of them are now considering detailed behavioural observations which they will correlate with their refined neurophysiological techniques; I would like to emphasize that this is certainly a necessary and important extension of their work.

Comparing premature and fullterm infants, in order to see whether extra-uterine experience makes a difference to the onset of function, turned out to be useful for distinguishing between different kinds of developmental processes. Everybody contributing to this discussion emphasized that one cannot generalize from isolated cases, nor can one assume that extra-uterine experience does, or does not, influence the general rate or direction of development. Again, we decided that every system has to be studied and analysed in its own right, because extra-uterine experience (learning?) seems to make a difference in some cases, but no obvious difference in others.

Bower's presentation was not intended as a contribution to the study of brain function; yet his results show us the high degree of sophistication which the visual system must have at birth. His studies immediately suggested parallel investigations on the organizing capacity of the auditory system in the young infant; I believe some such studies are now under way.

There was also a direct connection between Bower's "psychological" studies and the detailed neurophysiological investigations reported by Kuffler (1953) and Hubel and Wiesel (1962). This overlap indicates that brain-behaviour relationships can be studied very productively with the tools now at our disposal. The fascinating experiment reported by Lipsitt, and carried out by him and Ambrose, raised a very puzzling question: how can the naive infant anticipate events in real (physical) time? Even if some aspects of the results Lipsitt reported can be reduced to classical and reinforcement learning, that explanation would be insufficient. Probably we must postulate the existence of an "inborn" clocking mechanism, to account for the naive infant's capacity to anticipate events, since it is very hard to imagine how "real" time could be learned unless some neurophysiological substrate served as a clocking mechanism.

I doubt whether studying babies with gross brain abnormalities will in the long run yield a great deal of refined knowledge about brain-behaviour relations. The defect I studied was so gross that it would have been impossible to correlate observed abnormalities in behaviour with details of central nervous system disorganization, even with the invaluable assistance of Dr. Yakovlev and his neuroanatomy group. I undertook this study because our present knowledge of the relation between brain function and behavioural development in the human infant is still so primitive that there is room for elaboration on the pioneer studies by Gamper (1926), even by this crude model. Now, I understand, Dr. Bergström plans to apply his refined methods to the study of babies with congenital brain malformations; from such an approach we may indeed get more systematic knowledge of the problem we set ourselves.

In his report Ploog hit squarely on the point about interdisciplinary research, which I made at the beginning of this summary. He first combined anatomical considerations with detailed behavioural observations in a natural context (rather than an analysis of stimulus-response sequences); he then added a technique for modifying behaviour systematically by direct brain stimulation. By these techniques he is able to investigate the neurophysiological correlates of social behaviour in monkeys. I believe that many more studies in which one investigator uses a combination of methods are still needed. Here I would also like to mention Kaufman's studies on behaviour genetics, in which he compares social behaviour among related species of monkeys. This work has often been in the background of our papers, and it is unfortunate that lack of time precluded a detailed discussion on it at this session. The analysis of species-specific social behaviour patterns in different species, and subsequently of the F_1 generations resulting from cross-breeding, should become a very significant avenue to understanding brain-behaviour relations.

Permit me to put studies on learning at the end; the interesting reports on neonatal conditioning by Dr. Lipsitt implicitly indicated where his work will take him in the future. It also became clear that the *methods* of classical and reinforcement conditioning could be applied as a tool for investigating developmental processes in young infants without requiring us to subscribe to the assertions of learning theory itself. The distinction between using the *methods* of reinforcement conditioning, and investigating *learning* by this technique, was beautifully demonstrated both in Bower's and in Papoušek's studies. We saw how a technique born out of a radical empiricist tradition was applied to studies whose results forced upon us conclusions about development that were quite at odds with learning theory. In this connection, it remained an open question at the conference just how relevant the demonstration of conditioning in infancy is for understanding how the infant learns. All along we tried to distinguish levels of learning. We must continue to keep in mind that there are many such levels, of which conditioning may be one, albeit relatively non-complex, form. The analysis of behaviour in terms of stimulus-response sequences and reinforcement contingencies turned out not to be the kind of causal analysis to which Prechtl referred in his opening remarks.

Finally, Bronson's presentation, and the discussion that followed, indicated how useful speculations about brain and behaviour can be when they start from concrete data and end up with suggestions for concrete application to actual research questions. Bronson did just that. He outlined definite strategies for future research, and specified some of the problems that are urgently in need of resolution.

REFERENCES

GAMPER, E. 1926. Bau und Leistungen eines Menschlichen Mittelhirnwesens (Arhinocephalie mit Encephalocele) zugleich ein Beitrag zur Teratologie und Fasersystematik. *Z. ges. Neurol. Psychiat.* **102,** 154–235.

HUBEL, D. H. and WIESEL, T. N. 1962. Receptive fields, binocular interaction and functional architecture in the cat's visual cortex. *J. Physiol., Lond.* **160,** 106–154.

KUFFLER, S. W. 1953. Discharge patterns and functional organization of mammalian retina. *J. Neurophysiol.* **16,** 37–68.

WEISS, P. 1939. *Principles of development.* Holt, New York.

Discussion

KAUFMAN: It is a help in studying development to know that a human baby will grow into a human being. Development is increased complexity towards stability of a certain kind, which is species-characteristic. I feel it is useful to keep that in mind in whatever kind of study we plan. We can study the emergence of a function because we know in a broad way, at least, where it is going.

LIPSITT: We need to know so much more about the processes by which the individual becomes a characteristic member of his species, and to know what the determining developmental aspects of the child's history are, in order to find out what he is going to become. That is the way to understand individual differences within species.

PLOOG: I think one should divide all these studies into two kinds. First there is the more biological aspect of development in relation to time, whereby I know that if a child does not have certain capacities by a certain age then there is something wrong with it, wherever it has grown up. Research into this aspect raises problems which can be tackled by methods all the way from neuroanatomy to neurophysiology to the kind of perceptual investigations Dr. Bower presented to us. The other kind of study is looking for personal, individual differences and for the mechanisms of learning in detail. Here the conditioning method is the best way we can learn about newborn and young infants. All other ways are either not applicable or they are not controlled in their parameters. The two kinds of study can be combined and there is really no gap, but the one way is the more programmed way—looking at man as an animal that runs its course—and the other way is looking at man as embracing personalities of various capacities and faculties. It is apparent to all of us that every species has certain genetically encoded predispositions to behave in certain ways. But within those boundaries an enormous amount of variation is possible.

BRONSON: A further refinement is to sort out experientially labile systems from experientially stable ones. With development of the nervous system, more and more functioning is experientially labile. But how labile are the initial systems that we see at birth: we can condition them, but how enduring are the consequences of neonatal learning?

PLOOG: Methods are important. For example, if one is to do a learning study in a newborn, is there an approach other than conditioning studies? We also need a new anatomical technique which will enable us to follow the development of the nervous system.

WOLFF: What kinds of things would Humphrey do if she had another batch of fetuses?

HUMPHREY: One of the things I would mention to Wolff, because he is psychiatrically oriented, is that genital stimulation elicits early responses. That is one line of investigation I would like to follow, because I think it is both interesting and significant. We have two fundamental goals in the development of the individual—self-preservation and the preservation of the race. That reactions to genital stimulation should follow the avoiding type of reaction to stimulation of the perioral region in the order that I gave them is, I think, to be expected. Likewise many of the actions that we see later on in postnatal behavioural development should have some reflex counterpart during fetal life.

LIPSITT: Does the possibility of seeing if you can get conditioning in the fetus appeal to you?

HUMPHREY: No, it doesn't. I think there are many things more easily done, more practical, and more significant.

PLOOG: It would be very interesting to try to condition fetuses. Mothers often claim the child has developed in a particular way because the mother had some particular experience during pregnancy. Perhaps a fetus has responses to stimuli *in utero*; if that is true, then it should be possible to condition the fetus.

HUMPHREY: It has been claimed to have been done with auditory stimulations.

PLOOG: Yes, but you never know whether the auditory stimulus goes via the mother's sympathetic nervous system.

WOLFF: Don't extra-uterine fetuses live too short a time for conditioning studies?

LIPSITT: Not necessarily. I can conceive of getting habituation effects in the extra-uterine fetus during its viable period, and I can conceive also of our becoming sufficiently competent in head-turning conditioning for us to get that within a sufficiently short period of time to be applicable to the fetus. Moreover, new techniques might enable us to keep the fetus viable for a longer period of time than is now possible. I am fascinated by the possibility of fetal conditioning.

SCHULTE: Why not work first on the slightly older fetuses which are the prematures and which are available in much greater numbers and for a much longer period of time? You can get fetuses of 25 or 26 weeks' gestation.

LIPSITT: I should not want to do this merely for the feat of conditioning a fetus, however remarkable that might be, but I should want to go on and discover the parameters which control conditioned behaviour in the fetus. The more information of that sort we have, the better equipped neurophysiologists will be to tell us about structural aspects of the organism.

SCHULTE: Is there any other way of studying mechanisms of learning in the newborn than with these conditioning experiments?

PAPOUŠEK: No, but you need not use the classical models of conditioning. You can develop them, modify them in different directions and then you can just use them for moulding more complicated model situations.

SCHULTE: So, all that you do is to make the conditioning more complex.

PLOOG: No, conditioning is nothing but a means.

LIPSITT: It is a prototype. Many different kinds of conditioning processes are available for study even in the newborn child and some of them are more complicated than others, but they are all conditioning or learning techniques in that they all involve the development of a new association, or the intensification of an old one.

Author Index

Numbers in italics refer to pages where References are listed at the end of each article.

V

W

Y

Z

Subject Index

T

V

W